PROGRESS IN BRAIN RESEARCH

VOLUME 62

BRAIN ISCHEMIA:
QUANTITATIVE EEG AND IMAGING TECHNIQUES

Recent volumes in PROGRESS IN BRAIN RESEARCH

Volume 46: Membrane Morphology of the Vertebrate Nervous System. A Study with Freeze-etch Technique, by C. Sandri, J.M. Van Buren and K. Akert — *revised edition* — 1982

Volume 53: Adaptive Capabilities of the Nervous System, by P.S. McConnell, G.J. Boer, H.J. Romijn, N.E. Van de Poll and M.A. Corner (Eds.) — 1980

Volume 54: Motivation, Motor and Sensory Processes of the Brain: Electrical Potentials. Behaviour and Clinical Use, by H.H. Kornhuber and L. Deecke (Eds.) — 1980

Volume 55: Chemical Transmission in the Brain. The Role of Amines, Amino Acids and Peptides, by R.M. Buijs, P.Pévet and D.F. Swaab (Eds.) — 1982

Volume 56: Brain Phosphoproteins, Characterization and Function, by W.H. Gispen and A. Routtenberg (Eds.) — 1982

Volume 57: Descending Pathways to the Spinal Cord, by H.G.J.M. Kuypers and G.F. Martin (Eds.) — 1982

Volume 58: Molecular and Cellular Interactions Underlying Higher Brain Functions, by J.-P. Changeux, J. Glowinksi, M. Imbert and F.E. Bloom (Eds.) — 1983

Volume 59: Immunology of Nervous System Infections, by P.O. Behan, V. ter Meulen and F. Clifford Rose (Eds.) — 1983

Volume 60: The Neurohypophysis: Structure, Function and Control, by B.A. Cross and G. Leng (Eds.) — 1983

Volume 61: Sex Differences in the Brain: The Relation Between Structure and Function, by G.J. De Vries, J.P.C. De Bruin, H.B.M. Uylings and M.A. Corner (Eds.) — 1984

Volume 62: Brain Ischemia: Quantitative EEG and Imaging Techniques, by G. Pfurtscheller, E.J. Jonkman and F.H. Lopes da Silva — 1984

PROGRESS IN BRAIN RESEARCH

VOLUME 62

BRAIN ISCHEMIA: QUANTITATIVE EEG AND IMAGING TECHNIQUES

Edited by

G. PFURTSCHELLER

*Department of Computing, Institute of Biomedical Engineering, Technical University of Graz,
A—8010 Graz (Austria)*

E.H. JONKMAN

*Research Group for Clinical Neurophysiology, TNO, Westeinde Hospital, Lijnbaan, 32, 2512 VA The
Hague (The Netherlands)*

and

F.H. LOPES DA SILVA

*Neurophysiology Group, Department of Zoology, University of Amsterdam, Kruislaan 320, 1098 SM
Amsterdam (The Netherlands)*

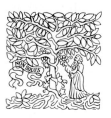

ELSEVIER

AMSTERDAM – NEW YORK – OXFORD

1984

PUBLISHED BY:
ELSEVIER SCIENCE PUBLISHERS B.V.
P.O. BOX 211
AMSTERDAM, THE NETHERLANDS

SOLE DISTRIBUTOR FOR THE U.S.A. AND CANADA:
ELSEVIER SCIENCE PUBLISHING CO., INC.
52 VANDERBILT AVENUE
NEW YORK, NY 10017, U.S.A.

Library of Congress Cataloging in Publication Data

Main entry under title:

Brain ischemia.

(Progress in brain research; v. 62)
"Most of the material in this book was presented at the Internatioal Symposium on Quantitative EEG and
Imaging Techniques in Brain Ischemia, held in Schladming, Austria, in September 1983 under the auspices
of the Austrian Academy of Sciences"—Acknowledgements.

Includes index.

1. Cerebral ischemia—Diagnosis—Congresses. 2. Electroencephalography—Data
processing—Congresses. 3. Tomography—Congresses. 4. Cerebral ischemia—Animal
models—Congresses. I. Pfurtscheller, Gert. II. Jonkman, E.J. (Erik Joost). III. Lopes da Silva, F.H.
(Fernando Henrique), 1935–   . IV. International Symposium on Quantitative EEG and Imaging
Techniques in Brain Ischemia (1983 : Schladming, Austria). V. Österreichische Akademie der
Wissenschaften. VI. Title: Brain ischemia : quantitative EEG and imaging techniques. VII. Series.
QP376.P7 vol. 62 612'.82 s [616.8'1075] 84-21161 [RC388.5]
ISBN 0-444-80582-6 (U.S.)

ISBN FOR THE SERIES 0-444-80104-9
ISBN FOR THE VOLUME 0-444-80582-6

WITH 130 ILLUSTRATIONS AND 48 TABLES

6-3-85

List of Contributors

G. Araki, Department of Neurology and Neurosurgery, Institute of Brain and Blood Vessels, Mihara Memorial Hospital, 366 Oota-Machi, Isesaki, Gunma, Japan

L.M. Auer, Department of Neurosurgery, University of Graz, A-8036 Graz, Austria

N.M. Branston, The Gough-Cooper Department of Neurological Surgery, Institute of Neurology, and National Hospital, Queen Square, London WC1 3BG, U.K.

M.S. Buchsbaum, Department of Psychiatry, University of California, Irvine, CA 92717, U.S.A.

J. Cappelletti, Section of Clinical Psychophysiology, NIMH, Bethesda, MD 20205, U.S.A.

G. Clincke, Department of Neuropharmacology, Janssen Pharmaceutica, B-2340 Beerse, Belgium

W.-D. Heiss, Max-Planck-Institut für Neurologische Forschung, Ostmerheimer Str, 200, D-5000 Köln 91, F.R.G.

L. Henriksen, Department of Neurology, Rigshospitalet, DK-2100 Copenhagen, Denmark

K. Herholz, Max-Planck-Institut für Neurologische Forschung, Ostmerheimer Str. 200, D-5000 Köln 91, F.R.G.

C. Hermans, Department of Neuropharmacology, Janssen Pharmaceutica, B-2340 Beerse, Belgium

G. Hoppe, Max-Planck-Institut für Neurologische Forschung, Ostmerheimer Str. 200, D-5000 Köln 91, F.R.G.

K.-A. Hossmann, Max-Planck-Institut für Neurologische Forschung, Ostmerheimer Str. 200, D-5000 Köln 91, F.R.G.

A. Hyodo, Department of Neurology and Neurosurgery, Institute of Brain and Blood Vessels, Mihara Memorial Hospital, 366 Oota-Machi, Isesaki, Gunma, Japan

K. Isobe, Department of Neurological Surgery, Chiba University, School of Medicine, Inohana 1-8-1, Chiba-Shi, Chiba, Japan 280

J. Johnson, Section of Clinical Psychophysiology, NIMH, Bethesda, MD 20205, U.S.A.

E.J. Jonkman, Research Group for Clinical Neurophysiology, TNO, Westeinde Hospital, Lijnbaan 32, 2512 VA The Hague, The Netherlands

R. Kessler, Department of Nuclear Medicine, NIH Clinical Center, Bethesda, MD 20205, U.S.A.

A. King, Section on Clinical Psychophysiology, NIMH, Bethesda, MD 20205, U.S.A.

V. Köpruner, Department of Computing, Institute of Biomedical Engineering, Technical University of Graz, A-8010 Graz, Austria

A. Ladds, The Gough-Cooper Department of Neurological Surgery, Institute of Neurology, and National Hospital, Queen Square, London WC1 3BG, U.K.

G. Ladurner, Department of Neurology and Psychiatry, University of Graz, A-8036 Graz, Austria

F.H. Lopes da Silva, Neurophysiology Group, Department of Zoology, University of Amsterdam, Kruislaan 320, 1098 SM Amsterdam, The Netherlands

H. Maresch, Department of Computing, Institute of Biomedical Engineering, Technical University of Graz, A-8010 Graz, Austria

W. Melis, Department of Neuropharmacology, Janssen Pharmaceutica, B-2340 Beerse, Belgium

G. Mies, Max-Planck-Institut für Neurologische Forschung, Ostmerheimer Str. 200, D-5000 Köln 91, F.R.G.

M. Mizukami, Department of Neurology and Neurosurgery, Institute of Brain and Blood Vessels, Mihara Memorial Hospital, 366 Oota-Machi, Isesaki, Gunma, Japan

K. Nagata, Department of Neurology, University of Colorado, Health Science Center, B-182, 4200 East Ninth Avenue, Denver, CO 80220, U.S.A.

T. Nakamura, Department of Neurological Surgery, Chiba University, School of Medicine, Inohana 1-8-1, Chiba-Shi, Chiba, Japan 280

O.B. Paulson, Department of Neurology, Rigshospitalet, DK-2100 Copenhagen, Denmark

G. Pawlik, Max-Planck-Institut für Neurologische Forschung, Ostmerheimer Str. 200, D-5000 Köln 91, F.R.G.

G. Pfurtscheller, Department of Computing, Institute of Biomedical Engineering, Technical University of Graz, A-8010 Graz, Austria.

L. Ponsen, Research Group for Clinical Neurophysiology, TNO, Westeinde Hospital, Lijnbaan 32, 2512 VA The Hague, The Netherlands

D.C.J. Poortvliet, TNO Research Unit for Clinical Neurophysiology, Westeinde Hospital, 32 Lijnbaan, 2512 VA The Hague, The Netherlands vi

R.E. Ramsay, Department of Neurology, University of Miami, Miami, FL, U.S.A.

S. Rehncrona, Department of Neurosurgery, University Hospital, S-221 85 Lund, Sweden

I. Rosén, Department of Clinical Neurophysiology, University Hospital, S-221 85 Lund, Sweden

M.-L. Smith, Department of Experimental Brain Research, University Hospital, S-221 85 Lund, Sweden

I. Sulg, University Hospital, Department of Clinical Neurophysiology, Trondheim, Norway

L. Symon, The Gough-Cooper Department of Neurological Surgery, Institute of Neurology, and National Hospital, Queen Square, London WC1 3BG, U.K.

A.M. Tielen[†], Institute of Medical Physics, TNO, Da Costakade 45, Utrecht, The Netherlands

H. Tolonen, Department of Clinical Neurophysiology, University of Oulu, SF-90220 Oulu 22, Finland

C.A.F. Tulleken, Department of Neurosurgery, University Hospital, P.O. Box 16250, 3500 CG Utrecht, The Netherlands

J. Vadja, National Institute of Neurosurgery, Amerikai 57, Budapest, 1145 Hungary

A. van Dieren, Institute of Medical Physics, TNO, Utrecht, The Netherlands

A.C. van Huffelen, TNO Research Unit for Clinical Neurophysiology, Westeinde Hospital, 32 Lijnbaan, 2512 VA The Hague, The Netherlands

J. van Loon, Department of Neuropharmacology, Janssen Pharmaceutica, B-2340 Beerse, Belgium

C.J.M. van der Wulp, TNO Research Unit for Clinical Neurophysiology, Westeinde Hospital, 32 Lijnbaan, 2512 VA The Hague, The Netherlands

W.A.E. van den Broeck, Department of Neuropharmacology, Janssen Pharmaceutica, B-2340 Beerse, Belgium

M.M. Veering, Research Group for Clinical Neurophysiology, TNO, Westeinde Hospital, Lijnbaan 32, 2512 VA The Hague, The Netherlands

R. Vollmer, Ludwig Boltzmann Institute of Clinical Neurobiology, A-1130 Vienna, Austria

S. Vorstrup, Department of Neurology, Rigshospitalet, DK-2100 Copenhagen, Denmark

R. Wagner, Max-Planck-Institut für Neurologische Forschung, Ostmerheimer Str. 200, D-5000 Köln 91, F.R.G.

A.D. Wang, The Gough-Cooper Department of Neurological Surgery, Institute of Neurology, and National Hospital, Queen Square, London WC1 3BG, U.K.

A. Wauquier, Department of Neuropharmacology, Janssen Pharmaceutica, B-2340 Beerse, Belgium

K. Wienhard, Max-Planck-Institut für Neurologische Forschung, Ostmerheimer Str. 200, D-5000 Köln 91, F.R.G.

P.K.H. Wong, Department of Paediatrics, University of British Columbia, Vancouver B.C., Canada

I. Yamakami, Department of Neurological Surgery, Chiba University, School of Medicine, Inohana 1-8-1, Chiba-shi, Chiba, Japan 280

A. Yamaura, Department of Neurological Surgery, Chiba University, School of Medicine, Inohana 1-8-1, Chiba-Shi, Chiba, Japan 280

K. Yunoki, Department of Neurology and Neurosurgery, Institute of Brain and Blood Vessels, Mihara Memorial Hospital, 366 Oota-Machi, Isesaki, Gunma, Japan

Preface

The EEG has been extensively used in the diagnosis of cerebrovascular disorders. The appearance of a focus of slow waves in an acute stroke is a well-known example of an EEG phenomenon, characteristic of an acute cerebrovascular accident. However, in some instances, the EEG changes may be slight as compared with the clinical picture.

In recent years, considerable interest has been given to transient ischemic attacks (TIAs) which may precede, in a proportion of cases, a more severe ischemic lesion. There has been considerable controversy about the value of the EEG for the evaluation of TIAs. EEGs of patients who suffered a TIA are often considered normal upon visual assessment.

Quantification of the EEG (qEEG), by way of computer analysis, has opened up new possibilities for the evaluation of slight EEG changes which may accompany cerebrovascular insufficiency. Moreover, qEEG allows us to perform an objective assessment of minor EEG changes both in the course of time and in response to specific forms of activation. It should be emphasized that the EEG is a non-invasive method which allows continuous monitoring of brain function.

One of the main aims of this book and of the scientific meeting at which the authors exchanged their experience and points of view, was to evaluate the value of qEEG in brain ischemia.

The EEG, whether quantified or not, is not the only diagnostic laboratory method of interest in cerebrovascular disorders. In the last decades a number of new techniques for revealing brain lesions have become available: clearance of xenon-133 to determine cerebral blood flow (CBF), computed tomography (CT) and nuclear magnetic resonance (NMR) for the demonstration of brain lesions, positron emission tomography (PET), mainly using $H^{18}F$-2-deoxy-D-glucose, for the study of brain metabolism. All CT, NMR and PET scans are based on the general principles of computed tomography by means of which slices of the brain can be visualized in vivo. These techniques are excellent for obtaining images of the brain and revealing local variations in metabolism or CBF, although not on a continuous time scale. These methods are of great interest for the diagnosis of cerebrovascular disorders.

Using modern computer facilities, methods for topographic displaying the qEEG have been recently developed. In this way, maps of the distribution of EEG variables over the scalp during rest and during different forms of activity can be constructed. Brain imaging is thus not any longer restricted to computed tomographic techniques but it is also becoming available for the electrical activity.

A momentous question of interest is to evaluate how far these different aids to the diagnosis of brain ischemic conditions are of utility and may have complementary or supplementary value. This is a question which played an important role in the discussions which led to the appearance of this book.

The problems discussed above are considered not only in relation to the general clinical evaluation of patients suffering from brain ischemia but also regarding those patients who are submitted to bypass surgery. The suggested beneficial effect of bypass surgery in patients with brain ischemia, is still controversial.

The role of animal experimentation is of paramount importance, not only for the study of the pathophysiology of brain ischemia but also for a better understanding of the significance and limitations of methods of functional analysis. Therefore, these aspects occupy also an important place in this book.

The book has been divided into four sections dealing with the following topics:
- quantitative EEG in brain ischemia;
- quantitative EEG follow-up studies;
- experimental models of ischemia;
- brain imaging techniques.

The material presented here will, we hope, be relevant for the future development of new concepts of diagnostics and treatment of brain ischemia.

G. Pfurtscheller
E.J. Jonkman
and
F.H. Lopes da Silva

Acknowledgements

Most of the material in this book was presented at the *International Symposium on Quantitative EEG and Imaging Techniques in Brain Ischemia*, held in Schladming, Austria, in September 1983 under the auspices of the Austrian Academy of Sciences.

This symposium was organized with the financial assistance of:
Wiener Medizinische Akademie für Ärztliche Fortbildung,
Bundesministerium für Wissenschaft und Forschung,
Steiermärkische Landesregierung,
Osterreichische Forschungsgemeinschaft,
Sandoz AG, Basel and
Janssen Pharmaceutica, Belgium.

The generous support of the Fonds zur Förderung der wissenschaftlichen Forschung in Österreich, made it possible to include color prints.

The editors gratefully acknowledge the valuable support by all organizations and institutions mentioned above.

The manuscripts were edited by Eugenia Lamont.

Contents

List of Contributors v

Preface vii

Acknowledgements ix

Section I — Quantitative EEG in Brain Ischemia

Quantitative electroencephalography in cerebral ischemia. Detection of abnormalities in "normal" EEGs
  A.C. van Huffelen, D.C.J. Poortvliet and C.J.M. van der Wulp (The Hague, The Netherlands) 3

Quantitative EEG in normals and in patients with cerebral ischemia
  V. Köpruner, G. Pfurtscheller and L.M. Auer (Graz, Austria) 29

Parametric relationships between four different quantitative EEG methods in cerebral infarction
  U. Tolonen (Oulu, Finland) 51

Quantitative EEG as a measure of brain dysfunction
  I. Sulg (Trondheim, Norway) 65

Limitations of EEG frequency analysis in the diagnosis of intracerebral diseases
  G. Mies, G. Hoppe and K.-A. Hossmann (Köln, F.R.G.) 85

Section II — Quantitative EEG Follow-up Studies

Non-invasive follow-up studies of stroke patients with STA-MCA anastomosis; computerized topography of EEG and 133-xenon inhalation rCBF measurement
  I. Yamakami, A. Yamaura, T. Nakamura and K. Isobe (Chiba, Japan) ... 107

Quantitative EEG follow-up study after extracranial-intracranial bypass operation for cerebral ischemia
  G. Pfurtscheller, L.M. Auer and V. Köpruner (Graz, Austria) 121

EEG and CBF in cerebral ischemia. Follow-up studies in humans and monkeys
  E.J. Jonkman, A. van Dieren, M.M. Veering, L. Ponsen, F.H. Lopes da Silva and C.A.F. Tulleken (The Hague, Amsterdam and Utrecht, The Netherlands) 145

Section III — Experimental Models of Ischemia

Quantitative EEG and evoked potentials after experimental brain ischemia in the rat; correlation with cerebral metabolism and blood flow
  I. Rosén, M.-L. Smith and S. Rehncrona (Lund, Sweden) 175

Somatosensory evoked potentials in experimental brain ischemia
N.M. Branston, A. Ladds, L. Symon, A.D. Wang and J. Vadja (London,
U.K. and Budapest, Hungary) 185

Cortical and thalamic somatosensory evoked potentials in brain ischemia in the
monkey
F.H. Lopes da Silva, A.M. Tielen, A. van Dieren, E.J. Jonkman and
C.A.F. Tulleken (Amsterdam, Utrecht and The Hague, The Netherlands) 201

Global incomplete ischemia in dogs assessed by quantitative EEG analysis.
Effects of hypnotics and flunarizine
A. Wauquier, G. Clincke, W.A.E. van den Broeck, C. Hermans, W. Melis
and J. van Loon (Beerse, Belgium) 217

A new technique for the revascularization of a chronic ischemic brain area in cats
and monkeys
C.A.F. Tulleken, A. van Dieren and E.J. Jonkman (Utrecht and The
Hague, The Netherlands) 235

Section IV — Brain Imaging Techniques

Regional cerebral blood flow measured by Xenon-133 and [123I]iodo-ampheta-
mine in patients with cerebrovascular diseases
L. Henriksen, S. Vorstrup and O.B. Paulson (Copenhagen, Denmark) ... 245

Positron emission tomography study of regional glucose metabolism in cerebral
ischemia — topographic and kinetic aspects
G. Pawlik, K. Wienhard, K. Herholz, R. Wagner and W.-D. Heiss (Köln,
F.R.G.) 253

Simultaneous cerebral glucography with positron emission tomography and
topographic electroencephalography
M.S. Buchsbaum, R. Kessler, A. King, J. Johnson and J. Cappelletti
(Irvine, CA and Bethesda, MD, U.S.A.) 263

Topographic electroencephalographic study of ischemic cerebrovascular disease
K. Nagata, K. Yunoki, G. Araki, M. Mizukami and A. Hyodo (Denver,
CO, U.S.A. and Gunma, Japan) 271

Brain electrical activity mapping in normal and ischemic brain
G. Pfurtscheller, G. Ladurner, H. Maresch and R. Vollmer (Graz and
Vienna, Austria) 287

Comparison of electrophysiologic and metabolic changes in the human epileptic
cortex
P.K.H. Wong and R.E. Ramsay (Vancouver, Canada and Miami, FL,
U.S.A.) 303

Subject Index 315

Quantitative EEG in Brain Ischemia

Brain Ischemia: Quantitative EEG and Imaging Techniques, Progress in Brain Research, Vol. 62, edited by
G. Pfurtscheller, E.J. Jonkman and F.H. Lopes da Silva

Quantitative Electroencephalography in Cerebral Ischemia.
Detection of Abnormalities in "Normal" EEGs

A.C. VAN HUFFELEN, D.C.J. POORTVLIET and C.J.M. VAN DER WULP

TNO Research Unit for Clinical Neurophysiology, Westeinde Hospital, 32 Lijnbaan, 2512 VA, The Hague
(The Netherlands)

INTRODUCTION

Clinical importance of minor ischemia

Neurologists are increasingly aware of the importance of minor degrees of cerebral ischemia. From a pathophysiological point of view attention is directed to the stage in which the ischemic tissue still may recover and can be saved from irreversible damage (Raichle, 1983), and to the restoration of the function of the tissue in the ischemic "penumbra" (Symon, 1980), the bordering zone of nonfunctioning but structurally preserved brain tissue around an infarct. From an anatomic, pathological and clinical point of view attention is focused on "lacunes", small, deep cerebral infarctions, most often encountered in hypertensive patients (Mohr, 1982).

The increasing number of methods of treatment excites the interest of neurologists and neurosurgeons concerned with the therapy of cerebral ischemia. Future stroke may be prevented in patients with atheromatous lesions of the carotid arteries by platelet aggregation inhibitors or anticoagulants. Antihypertensive treatment may benefit hypertensive patients threatened by new lacunar strokes. Once prevention of ischemia has failed, intervention in the ongoing process of ischemic damage is important to diminish or even to avert irreversible cellular damage. Several drugs, such as calcium entry blockers and prostaglandins are now being intensely studied. Surgical methods, e.g. carotid endarterectomy and extra-intracranial arterial bypass operations are applied widely. No consensus, however, concerning the indications for these operations has yet been reached.

The patients selected for most of these established or experimental methods of treatment have only suffered transient or minor neurological deficits ("minor ischemia") and are threatened by recurrence of an ischemic episode that could cause a severe deficit or even death.

Diagnostic studies therefore should be focused on patients with minor ischemia. Ischemia is called "minor" in patients whose deficit is reversible within 24 h (transient ischemic attack, TIA) or within 3 weeks (reversible ischemic neurological deficit, RIND) or who have only such a small residual deficit that they are fully independent as far as activities of daily living are concerned, and that they are able to return to their previous occupation without any modification (partial nonprogressing stroke, PNS) (Ad hoc Committee on Cerebrovascular Disease, 1975; Joint Committee for

Stroke Resources, 1977). There are several fields of study concerned with the diagnosis of minor ischemia. Few studies have been devoted to the reliability of the neurological diagnosis in patients with reversible ischemia. The results of computer tomographic studies have been evaluated in several series of patients. The results of EEG examination and CT scans have been compared in some of these studies. Recently, several reports have been published on EEG and especially on quantitative EEG (qEEG) in patients with cerebral ischemia. A short survey of these methods, all of which are noninvasive, will be presented. Studies involving NMR, PET scan, rCBF measurements and angiographic studies will not be considered in this survey.

Reliability of clinical diagnosis in minor ischemia

The clinical diagnosis of TIA or RIND may be uncertain because objective neurological signs often have vanished by the time the patient is examined by the neurologist, who consequently has to depend on the subjective medical history of the patient. This explains why there is only moderate agreement among neurologists concerning the diagnosis of reversible ischemia. Sisk et al. (1970) found about 80% agreement on symptoms or signs of paresis between two staff neurologists in the same hospital examining patients with transient ischemia (history 75%, examination 83%). Calanchini et al. (1977) reviewed patient charts in a large series of patients suspected of having suffered from TIAs. A definite diagnosis of TIA was only approved in 39% of these patients. In a multi-center cooperative study on reversible cerebral ischemia, Tomasello et al. (1982) found an inter-observer index of agreement of about 60% (medical history 62%, examination 55%). Far better results are reported in patients with completed stroke. In a series of 821 consecutive stroke patients including only 96 TIA patients, Norris and Hachinski (1982) found an overall percentage of 13% of patients whose initial diagnosis proved to be incorrect. These results clearly show the importance of confirmatory tests, especially in patients with minor ischemia.

CT findings in minor cerebral ischemia

Cerebral lesions due to ischemia may be shown in computer tomography as hypodense areas. Such lesions are found in a small percentage of TIA patients (Ottonello et al., 1980: 0%; Biller et al., 1982: 2.2%; Ladurner et al., 1979: 18%; Perrone et al., 1979: 34%). Higher percentages of ischemic lesions are obtained in RIND patients (Logar et al., 1979: 9%; Ladurner et al., 1979: 76%). Still higher figures are reported in patients with completed stroke (Logar et al., 1979: 79%; Ottonello et al., 1980: 84%; Ladurner et al., 1979: 95%). Nevertheless, CT scans may appear remarkably normal in patients with completed stroke, despite extensive clinical and EEG abnormality (Yanagihara et al., 1981).

False negative CT scan results may be explained in several ways. Even the most modern CT scanner may miss lacunes smaller than a few mm^3 situated in the internal capsule or the thalamus (Mohr, 1982; Pullicino et al., 1982). Absence of hypodense areas may be due to the "fogging effect" (Becker et al., 1979). In patients with minor ischemia, the ischemic process may cause selective neuronal loss and leave glial cells and vessels alive. Thus no hypodense area develops despite severe functional and microscopic structural loss (Lassen, 1982).

An important factor in CT scanning is the time course between the stroke and the moment of scanning. It may take days or even weeks before the hypodense areas become clearly visible. This is a serious disadvantage in ischemic patients, where immediate treatment is considered useful. In the first weeks the study of contrast medium enhancement may improve the diagnostic results. This, however, renders CT an invasive examination (Pullicino et al., 1982). The use of the CT scan as a confirmatory test in patients with minor ischemia thus appears to be rather unsatisfactory.

EEG in minor ischemia

There is an extensive literature on the EEG in patients with cerebral ischemia. Reviews have been given by Van der Drift (1972), Van der Drift and Kok (1972) and Van Huffelen et al. (1980). Only data pertaining to minor ischemia will be dealt with here.

Absence of EEG changes

Absence of EEG changes in cerebral ischemia has been reported by many authors. The percentage of patients showing a "normal" EEG depends on many factors. These include the age of the patient, the clinical classification of the cerebral ischemia, the vascular territory involved, the location and extent of the ischemic lesion, the time interval between the stroke and the EEG, the EEG recording technique, the interpretative criteria, and the expertise and experience of the EEG interpreter. In TIA patients a normal EEG is often found, in contrast to patients with completed stroke. For this reason, TIA patients were excluded from several EEG studies on cerebral ischemia (e.g. Kayser-Gatchalian and Neundörfer, 1980). In a large series of 295 TIA patients, Enge et al. (1980) found a normal EEG in 44% of their patients (in 51% of patients up to 50 years of age and in 41% of older patients). In two small series of TIA patients (Ott et al., 1980; Ottonello et al., 1980) the EEG was interpreted as normal in 29% and 14% of the cases, respectively. Logar et al. (1979) found EEG abnormalities in 64% of a series of RIND patients. Still higher values (80–90%) were obtained in patients with completed stroke (Logar et al., 1979; Otto et al., 1980; Ottonello et al., 1980). The amount of abnormality found is maximal immediately after the stroke and decreases in the course of time after the stroke. Superficial cortical lesions give rise to extensive EEG changes, in contrast to small deep lesions (lacunes) that generally cause no EEG abnormalities.

EEG changes

Cerebral ischemia may produce several types of changes in the EEG. The rhythms and activities normally present may change in several ways. Their frequency, amplitude, abundance, topology, reactivity and variability may change. The rhythms and activities normally present, such as the alpha rhythm, the mu rhythm, delta activity and photic driving reactions will be considered here. The appearance of activities that are normally absent, e.g. frontal intermittent rhythmic delta activity (FIRDA), periodic lateralized epileptiform discharges (PLEDs) etc., will not be considered because they are rare in patients with minor ischemia.

The alpha rhythm. The alpha rhythm may be changed in cerebral ischemia in several ways. It may be absent on the ischemic side. There may be a decrease of abundance or an amplitude asymmetry with smaller amplitudes on the affected side. In some cases, however, larger amplitudes are found on the ischemic side. In contrast

6

to the amplitude asymmetries, frequency asymmetries, when present, have a rather constant character. Unilateral slowing of the alpha rhythm indicates the ischemic side. The alpha rhythm asymmetries, however, have to exceed 0.6 Hz before they can be distinguished by visual assessment, as was found by the present authors in an investigation among 82 qualified electroencephalographers. The reactivity of the alpha rhythm may be changed. The reaction to opening of the eyes ("alpha blocking") may be diminished or even absent on the ischemic side (Castorina and Marchini, 1958). The alpha squeak phenomenon after eye closure may disappear (Farbrot, 1954). The variability of the alpha rhythm may decrease or increase.

The mu rhythm. The mu rhythm is observed in a minority of patients with ischemia. Van der Drift and Magnus (1961) found a mu rhythm in 20% of their patients, mainly on the nonischemic side. This was interpreted as an absence or a decrease of mu rhythm on the ischemic side. A unilaterally increased mu rhythm was found by Pfurtscheller et al. (1981) in deep lesions. Thus both mu attenuation and mu enhancement have been reported. The reactivity of the mu rhythm has been observed to diminish in ischemia (Pfurtscheller et al., 1980, 1981). Frequency asymmetries of the mu rhythm have not been reported as yet.

Delta activity. Delta activity has been studied extensively in cerebral ischemia. It may be diffusely present over the ischemic hemisphere and/or locally dominant in the anterior and mid-temporal regions.

Photic stimulation. Photic stimulation in patients with cerebral ischemia has been investigated by several authors (Farbrot, 1953; Kooi et al., 1957; Van Huffelen et al., 1980). Decreased photic driving may be found on the ischemic side, particularly at higher flash frequencies. Enhanced photic driving on the ischemic side may occur when flash frequencies in the delta range are applied.

EEG and CT scan

The EEG appeared to be superior from a diagnostic point of view in those studies on minor ischemia in which EEG and CT scan results were compared. In TIA patients the diagnostic yield of EEG was about twice that of CT (Enge et al., 1980; EEG 60%, CT 34%; Ott et al., 1980; EEG 29%, CT 14%; Ottonello et al., 1980; EEG 14%, CT 0%). The same trend was found by Logar et al. (1979) in RIND patients (EEG 64%, CT 9%). In patients with completed stroke (CS) the diagnostic results of CT and EEG are nearly equal (80–90%). The amount of EEG abnormality found is maximal immediately after the stroke and decreases in the course of time after the stroke, which is in contrast to the evolution of CT abnormalities. Considering these data, the question arises whether the diagnostic significance of the EEG in minor cerebral ischemia can be further improved by the application of the computer analysis.

Quantitative EEG (qEEG)

EEG data processing by computers can be applied to *support* the EEG interpreter. It can also be used to *extend* the faculties of the EEG interpreter (Lopes da Silva, 1976). Thus information can be obtained that escapes visual analysis (Binnie et al., 1978; Van Huffelen et al., 1980).

Several reviews on data processing of the EEG have been published in recent years (Barlow, 1979; Lopes da Silva, 1981; Bickford, 1981; Ellingson and Peters, 1981). Many methods of EEG data processing have been used and evaluated. The most common technique in this field is the Fourier analysis technique or power spectral density estimation based on discrete Fourier transformation. Other methods are period analysis (Cohen, 1975), combined period and amplitude analysis (Stigsby et al., 1973) and the normalized slope descriptor technique (Hjorth, 1970, 1973). Several authors evaluated different diagnostic techniques independently and found spectral analysis superior to other methods (Binnie et al., 1978; Sotaniemi et al., 1980; Tolonen and Sulg, 1981). Spectral results have been used in several different ways. A simple graphical presentation of the time variation in the spectral components – the compressed spectral array – was introduced by Bickford et al. (1973).

qEEG data on spontaneous activity

The power spectrum has been divided into certain frequency bands (delta, theta, alpha, beta) and the total power in these bands has been estimated. The absolute power in these individual bands appeared to vary considerably. A substantial reduction of variance was obtained by considering the power in a given band in relation to the power in other bands. For this reason several ratios have been created, for instance, the percentage of alpha power in the total power (Tolonen and Sulg, 1981) or (alpha + beta)/(theta + delta) (Sotaniemi et al., 1980), or the reverse (theta + delta)/(alpha + beta) for the construction of canonograms for the localization of brain lesions (Gotman et al., 1975). Right/left quotients have been calculated (Binnie et al., 1978). A relative asymmetry ratio (right − left)/(right + left) was applied by Van Huffelen et al. (1980).

Data on spectral power in predetermined bands were also used for the construction of computed EEG mapping, a topographic display of EEG analysis results comparable to CT displays (Duffy et al., 1979, 1981; Nagata et al., 1982; Pidoux et al., 1983).

Several authors determined power maxima or peaks in certain frequency bands of the power spectrum, especially in the alpha band (Hébert et al., 1980; Van Huffelen et al., 1980; Wieneke et al., 1980). Others studied mean spectral frequency or mean alpha frequency (Matejcek, 1980; Sotaniemi et al., 1980; Tolonen and Sulg, 1981).

qEEG data on reactivity

Reactivity of the EEG is usually studied by comparing the spontaneous EEG activity in the eyes closed condition with EEG activity in other conditions, e.g. with eyes open ("alpha blocking"), during hand movements (suppression of mu rhythm) and during photic stimulation.

The reactivity to opening of the eyes ("alpha blocking") was mentioned as one of several parameters by Binnie et al. (1978) and Hébert et al. (1980), but no details were published.

The mu rhythm was investigated by Kuhlman (1977), Schoppenhorst et al. (1977) and Storm van Leeuwen et al. (1978). The reactivity of central alpha activity to hand movements was investigated by Pfurtscheller et al. (1980, 1982, 1983) in the eyes closed condition.

The reactivity to photic stimulation was studied by Celesia et al. (1978, 1983) using the compressed spectral array technique. Relative power asymmetry ratios for symmetrical derivations in small bands centered on the photic stimulation frequency and the normalized cross power in these bands ("conformation") were investigated by Van Huffelen et al. (1980).

Combinations of several of these approaches have been used. Most investigators, however, focused on one single parameter or a very restricted number of parameters. Moreover, most authors applied these parameters to one or two pairs of channels to reduce the quantity of data. It remains to be seen whether such a complicated signal as the EEG signal, with its regional differences, can be reduced to one or two parameters from one or two channels without significant loss of information.

qEEG in minor ischemia

Several authors explicitly excluded patients with TIAs or RINDs from their studies and restricted themselves to the study of visibly abnormal EEGs (Tolonen and Sulg, 1981; Tolonen et al., 1981; Nagata et al., 1982). Pfurtscheller et al. (1981) investigated a group of patients, including a small number with TIAs in which a high percentage of CT abnormalities was found. No comparison was made between visual assessment of the EEG and qEEG analysis in these patients. These investigations can hardly substantiate the superiority of qEEG over the visually assessed EEG or CT scan, and the specific role of qEEG as a diagnostic aid in patients with minor ischemia. Van Huffelen et al. (1980) studied the results of qEEG exclusively in patients in which the EEGs had been interpreted as normal according to conventional clinical criteria. In this first study abnormal qEEG results were obtained in 11 of 20 patients with minor ischemia and a "normal" EEG on visual assessment. Similar results were obtained in a second study with 20 patients (Van Huffelen et al., 1982). The same approach was chosen in the present study with another group of 20 patients with minor ischemia, and a strictly normal EEG assessed visually. For this study, however, data on a reference group of 50 healthy volunteers were available. Some new EEG parameters were added to those previously studied.

The objective of this study was to substantiate the diagnostic superiority of the qEEG over the conventional EEG in cerebral ischemia and to establish the clinical significance of this diagnostic gain in relation to CT findings and clinical data.

MATERIAL AND METHODS

Reference subjects

Two groups of subjects were formed: a reference group (R), consisting of healthy remunerated volunteers, and a study group including patients with acute unilateral cerebral ischemia and a normal EEG on visual assessment (SN). The R group consisted of 50 healthy subjects with ages between 20 and 70 years ($\overline{X}$ 40 years). Thirty subjects were males and 20 females. In all subjects a standardized questionnaire was used and a medical and neurological examination performed. Subjects with a history of CNS disorder or any sign or symptom of neurological disease were excluded from this reference group. Other reasons for exclusion were hypertension, diabetes or the use of any kind of medication known to influence the EEG. The subjects were admitted to the R group irrespective of their EEG findings. EEG studies in all subjects included spontaneous EEG with eyes closed (EC) and eyes open (EO), and during photic stimulation. In most subjects tactile stimulation to the hands was applied in the EO condition.

Patients

Patients were admitted to the study group SN if their age did not exceed 70 years and they had signs or symptoms of an acute unilateral cerebral ischemic episode in the territory of the middle cerebral artery, and if the EEG recorded within one month of the ischemic episode did not show any abnormality upon visual assessment. CT scans were obtained from nearly all patients. Patients with intracerebral hemorrhage were excluded from the SN group. These criteria were used for the selection of three groups, each consisting of 20 patients. The present study group is indicated as SN_3 to distinguish it from two similar groups SN_1 and SN_2 investigated in former studies (Van Huffelen et al., 1980, 1982).

The SN_3 group consisted of 12 males between 27 and 68 years ($\bar{x}$ 54 years) and 8 females between 38 and 57 years ($\bar{x}$ 46 years) (group $\bar{x}$: 52 years) (Table I). All SN_3 patients were examined within one month of the onset of the ischemic episode ($\bar{x}$ 7 days). Most patients (16 out of 20) were examined within the first 10 days of the Transient Ischemic Attack (TIA) or Stroke. The patients were classified according to the system of the Ad hoc Committee on Cerebrovascular Disease (1975) and the Joint Committee for Stroke Resources (1977) as having TIAs, RIND or PNS. Patients with CS were not found in the three SN groups, although this had not been a reason for exclusion. The three classifications TIA, RIND and PNS were taken together as "minor" ischemia. Eight patients had suffered from one or more TIAs, three from a RIND and the other nine from a PNS. All patients had presented signs and/or symptoms of unilateral cerebral vascular disease in the supply area of the middle cerebral artery. The left hemisphere was affected in 12 patients, in the remainder the right hemisphere.

TABLE I

COMPARISON OF DATA FROM GROUP SN_1, SN_2
AND SN_3

m = male, f = female, l = left hemisphere ischemia, r = right hemisphere ischemia. Numbers in parentheses = number of abnormal CT scans

Group	SN_1	SN_2	SN_3	SN_{1-3}
n	20	20	20	60
Classification				
TIA	4(0)	8(3/7)	8(1/7)	20(4/18)
RIND	3(0)	5(1)	3(0)	11(1)
PNS	13(5)	7(5)	9(6)	29(16)
$\bar{x}$ age (yrs)	55	56	52	54
m/f	15/5	17/3	12/8	44/16
l/r	10/10	11/9	12/8	33/27
recording 10 days after ischemia	19	14	16	49

In all patients except one, CT scans were performed with a Siemens Somatom SF with a 512×512 matrix. Generally, no contrast medium was administered to maintain the strictly noninvasive character of the study. CT scans were performed 5 days or more following onset of the ischemic episode. The brain CT scans were evaluated for the presence of mass effects due to edema and/or hypodense areas due to edema or infarction in the supply area of the middle cerebral artery. In one out of seven TIA patients the CT scan showed a hypodense area; in none of the RIND patients and in six out of nine PNS patients ischemic abnormality was found (Table I).

The SN_1 group, also consisting of 20 patients with acute unilateral cerebral ischemia and having a normal EEG on visual assessment, was highly comparable to the SN_3 group. In these patients, however, CT scans were performed with a first-generation EMI scanner. Abnormalities were found in none of the TIA or RIND patients. In five out of 13 PNS patients the CT scan showed abnormality compatible with ischemia (Table I).

The SN_2 group, consisting of 20 patients with acute unilateral cerebral ischemia and a normal EEG according to conventional clinical criteria was similar to the SN_3 group. In this group the same CT scanner (512×512 matrix) was used as in the SN_3 group. In three out of seven TIA patients and in one out of five RIND patients the CT scan showed an ischemic lesion. In five out of seven PNS patients such an abnormality was found (Table I).

Data acquisition

In patients with acute unilateral cerebral ischemia the EEG was recorded within one month from the onset of the ischemic episode (mean SN_1: 6 days, SN_2: 10 days, SN_3: 7 days). In 49 out of 60 patients the EEG was obtained within 10 days (Table I). Ag-AgCl electrodes with a diameter of 10 mm were used. These were fixed to the scalp by means of collodion and placed according to the international 10–20 system. Contact resistance was always less than $5k\Omega$.

It was attempted to keep the patient in a state of quiet attentiveness while lying as comfortably as possible on a stretcher. During one part of the recording the patient's eyes were closed (EC), during another part the eyes were open (EO). In most patients, particularly in those showing a mu rhythm, tactile stimulation to the hands was applied in the EO condition. Photic stimulation (PS) was applied by means of an externally triggered, quartz controlled Van der Camp stroboscope. Each PS frequency was presented for 14 sec; the interval between PS series was 16 sec. The following PS frequency sequence was applied: 1,2,3,4,5,6,7,8,9,10,11,12,14 and 16 Hz.

The EEG apparatus was a 20-channel Van Gogh 50.000 electroencephalograph. Filter settings were: highpass filter $-3dB$ at 0.16 Hz and lowpass filter $-3dB$ at 75 Hz. The sensitivity used for the recording on paper generally was 70 microvolt/cm. A special montage was used with C_z as a common reference electrode; a midline reference was preferred because this study was based on left to right comparison or evaluation of asymmetries. C_z registers little EMG, EKG and EOG activity. It is an attractive reference for both mu rhythm (Pfurtscheller et al., 1980), alpha rhythm (Van Huffelen et al., 1980), temporal delta activity and reactions to photic stimulation. The following seven pairs of electrodes were used for the evaluation of asymmetries: F_4/F_3, C_4/C_3, P_4/P_3, O_2/O_1, F_8/F_7, T_4/T_3, T_6/T_5.

Spontaneous EEG activity was recorded for at least 10 min using the conventional bipolar and common average montages. The reactivity to opening and closing of the eyes and to tactile stimulation of the hands was tested. The special C_z montage was selected when the patient was in a stable condition. Thereafter, 120 sec of spontaneous EEG activity EC and 120 sec EO were recorded. The PS series were then recorded consecutively. Utmost care was taken to reduce the occurrence of artifacts. In most patients with a mu rhythm 120 sec EEG activity EO during tactile stimulation of the hands were recorded.

The EEG recorded on paper was independently studied and interpreted by three interpreters according to conventional clinical standards. EEGs were only considered normal if all three interpreters had independently assessed them as normal. The EEG signals were transferred to the A/D converter after filtering with an anti-aliasing filter -3 dB at 40 Hz. The sample frequency was 102.4 Hz. Data were stored on magnetic tape and analyzed offline.

Data processing

A PDP 15/76 DEC computer system was used. Periods with artifacts were excluded. Data from 100 sec spontaneous EEG activity were subdivided into 19 segments of 10 sec each, with overlap of 50% each to reduce the variance in the spectral estimates. Discrete Fourier Transformation using FFT was applied. The spectral estimates of the 19 segments were averaged and smoothed by a seven points normalized elliptic window. The coherence function was estimated for two symmetrical channels and smoothed by a similar window. Significant differences between the spectra of two symmetrical channels were calculated as function of frequency, taking into account the values of the coherence estimates. The significance of differences was determined by the F-test ($p<0.001$).

Several data on the spectral maxima, viz. frequency, amplitude, coherence and -3 dB frequency values of the spectral peak, were calculated. Maxima were determined by a "hill climbing" procedure (Van der Wulp in: Van Huffelen et al., 1980).

The autospectrum was divided into nine frequency bands ($delta_1$, $delta_2$, $theta_1$, $theta_2$, $alpha_1$, $alpha_2$, $beta_1$, $beta_2$, $beta_3$). In this study the following bands were used: $delta_2$ (2.0–3.4 Hz), $alpha_1$ (7.5–9.9 Hz) and $alpha_2$ (10.0–12.4 Hz). The total power for each frequency band was calculated. The amount of asymmetry between homologous/symmetrical channels was computed for each frequency band and expressed as relative deviation from the mean of both channels, the relative asymmetry R_A:

$$R_A = (P_R - P_L)/(P_R + P_L),$$ in which P_R indicates the total power from the right channel and P_L that from the left.

The amount of reactivity to opening of the eyes was calculated for each channel and each frequency band and expressed as relative deviation from the mean of both conditions: the relative reactivity ratio R_R:

$$R_R = (P_{EC} - P_{EO})/(P_{EC} + P_{EO})$$ in which P_{EC} indicates the total power for a given channel and a given band in the EC condition and P_{EO} that for the EO condition.

The actitivity related to photic stimulation (PS) was studied in bands of 0.7 Hz centered upon the PS fundamental frequency and its two higher harmonics. The

12

power in these three bands of 0.7 Hz was summated. A relative power ratio (R − L)/(R + L) was calculated. Another measure was defined to express the similarity of the signals of two symmetrical channels within the mentioned frequency bands. The normalized cross power was calculated for symmetrical sets of 21 spectral points (three bands of 0.7 Hz). The term "conformation" was introduced for this measure (Poortvliet and Van Huffelen, 1981). Another measure was the phase of the cross power, which was computed for the same sets of data.

Data presentation

The autospectra from symmetrical channels are presented graphically (Fig. 1). The spectrum of the right channel is plotted upwards, that from the left channel is plotted downwards. The difference of both spectra is plotted in between. The difference curve is plotted with cross hatchings where there are significant differences (F-test, $p<0.001$) between right and left. The x-axis is calibrated in 5 Hz steps from 0 to 40 Hz, the y-axis is calibrated in steps of 5 microvolt/$\sqrt{\text{Hz}}$, to decrease the dynamic range of the data presented. The coherence function is plotted above the autospectra, with a y-axis ranging from 0 to 1.

Numerical results are printed separately. For the spectral peaks these are: peak frequency, −3dB values, amplitude in microvolt/$\sqrt{\text{Hz}}$ and coherence values at the peak frequency. Summated power from the right and left channels is given for the

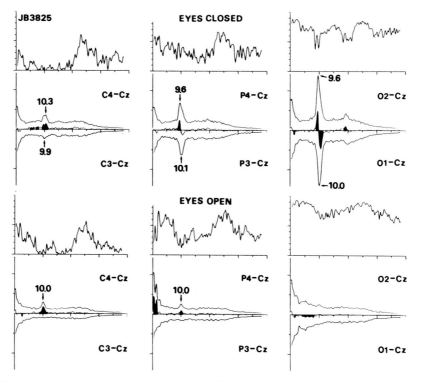

Fig. 1. Spectra from male patient, 59 years of age with PNS in the right hemisphere. CT scan: small ischemic lesion in the anterior limb of the internal capsule. Alpha peak frequency asymmetry with lower frequency on the ischemic side. Mu peak only present (augmented) on the same side.

nine bands. In addition, separate data for combined theta$_1$ and theta$_2$, alpha$_1$ and alpha$_2$, beta$_1$ and beta$_2$ bands were presented. For symmetrical channels the relative asymmetry ratio R_A and for individual channels the reactivity ratio R_R were printed. All numerical results were also stored on disk for further statistical investigations.

Parameters

Spectral peak parameters

Alpha peak frequency. From the many detected maxima in each spectrum only one peak was considered as the alpha peak, i.e. the peak with the largest amplitude in the alpha range and a value $\geqslant 1$ microvolt/$\sqrt{Hz}$. In questionable cases, when some maxima had equal amplitudes, data from neighboring electrodes were also taken into account for the decision on the peak to be identified as the alpha peak. Alpha peaks were determined in the occipital, parietal, posterior and mid-temporal regions, both in the EC and in the EO condition.

Alpha peak frequency asymmetry. Because symmetrical derivations were always considered, the occurrence of differences between alpha peak frequencies from the right and left hemisphere could be studied in homologous regions. These absolute frequency differences were called alpha peak frequency asymmetries.

Alpha peak frequency shift EC–EO. In the majority of cases the alpha rhythm did not completely disappear when the eyes were opened. In many of these cases an alpha peak frequency EO could be distinguished in addition to the alpha peak frequency EC. In most cases the alpha peak frequencies EC and EO were slightly different. There was thus a frequency change, Δf (EC–EO), called the alpha peak frequency shift.

Alpha peak frequency shift asymmetry. The occurrence of alpha peak frequency shift differences between homologous derivations was investigated. These absolute differences were called peak frequency shift asymmetries.

Mu peak frequency. Mu peaks were studied in the central derivations. Peaks were called mu peaks only if the amplitude was 1 microvolt/$\sqrt{Hz}$ or more, if the peak frequency differed from the alpha peak frequency, if the bilateral coherence was very low and if the mu peak was not suppressed by opening of the eyes. It had, however, to be suppressed by tactile stimulation of the hands.

Mu peak frequency asymmetry. If mu peaks were discerned on both sides, absolute peak frequency differences could be determined. These were called mu peak frequency asymmetries.

Band power parameters

Relative delta$_2$ power asymmetry. The relative delta$_2$ power asymmetry ratio R_A was studied in the posterior and mid-temporal regions.

Relative alpha power asymmetry EC. The relative alpha power asymmetry ratio R_A was calculated for the occipital, parietal, and posterior temporal derivations in the EC condition. Three bands were studied: alpha$_1$, alpha$_2$ and alpha$_{1+2}$.

Relative alpha power asymmetry EO. The same parameter was studied for the same regions and bands in the EO condition.

The alpha power reactivity. The relative suppression of alpha power EO in respect to the power EC was determined as the reactivity ratio R_R. This ratio was investigated in the posterior temporal and mid-temporal regions. It was calculated for the alpha$_1$,

14

alpha$_2$ and alpha$_{1+2}$ bands.

Photic stimulation parameters
Relative power asymmetry. The asymmetry ratio R$_A$ was calculated for 0.7 Hz bands centered on the fundamental PS frequencies and two higher harmonics. It was determined for all symmetrical derivations except Fp$_2$/Fp$_1$.
Conformation. The normalized cross power was computed for the same frequency bands and pairs of derivations.
Phase of the cross power. The phase of the cross power was calculated for the same frequency bands and pairs of derivations.

RESULTS

Reference group

(a) *Spectral peak parameters in the reference group*
(i) *Alpha peak frequency EC.* Alpha peaks were identified in all 50 subjects from the reference group R in the eyes closed (EC) condition in the occipital and posterior temporal regions. Parietal and mid-temporal alpha peaks could be discerned in 96% of the subjects. There appeared to be a considerable variance of the alpha peak frequency values. An age dependence of the alpha peak frequencies was only indicated in the highest age group (Fig. 2). In only two subjects (4%) aged 64 and 67 years were alpha peaks below 8.0 Hz found. This frequency was determined as the lower limit of normality, aiming at a 5% confidence limit.
In the EO condition alpha peaks could still be identified in 69% of the subjects in

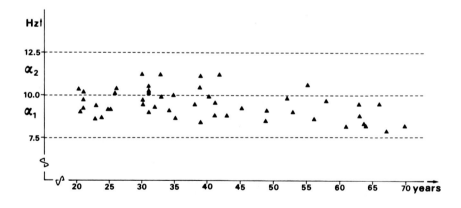

Fig. 2. Alpha peak frequencies in 50 normal subjects. Condition: eyes closed. Derivation: O$_2$–C$_z$.

the occipital, in 61% in the posterior temporal, in 53% in the mid-temporal and in 45% in the parietal regions (overall 57%).
(ii) *Alpha peak frequency asymmetry.* Alpha peak frequency asymmetries were calculated in the EC condition in the occipital and posterior temporal regions (100%

of subjects) and in the parietal and mid-temporal regions (96% of subjects). Peak asymmetry values differed per region (Table II). The least asymmetry was found in the occipital region: 2% of the subjects had an asymmetry of >0.3 Hz. In the parietal region, 2% of the subjects had an asymmetry >0.4 Hz. In the posterior temporal regions no subject had an asymmetry >0.5 Hz and in the mid-temporal region an asymmetry >0.6 Hz was found in 4% of the subjects. These values were determined as limits of normality. Combining the data of these four derivations and accepting no values exceeding these limits, abnormality was found in 8% of the reference subjects. This means that this parameter when applied to patients had a specificity of 92%.

TABLE II

SUBJECTS WITH ALPHA PEAK FREQUENCY ASYMMETRIES
>0.2 Hz (EC) ($N = 50$)

Limits of normality are indicated

	Δf_α	>0.2	>0.3	>0.4	>0.5	>0.6	>0.7
O		2	1	1	0	0	0
P		4	3	1	0	0	0
T_P		11	6	3	0	0	0
T_M		8	5	4	3	2	2

(iii) *Alpha peak frequency shift.* An alpha peak frequency shift was observed in nearly all subjects (Fig. 3). These shifts showed a considerable variance. Yet there was a tendency for the alpha peaks to have a higher frequency in the EO condition. The mean frequency increase Δf (EO–EC) was 0.3 Hz.

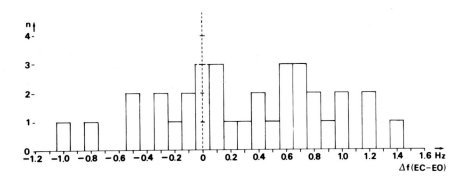

Fig. 3. Alpha peak frequency shift from condition eyes closed to condition eyes open. Derivation: O_2–C_z.

(iv) *Alpha peak frequency shift asymmetry.* The variance of the shift asymmetries was considerably less than the variance of the absolute shift values for each individual region. Only 4% of the subjects showed a frequency shift asymmetry of the alpha peak frequency >0.6 Hz. This value was determined as a limit of normality. Consequently, this parameter has a specificity of 96%.

(v) *Mu peak frequency.* Mu peaks were identified in 20% of the reference subjects. All but one of these subjects were less than 40 years of age ($\bar{x}$ 30 years). In all 10 cases mu peaks were discovered in both central regions. In nine out of 10 subjects the mu rhythm had a higher frequency than the alpha rhythm (mean difference 1.4 Hz).

(vi) *Mu peak frequency asymmetry.* In all 10 subjects mu peaks occurred bilaterally. A frequency difference between the mu peaks from the right and left central area >0.2 Hz was not found. Asymmetries >0.2 Hz were considered as abnormal, as was unilateral absence or presence of the mu rhythm. The absence of such abnormalities in the reference groups leads to a specificity of this parameter of 100%.

(b) *Band power parameters in the reference group*

Confidence limits of 5% were observed for the determination of the limits of normality for each band parameter. For each parameter, these limits of normality were applied to all mentioned derivations. The criterion of abnormality for each parameter was an abnormal result in at least one of the derivations studied; thus no degrees of abnormality were distinguished per derivation or per set of derivations. Here only data for the $alpha_1$ band concerning the $R_A(EC)$ and $R_A(EO)$ parameter are presented, as are only data for the $alpha_{1+2}$ band concerning the R_R parameter. The other alpha bands appeared to provide parameters with less sensitivity and specificity than those presented.

(i) *Relative delta$_2$ power asymmetry.* R_A limits were calculated for the posterior temporal and mid-temporal regions in the EC condition. These were: T_6/T_5: $-0.138 \div 0.213$ and T_4/T_3: $-0.188 \div 0.163$. The specificity of this parameter concerning two pairs of derivations appeared to be 95% when applied to the reference group.

(ii) *Relative alpha$_1$ power asymmetry EC.* The following limits of normality considering 5% confidence limits were found for the $alpha_1$ band:

O_2/O_1: $-0.213 \div 0.438$ (mean: 0.069)
P_4/P_3: $-0.288 \div 0.438$ (mean: 0.032)
T_6/T_5: $-0.300 \div 0.563$ (mean: 0.067)

These data show that in the reference group there is a tendency toward a higher $alpha_1$ power in the temporo-occipital region on the right hemisphere. The specificity of this parameter for three pairs of derivations, when applied to the reference group, appeared to be 92%.

(iii) *Relative alpha$_1$ power asymmetry EO.* The following ranges of R_A EO were found, with confidence limits of 5% for the $alpha_1$ band:

O_2/O_1: $-0.163 \div 0.163$
P_4/P_3: $-0.238 \div 0.188$
T_6/T_5: $-0.213 \div 0.288$

The specificity of this parameter for three pairs of derivations was 94%.

(iv) *Alpha$_{1+2}$ power reactivity.* The limits for the reactivity of the $alpha_{1+2}$ band were determined with a single sided test, confidence limits 5%. They were:

T_6: 0.213 T_5: 0.188
T_4: 0.113 T_3: 0.065

The specificity of this parameter for two pairs of derivations was 98%.

(c) *Photic stimulation parameters*

A multivariate F-test was applied to the PS parameters, taking into account the correlation between adjacent regions, with confidence limits of 5%. The combination of three parameters resulted in a specificity of 85%. Detailed data will not be presented here.

Study group (SN₃)

(a) *Spectral peak parameters in the study group*

(i) *Alpha peak frequency values* EC <8.0 Hz were not found in the study group (sensitivity 0%).

(ii) *Alpha peak frequency asymmetries.* In six patients, alpha peak frequency asymmetries were obtained exceeding the normal ranges (sensitivity 30%, specificity 92%).

(iii) *Alpha peak frequency shift.* Alpha peaks EO could be distinguished in 55% of the patients in the occipital, in 52% in the mid-temporal, in 50% in the posterior temporal and in 38% in the parietal regions (overall 49%). Thus in this patient group there were generally less alpha peaks EO than in the reference group. In the study group, shifts toward a higher and shifts toward a lower frequency were in balance. A mean alpha frequency increase EO was not observed.

(iv) *Alpha frequency shift asymmetry.* In three patients a shift asymmetry >0.6 Hz was found. The affected hemisphere generally showed a less pronounced shift than the normal one, thus giving rise to a shift asymmetry (sensitivity 15%, specificity 96%).

(v) *Mu peak asymmetry.* Mu peaks were identified in five patients. All patients but one were >55 years old ($\bar{x}$ 58 years), which is in contrast to the data on the reference group. In four patients the mu rhythm had a higher frequency than the alpha rhythm. In the fifth patient the symmetrical mu rhythm held an intermediate position between the two asymmetrical alpha peaks. It was slower than the alpha rhythm of the normal hemisphere, but faster than the alpha rhythm of the affected hemisphere. In two patients the mu rhythm showed an abnormal frequency asymmetry (0.4 and 0.6 Hz) and was slower on the ischemic side (Fig. 4). In two patients the mu rhythm occurred on only one side. In one of these patients it was absent on the affected side (depressed), in the other patient it was only present on the ischemic side (enhanced) (Fig. 1). Thus in four out of five patients the mu rhythm was abnormal. The sensitivity for the whole group of patients was 20%, specificity 100%. The combination of the parameters (a) (ii), (iv) and (v) applied both to the reference group and the study group resulted in a combined sensitivity of 50% and a combined specificity of 90%.

(b) *Band power parameters in the study group*

(i) *Delta₂ power asymmetry.* Only one patient had an abnormal ratio value for one region (sensitivity 5%, specificity 95%).

(ii) *Relative alpha₁ power asymmetry EC.* Seven patients had abnormal values in one or more of the derivations studied (sensitivity 35%, specificity 92%).

18

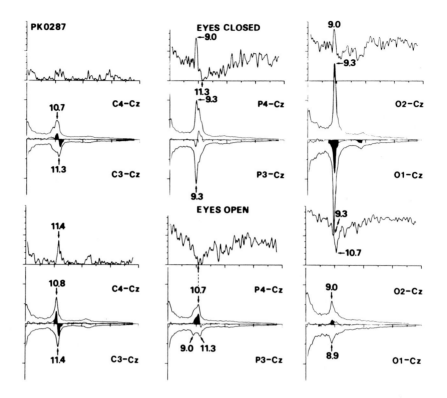

Fig. 4. Spectra from male patient, 30 years of age with RIND in the right hemisphere. CT scan: repeatedly normal with normal contrast studies; angiography: occlusion of the middle cerebral artery at 2 cm distance from the bifurcation. Alpha rhythm slightly depressed on the ischemic side. Mu peak frequency asymmetry of 0.6 Hz with lower frequency on the ischemic side.

(iii) *Relative alpha₁ power asymmetry EO*. Six patients had values outside the normal range in one or more of the regions considered (sensitivity 30%, specificity 94%).

(iv) *Alpha₁₊₂ power reactivity*. Five patients had abnormal reactivity ratio results, i.e. their alpha rhythm was less suppressed in the EO condition in one or more of the temporal derivations (sensitivity 25%, specificity 98%). The combination of three parameters (b) (ii), (iii) and (iv) and applied to both the reference group and the study group led to a combined sensitivity of 55% and a combined specificity of 86%.

(c) *Photic stimulation parameters in the study group*

Each of the three PS parameters enabled the detection of two patients in the study group (sensitivity 10%, specificity 95%). The combination of three PS parameters revealed six patients (sensitivity 30%, specificity 85%). These six patients were already identified as patients by one or more of the spontaneous EEG parameters. The sensitivity and the specificity for each of the parameters used are summarized in Table III.

TABLE III

SENSITIVITY AND SPECIFICITY FOR NINE qEEG PARAMETERS

	Sensitivity[a] (%)	Specificity[b] (%)
Alpha peak frequency	0	96
Alpha peak frequency asymmetry EC	30	92
Alpha peak frequency shift asymmetry	15	96
Mu asymmetry	20	100
Delta$_2$ power R$_A$	5	95
Alpha$_1$ power R$_A$EC	35	92
Alpha$_1$· power R$_A$EO	30	94
Alpha$_{1+2}$ power R$_R$	25	98
Photic stimulation parameters	30	85

[a]Sensitivity: $\dfrac{\text{true positives}}{\text{true positives + false negatives}} \times 100\%$.

[b]Specificity: $\dfrac{\text{true negatives}}{\text{true negatives + false positives}} \times 100\%$

(d) *Combination of parameters in the study group*

Several combinations of parameters can be used, resulting in both sensitivity increase and specificity decrease. The combination of five parameters (alpha peak frequency asymmetry, alpha peak frequency shift asymmetry, mu asymmetry, alpha$_1$ power asymmetry EC and alpha$_{1+2}$ power reactivity) provided the following data: combined sensitivity 70%, combined specificity 80%. When using seven parameters (all parameters except alpha peak frequency and delta$_2$ power R$_A$) and demanding that two parameters or more provide abnormal results, the result is: combined sensitivity 50%, combined specificity 100% (Table IV).

TABLE IV

ABNORMAL qEEG RESULTS IN GROUP SN$_3$

	n	*	**
TIA	8	6	4
RIND	3	2	1
PNS	9	6	5
Total	20	14	10

* 1 of 5 parameters abnormal.
** ≥2 of 7 parameters abnormal.

(e) *Comparison of qEEG results with clinical classification and CT scan findings*

The abnormal qEEG results (five-parameter score and seven-parameter score with more than one parameter abnormal) are related to the clinical classification in Table

IV. The relation between clinical classification and CT scan findings is presented in Table I. From these data, it appears that qEEG results are not clearly related to clinical classification, in contrast to CT scan findings. The discrepancy between qEEG and CT scan findings is most striking in the group of patients with reversible ischemia (TIA, RIND). In this group, qEEG was abnormal in 8 out of 11 patients, whereas CT scan revealed abnormality in only 1 out of 10 patients with transient ischemia. Thus the superiority of qEEG over visually assessed EEG and CT scan is most clearly demonstrated in patients with transient ischemia.

DISCUSSION

From a therapeutical point of view, the minor degrees of cerebral ischemia (TIA, RIND, PNS) are most important. Future stroke in these patients may be prevented by several methods of treatment. Especially in the transient forms of ischemia and to a lesser degree in those with minimal deficit, the neurological diagnosis may be questionable. The interobserver index of agreement among neurologists diagnosing patients with reversible ischemia is restricted. In such cases a confirmatory laboratory test would be advantageous. CT scans, however, are mostly normal in minor ischemia, especially in transient ischemia.

In addition, when considering prompt diagnosis and treatment to prevent further disability, CT has a serious advantage. It may take days or even weeks before small ischemic lesions become visible. The opposite is true for the EEG. Most EEG abnormalities are found during and immediately after the ischemic episode, decreasing in the course of time. In patients with transient ischemia, the EEG signs of ischemia may be more protracted than the clinical signs and symptoms. Absence of EEG signs in minor ischemia, however, is widely reported. In patients with TIAs, the EEG may be normal in up to 50% of these patients (Enge et al., 1980), whereas CT may be normal in up to 100% of these patients (Ottonello et al., 1980). In studies comparing EEG and CT in patients with TIAs and RINDs, the sensitivity of the EEG is about twice that of the CT scan. Under these circumstances the question arises whether computer analysis can improve the results of EEG assessed by the human interpreter.

Many forms of computer analysis have been used and evaluated in recent years. Some of these forms have been applied to EEGs from patients with cerebral ischemia. In general, however, qEEG studies have been performed on EEGs that were already abnormal on visual assessment, recorded as they were in patients with cerebral infarction and/or CT scan abnormality (Tolonen and Sulg, 1981; Tolonen et al., 1981; Pfurtscheller et al., 1981; Nagata et al., 1982).

The present authors investigated qEEG exclusively in patients with minor ischemia, whose EEGs were "normal" on visual assessment (Van Huffelen et al., 1980, 1982). In studies of this kind data processing is aimed at extension of the faculties of the EEG interpreter by acquisition of information which escapes visual analysis. Here, the presence of a major group of normal reference subjects is of paramount importance. In two previous studies (SN_1, SN_2) two groups of 20 patients were compared with 20 reference subjects and qEEG appeared to be abnormal in contrast to visual assessment in 55% of the patients, (sensitivity 55%, specificity 95%). The present study had at its disposal a reference group of 50 healthy volunteers in the same age range as the patients. The present series of 20 patients SN_3 was highly comparable with the former two SN_1 and SN_2 groups. Yet there were some differences. In the first series SN_1 only 7 patients out of 20 had transient ischemia, whereas in the last two series there were 13 (SN_2) and 11 (SN_3) patients with TIA or RIND. Thus the last series contained more patients with transient ischemia, decreasing the probability that any EEG abnormality could be found. In the first series SN_1 a first-generation CT scanner was used, which may explain the small number of abnormal scans (25%) obtained. In the last two series SN_2 and SN_3, more CT abnormality was discovered (SN_2: 47%, SN_3: 37%) (Table I), although less abnormality was expected on the basis of clinical classification of the patients. The last series SN_3 contained less patients with CT scan abnormality than the former series SN_2, while both were studied with the same scanner, indicating that the SN_3 series included more patients with minimal ischemia. In the last series SN_3, CT scan was abnormal in only 10% of the TIA/RIND patients.

Nevertheless, the three groups SN_1, SN_2, SN_3 had many findings in common. All patients had the same mean age (54 years), the same age range (27–70 years) and were examined in the acute phase (82% within the first 10 days). In all three groups there was a preponderance of male patients (73%) and of left-sided ischemia (55%). Thus some general trends may be outlined on the basis of the study of the SN_{1-3} group of 60 patients. In patients with a normal EEG the prognosis for recovery is favorable, in accordance with much literature data (e.g. Kayser-Gatchalian and Neundörfer, 1980). Recurrence of stroke, however, remains threatening. In patients with transient ischemia, CT scan reveals abnormality in only 17% in accordance with data from Ladurner et al. (1979), and other authors. Therefore the finding of abnormal qEEG results in these cases is of considerable clinical diagnostic importance.

For an evaluation of the superiority of qEEG over conventional EEG, the reliability of EEG interpretation according to conventional clinical criteria has to be discussed. It cannot be denied that personal experience of the individual interpreter plays a role and that different EEG interpreters may come to various interpretations of the same EEG. Thus different series of EEGs interpreted as "normal" may be dissimilar. This in itself is an argument in favor of objective EEG analysis. The present series of EEGs (SN_3) was independently assessed by three interpreters who have special experience and expertise in the interpretation of EEGs in cerebral ischemia. Thus the SN_3 series is more strictly selected than the SN_1 and SN_2 series and this explains why some parameters revealed abnormality in the SN_1 and SN_2 series and did not in the SN_3 series. An alpha rhythm frequency <8.0 Hz was found in 5 patients, 2 patients and no patients in the SN_1, SN_2 and SN_3 series, respectively and an abnormal $delta_2$ asymmetry ratio in temporal regions was found in 9, 5 and 1 patient in the same groups, respectively. Thus the SN_3 group of patients fulfills many criteria for selection, rendering it improbable that any EEG abnormality could be expected. These criteria are: clinical classification (preponderance of transient ischemia), CT scan findings (absence of abnormality) and strict EEG interpretation by different interpreters.

Data processing of the EEG may be based on several kinds of approaches to the EEG signal. In many studies, qEEG is restricted to one or two pairs of derivations and to one parameter or a restricted set of parameters. In this study, a multi-derivation and multi-parameter approach was chosen to improve the sensitivity of the qEEG. Analysis was applied to seven pairs of symmetrical derivations in a montage with C_z as a common reference. Thus the major part of the scalp was covered, rendering it improbable that local abnormalities could be overlooked. In addition, many parameters were investigated, both spectral maxima or peaks and band power data were studied. In general, mean frequency values are determined in whole spectra or bands (Tolonen and Sulg, 1980; Tolonen et al., 1980, 1981), whereas in this study individual spectral peaks were determined. The absolute power in individual bands has been studied by many authors and appears to have a considerable variance. In this study, ratios showing considerably less variance, i.e. asymmetry ratios and reactivity ratios were investigated on which there is no detailed data in the literature. Photic stimulation data have not been studied so far using the parameters in the present study.

Here, some parameters used in former studies appeared to be ineffective. These parameters, i.e. alpha peak frequency (<8.0 Hz) and $delta_2$ power ratio, being insensitive to minor ischemia, are important for objective assessment of abnormalities found in EEGs scored as abnormal. In the present study some parameters used in previous studies again appeared to be of importance, i.e. the alpha peak frequency asymmetry and the photic stimulation parameters, although the latter were considerably less so than in previous studies.

The photic stimulation parameters in the present study revealed less abnormality than in the previous series. For the power asymmetry ratio abnormal results were: SN_1: 25%, SN_2: 60%, SN_3: 10%. The conformation parameter results were: SN_1: 55%, SN_2: 60%, SN_3: 10%. The introduction of a new parameter for the phase of the cross power gave only a slight improvement of the sensitivity of 10%; thus the combination of three PS parameters resulted in a sensitivity of 30% with a specificity of 85%. The differences between the results from the previous studies and the present one are caused by two independent factors: the SN_3 group was more strictly selected than the SN_1 and SN_2 groups, resulting in a lower sensitivity in the SN_3 group. The statistics used in the present series took into account the correlation between adjacent regions (multivariate F-test). The now more reliable results revealed less impressive data than the former ones. The PS parameters detected no patients not already identified as patients with the spontaneous EEG parameters. Consequently, full attention was directed to the spontaneous EEG parameters. In addition to the alpha peak frequency asymmetry used in previous studies, several new parameters were studied, i.e. alpha peak frequency shift asymmetry, mu peak frequency asymmetry, alpha power asymmetry EC, EO and alpha band power reactivity.

The alpha peak frequency asymmetry in this study was slightly different from the one previously used (abnormal > 0.4 Hz). Due to the larger reference group, limits of normality could be differentiated per region (>0.3 Hz – >0.6 Hz) and a higher specificity obtained (92% instead of 85%). Using these differentiated limits of normality, abnormal values were found in 30% of the patients (SN_1: 55%, SN_2: 45%). Thus this parameter appeared to be of major importance in the three series of patients. The question arises whether this qEEG parameter cannot be used in visual assessment of the EEG. If the EEG interpreter could distinguish these asymmetries in alpha frequencies, data processing would be redundant. In an investigation among 82 qualified electroencephalographers assessing computer generated EEG signals, the present authors found that only frequency differences >0.6 Hz between alpha peak frequencies could reliably be detected by the interpreters. This shows that computer analysis is superior to visual assessment of the EEG, enabling the detection of asymmetries of 0.3 Hz and more and consequently by increasing diagnostic sensitivity, enabling more patients to be identified.

The alpha peak frequency shift asymmetry due to opening of the eyes has not been studied by qEEG, as yet. It has been described implicitly by Farbrot (1954) in the visually assessed EEG. The finding that the alpha rhythm still could be detected in the EEG spectra in the EO condition in about 60% of the subjects and that it generally had a higher frequency than the alpha rhythm EC has not yet been published. The shift asymmetry parameter appeared to have a restricted sensitivity (15% with a specificity of 96%), partly due to the fact that it can be used in only 50% of the patients, permitting the detection of some patients not found with the aid of the other alpha rhythm parameters.

A more sensitive parameter was provided by several aspects of the mu rhythm. Initially, one serious drawback was thought to be present. The mu rhythm is seldom found in older subjects (Magnus and Beek, 1959; Niedermeyer and Koshino, 1975). When using computer analysis a higher percentage may be found, especially in young adults (Storm van Leeuwen et al., 1978; Schoppenhorst et al., 1980). In accordance with the literature, in the present reference group of 50 subjects a mu rhythm was found in the younger age group (mean age of 10 subjects with mu rhythm 30 years). Consequently, the clinical significance of the mu rhythm for the detection of ischemia in older patients was open to question. An interesting finding, however, was that in the study group a mu rhythm was discovered in older patients (mean age 58 years). When present, the mu rhythm appeared to be very sensitive to ischemia. In four out of five patients the mu rhythm appeared to be very asymmetrical. Mu augmentation due to deep lesions and mu depression due to more widely spread ischemia were found in accordance with the findings of Pfurtscheller (1981). Due to the peak detection technique, subtle frequency differences could also be studied in the present series. This permitted detection of unilateral slowing of mu rhythm on the ischemic side. This also permitted a clear differentiation between alpha and mu rhythm. In this study the mu rhythm was studied in the EO condition and reactivity was tested with tactile stimulation of the hands. The low coherence between bilateral mu rhythms (Storm van Leeuwen et al., 1978) was observed. Thus, based on criteria of frequency, coherence, persistence in EO condition and reactivity to tactile stimulation the mu rhythm could be more clearly differentiated from alpha activity than in the studies of Pfurtscheller et al. (1981). The mu rhythm parameter added to the above-mentioned parameters increased the sensitivity of the qEEG. Mu abnormality was found in some patients with normal alpha rhythm parameters. The combination of the three discussed peak parameters (alpha peak frequency asymmetry, alpha peak frequency shift asymmetry and mu asymmetry) resulted in a sensitivity of 50% and a specificity of 90%. This underscores the importance of multi-parameter, multi-derivation studies.

Two band power ratios were used in the present study: an asymmetry ratio and a reactivity ratio on which there are no detailed normative data in the literature. These two parameters cannot be studied visually (Binnie et al., 1978). It is difficult to get more than a general impression on the energy in a given band over a period of 100 sec and to assess its reactivity and asymmetry when studying symmetrical derivations. Frequently, the alpha rhythm shows larger amplitudes in the right temporo-occipital region. In the present study results of investigations of a reference group were used to determine the range of normality with 5% confidence limits. The asymmetry ratio clearly showed a tendency toward asymmetry with higher values on the right side in temporo-occipital regions. The relative $alpha_1$ band power asymmetry ratios EC and EO yielded 35% and 30% of abnormal values, respectively (specificity 92% and

94%). The alpha power reactivity ratio revealed 25% of abnormal values with a specificity of 98%. The combination of the last three band power parameters resulted in a combined sensitivity of 55% (specificity 86%). Here, too, multiple parameters in multiple derivations are superior to one single parameter in one single pair of derivations.

One is tempted to add more and more parameter results to combine scores and to obtain an even higher sensitivity. Yet there is a limitation because in the present study in six patients (30%) none of the parameters studied resulted in an abnormal score. In many of the patients identified with one parameter, however, several parameters gave abnormal results. Another drawback of accumulating parameter scores is the fact that with increasing sensitivity, the specificity decreases due to the increasing number of false positives found in the reference group. When using five selective parameters (alpha frequency asymmetry, alpha peak frequency shift asymmetry, mu asymmetry, power asymmetry in the $alpha_1$ band EC, alpha power reactivity), a sensitivity of 70% was obtained with a specificity of 80%. Most striking is the fact that this combination of parameters showed abnormality in eight out of 11 patients with transient ischemia, whereas the CT scan showed abnormality in only one out of 10 patients with transient ischemia. These figures are superior to the results of previous investigations. In addition, one has to consider the fact that in the present study less abnormality could be expected to be present in the EEGs.

The results of the present study can be expressed in still another way. When demanding that at least two parameters provide abnormal results for the identification of patients, the specificity increases to 100%. The sensitivity, however, decreases to 50%. Thus expressed, the results are still better than those of previous studies.

In the present study significant results were gained using only two files of 100 sec spontaneous EEG activity, one in the EC condition and one in the EO condition. The application of photic stimulation gave no increase in sensitivity. When using a multiple parameter, multiple derivation approach, the analysis of two files of 100 sec of EEG activity results in a considerable extension of the diagnostic sensitivity of the EEG. This increase in diagnostic sensitivity of the EEG is of utmost importance in patients with transient cerebral ischemia. In many of these patients the neurologist is unable to detect objective neurological signs and his presumption that the patient suffers from ischemia has to be substantiated by a confirmatory test. In most of these cases, however, CT scan or conventional EEG show no abnormalities and the neurologist remains in doubt whether invasive investigations should be performed or treatment to prevent recurrence should be stopped. In such circumstances the qEEG may prove to be the only objective noninvasive method to confirm the diagnosis of transient ischemia.

SUMMARY

The acquisition of information which escapes visual analysis, is one of the objectives of computer analysis of the EEG. In patients with minor ischemia (TIA, RIND, PNS) the EEG is often "normal" on visual assessment, whereas CT is normal in the majority of these patients. Especially in the transient forms of ischemia the neurologist is unable to detect objective neurological signs. A confirmatory test to substantiate such a diagnosis would be advantageous.

Quantitative EEG (qEEG) was investigated exclusively in 20 patients with minor ischemia, whose EEGs were "normal" on visual assessment. A group of 50 healthy volunteers in the same age range was studied to obtain reference data.

Data processing of the EEG was applied to seven pairs of symmetrical derivations. Departing from power spectrum analysis using FFT many parameters were determined. Both spectral maxima or peaks and band power data were studied. The influence of several conditions, i.e. eyes closed (EC), eyes open (EO), tactile stimulation of the hands and photic stimulation was investigated.

The most sensitive parameters with highest specificity appeared to be: the alpha peak frequency asymmetry EC, the alpha peak frequency shift asymmetry due to opening of the eyes, the mu rhythm asymmetry EO, the power asymmetry in the $alpha_1$ EC and the alpha power reactivity to opening of the eyes.

With the combination of these five selective parameters a sensitivity of 70% was obtained with a specificity of 80%. This combination showed abnormality in 72% of the patients with transient ischemia, whereas the CT scan showed abnormality in only 10% of these patients.

In these circumstances qEEG is far superior to the conventional EEG and CT and it may prove to be the only objective noninvasive method to confirm the diagnosis of transient ischemia.

REFERENCES

Ad hoc Committee on Cerebrovascular Diseases (1975) A Classification and outline of cerebrovascular diseases. II. *Stroke*, 6: 564–616

Barlow, J.S. (1979) Computerized clinical electroencephalography in perspective. *IEEE Trans. Biomed. Eng. BME*, 26: 377–391.

Becker, H., Desch, H., Hacker, H. and Perez, A. (1979) CT fogging effect with ischemic cerebral infarcts. *Neuroradiology*, 18: 185–192.

Bickford, R.G. (1981) A combined EEG and evoked potential procedure in clinical EEG (Automated cerebral electrogram – Ace test). In N. Yamaguchi and K. Fujisawa (Eds.), *Recent Advances in EEG and EMG Data Processing*, Elsevier/North-Holland Biomedical Press, Amsterdam–New York–Oxford, pp. 217–235.

Bickford, R.G., Brimm, J.E., Berger, L. and Aung, M. (1973) Application of compressed spectral array in clinical EEG. In P. Kellaway and I. Petersén (Eds.), *Automation of Clinical Electroencephalography*, Raven, New York, pp. 55–64.

Biller, J., Laster, D.W., Howard, G., Toole, J.F. and McHenry, L.C. (1982) Cranial computerized tomography in carotid artery transient ischemic attacks. *Europ. Neurol.*, 21: 98–101.

Binnie, C.D., Batchelor, B.G., Bowring, P.A., Darby, C.E., Herbert, L., Lloyd, D.S.L., Smith, D.M., Smith, G.F. and Smith, M. (1978) Computer-assisted interpretation of clinical EEGs. *Electroenceph. clin. Neurophysiol.*, 44: 575–585.

Calanchini, P.R., Swanson, P.D., Gotshall, R.A. Haerer, A.F., Poskanzer, D.C., Price, T.R., Conneally, P.M., Dyken, M.L. and Futty, D.E. (1977) Cooperative study of hospital frequency and character of transient ischemic attacks. IV. The reliability of diagnosis. *J. Amer. med. Ass.* 238: 2029–2033.

Castorina, G. and Marchini, E. (1958) Le alterazione elettroencefalografiche da occlusione delle arterie carotide interna e cerebrale media. *Lav. Neuropsichat.*, 22: 3–67.

Celesia, G.G., Soni, V.K. and Rhode, W.S. (1978) Visual evoked spectrum array (VESA) and interhemispheric variations. *Arch. Neurol. (Chic.)*, 35: 678–682.

Celesia, G.G., Meredith, J.T. and Pluff, K. (1983) Perimetry, visual evoked potentials and visual evoked spectrum array in homonymous hemianopsia. *Electroenceph. clin. Neurophysiol.*, 56: 16–30.

Cohen, B.A. (1975) *Computer analysis of serial electroencephalograms from patients with cerebrovascular accidents. Dissertation*, Marquette University, Milwaukee, Wisconsin, p.366.

Duffy, F.H., Burchfiel, J.L. and Lombroso, C.T. (1979) Brain Electrical Activity Mapping (BEAM): a

26

method for extending the clinical utility of EEG and evoked potential data. *Ann. Neurol.*, 5: 309–321.

Duffy, F.H., Bartels, P.H. and Burchfiel, J.L. (1981) Significance probability mapping: an aid in the topographic analysis of brain electrical activity. *Electroenceph. clin. Neurophysiol.*, 51: 455–462.

Ellingson, R.J. and Peters, J.F. (1981) Contributions of data processing to clinical electroencephalography. In N. Yamaguchi and K. Fujisawa (Eds.), *Recent Advances in EEG and EMG Data Processing*, Elsevier/North-Holland Biomedical Press, Amsterdam–New York–Oxford, pp.247–260.

Enge, S., Lechner, H., Logar, Ch. and Ladurner, G. (1980) Clinical Value of EEG in Transient Ischemic Attacks. In H. Lechner and A. Aranibar (Eds.), *EEG and Clinical Neurophysiology*. Excerpta Medica, Amsterdam–Oxford–Princeton, pp.173–180.

Farbrot, Ö. (1953) Renseignements apportés par la stimulation lumineuse intermittente à l'étude électroencéphalographique des accidents vasculaires cérébraux. *Acta psychiat. scand.*, 28: 275–286.

Farbrot, Ö (1954) Electroencephalographic study in cases of cerebrovascular accidents (preliminary report) *Electroenceph. clin. Neurophysiol.*, 6: 678–681.

Gotman, J. Gloor, P. and Ray, W.F. (1975) A quantitative comparison of traditional reading of the EEG and interpretation of computer-extracted features in patients with supratentorial brain lesions. *Electroenceph. clin. Neurophysiol.*, 38: 623–639.

Hébert, F., Touraine, A., Bertolidi, I. and Samson-Dollfus, D. (1980) Résultats concernant l'analyse spectrale de l'EEG au cours du vieillissement cérébral chez des sujets témoins et des sujets cardiovasculaires. *Rev. EEG. Neurophysiol.*, 10: 131–135.

Hjorth, B. (1970) EEG analysis based on time domain properties. *Electroenceph. clin. Neurophysiol.*, 29: 306–310.

Hjorth, B. (1973). The physical significance of time domain descriptors in EEG analysis. *Electroenceph. clin. Neurophysiol.*, 34: 321–325.

Joint Committee for Stroke Resources (1977) Report XIV: Cerebral ischemia: the role of thrombosis and of anti-thrombotic therapy. *Stroke*, 8: 147–175.

Kayser-Gatchalian, M.C. and Neundörfer, B. (1980) The prognostic value of EEG in ischemic cerebral insults. *Electroenceph. clin. Neurophysiol.*, 49: 608–617.

Kooi, K.A., Eckman, H.G. and Thomas, M.H. (1957) Observations on the response to photic stimulation in organic cerebral dysfunction. *Electroencepn. clin. Neurophysiol.*, 9: 239–250.

Kuhlman, W.M. (1978) Functional topography of the human mu rhythm. *Electroenceph. clin. Neurophysiol.*, 44: 83–93.

Ladurner, G., Sager, W.D., Iliff, L.D. and Lechner, H. (1979) A correlation of clinical findings and CT in ischaemic cerebrovascular disease. *Europ. Neurol.*, 18: 281–288.

Lassen, N.A. (1982) Incomplete cerebral infarction – focal incomplete ischemic tissue necrosis not leading to emollision. *Stroke*, 13: 522–523.

Logar, Ch., Martischnig, R., Enge, S., Sager W.D. and Ladurner G. (1979) Zur Wertigkeit von EEG und Computertomographie bei ischämischen Insulten. *Z. EEG-EMG*, 10: 161–166.

Lopes da Silva, F.H. (1976) Computers in neurophysiology – methods in analysis. *Hoofdlijnen*, 11: 67–80.

Lopes da Silva, F.H. (1981) Analysis of EEG ongoing activity: Rhythms and nonstationarities. In N. Yamaguchi and K. Fujisawa (Eds.), *Recent Advances in EEG and EMG Data Processing*, Elsevier/ North-Holland Biomedical Press, Amsterdam–New York–Oxford, pp. 95–115.

Magnus, O. and Beek, H. (1959) Le rythme en arceau et l'âge. *Rev. neurol.*, 100: 382.

Matejcek, M. (1980) Application de l'analyse spectrale pour l'étude de certaines relations entre l'activité EEG occipitale et l'âge. *Rev. EEG Neurophysiol.*, 10: 122–130.

Mohr, J.P. (1982) Lacunes. *Stroke.*, 13: 3–11.

Nagata, K., Mizukami, M., Araki, G., Kawase, T. and Hirano, M. (1982) Topographic electroencephalographic study of cerebral infarction using computed mapping of the EEG. *J. Cereb. Blood Flow Metab.*, 2: 79–88.

Niedermeyer, E. and Koshino, Y. (1975) My-Rhythmus: Vorkommen und klinische Bedeutung. *Z. EEG-EMG*, 6: 69–78.

Norris, J.W. and Hachinski, V.C. (1982) Misdiagnosis of stroke. *Lancet*, i: 328–331.

Ott, E., Lechner, H., Marguc, K., Bertha, G., Aranibar, A., Ladurner, G. and Sager, W.D. (1980) Correlation of EEG and CT findings with cerebral blood flow measurements in patients with cerebrovascular disorders. In H. Lechner and A. Aranibar (Eds.), *EEG and Clinical Neurophysiology*, Excerpta Medica, Amsterdam–Oxford–Princeton, pp. 143–147.

Ottonello, G.A., Regesta, G. and Tanganelli, P. (1980) Correlation between computerized tomography and EEG findings in acute cerebrovascular disorders. In H. Lechner and A. Aranibar (Eds.), *EEG and Clinical Neurophysiology*, Excerpta Medica, Amsterdam–Oxford–Princeton, pp. 148–162.

Perrone, P., Candelise, L., Scotti, G., De Grandi, C. and Scialfa, J. (1979) CT evaluation in patients with transient ischemic attack. Correlation between clinical and angiographic findings. *Europ. Neurol.*, 18: 217–221.

Pfurtscheller, G and Auer, L.M. (1983) Frequency changes of sensorimotor EEG rhythm after revascularization surgery. *Electroenceph. clin. Neurophysiol.*, 55: 381–387.

Pfurtscheller, G., Wege, W. and Sager, W. (1980) Asymmetrien in der zentralen Alpha-Aktivität (My-Rhythmus) unter Ruhe- und Aktivitätsbedingungen bei zerebrovaskulären Erkrankungen. *Z.EEG-EMG.*, 11: 63–71.

Pfurtscheller, G., Sager, W. and Wege, W. (1981) Correlation between CT scan and sensorimotor EEG rhythms in patients with cerebrovacular disorders. *Electroenceph. clin. Neurophysiol.*, 52: 473–485.

Pidoux, B., Etevenon, P., Campistron, D., Peron-Magnan, P., Bisserbe, J-C., Verdeaux, G. and Deniker, P. (1983) Topoélectroencéphalographie quantitative par ordinateur. *Rev. EEG Neurophysiol.*, 13: 27–34.

Poortvliet, D.C.J. and Van Huffelen, A.C. (1981) *Evaluation of the relative asymmetry and conformation during photic stimulation.* In J. Baal-Schem, Z. Kohari, E.N. Protonotarios and J. Shamir (Eds.), Proceedings Melecon '81, 9,2,4.1–5.

Pullicino, P., Nelson, R.F., Kendall, B.E. and Marshall J. (1980) Small deep infarcts diagnosed on computed tomography. *Neurology*, 30: 1090–1096.

Raichle, M.E. (1983) The pathophysiology of brain ischemia. *Ann. Neurol.*, 13: 2–10.

Schoppenhorst, M., Brauer, F., Freund, G and Kubicki, St. (1980) The significance of coherence estimates in determining central alpha and mu activities. *Electroenceph. clin. Neurophysiol.*, 48: 25–33.

Sisk, Ch., Ziegler, D.K. and Zileli, T. (1970) Discrepancies in recorded results from duplicate neurological history and examination in patients studied for prognosis in cerebrovascular disease. *Stroke*, 1: 14–18.

Sotaniemi, K.A., Sulg, I.A. and Hokkanen, T.E. (1980) Quantitative EEG as a measure of cerebral dysfunction before and after open-heart surgery. *Electroenceph. clin. Neurophysiol.*, 50: 81–95.

Stigsby, B., Obrist, W.D. and Sulg, I.A. (1973) Automatic data acquisition and period-amplitude analysis of the EEG. *Comput. Progr. Biomed.*, 3: 93–104.

Storm van Leeuwen, W., Wieneke, G., Spoelstra, P. and Versteeg, H. (1978) Lack of bilateral coherence of mu rhythm. *Electroenceph. clin. Neurophysiol.*, 44: 140–146.

Symon, L. (1980) The relationship between CBF, evoked potentials and the clinical features in cerebral ischaemia. *Acta neurol. scand.*, (Suppl. 78), 62: 175–190.

Tolonen, U. and Sulg, I.A. (1981) Comparison of quantitative EEG parameters from four different analysis techniques in evaluation of relationships between EEG and CBF in brain infarction. *Electroenceph. clin. Neurophysiol.*, 51: 177–185.

Tolonen, U., Ahonen, F., Sulg, I.A., Kuikka, J., Kallanranta, T., Koskinen, M. and Hokkanen, E. (1981) Serial measurements of quantitative EEG and cerebral blood flow and circulation time after brain infarction. *Acta neurol. scand.*, 63: 145–155.

Tomasello, F., Mariani, F., Fieschi, C., Argentino, C., Bono, G., De Zanche, L., Inzitari, D., Martini, A., Perrone, P. and Sangiovanni, G. (1982) Assessment of inter-observer differences in the Italian multicenter study on reversible cerebral ischemia. *Stroke*, 13: 32–35.

Van der Drift, J.H.A. (1972) The EEG in cerebrovascular disease. In P.J. Vinken and G.W. Bruyn (Eds.), *Handbook of Clinical Neurology, Vol. 11: Vascular Disease of the Nervous System*, Elsevier North-Holland, Amsterdam, pp.267–291.

Van der Drift, J.H.A. and Kok, N.K.D. (1972) The EEG in cerebrovascular disorders in relation to pathology. In A. Rémond (Ed.), *Handbook of Electroencephalography and Clinical Neurophysiology, Vol 14A: Cardiac and Vascular Diseases*, Elsevier, Amsterdam, pp.12–64.

Van der Drift, J.H.A. and Magnus, O. (1961) The EEG in cerebral ischemic lesions: correlations with clinical and pathological findings. In J.S. Meyer and H. Gastaut (Eds.), *Cerebral Anoxia and the Electroencephalogram*, C.C. Thomas, Springfield, Ill., pp.180–196.

Van Huffelen, A.C., Poortvliet, D.C.J. and Van der Wulp, C.J.M. (1980a) *Quantitative electroencephalography in cerebral ischemia*, TNO, The Hague, p.161.

Van Huffelen, A.C., Poortvliet, D.C.J. and Van der Wulp, C.J.M. (1980b) Quantitative EEG in cerebral ischemia. A. Parameters for the detection of abnormalities in "normal" EEGs in patients with Acute Unilateral Cerebral Ischemia. (A.U.C.I.). In H. Lechner and A. Aranibar (Eds.), *EEG and Clinical Neurophysiology*, Excerpta Medica, Amsterdam–Oxford–Princeton, pp.125–130.

Van Huffelen, A.C., Poortvliet, D.C.J. and Van der Wulp, C.J.M. (1980c) Quantitative EEG in cerebral

28

ischemia. B. Parameters valuable for follow-up of patients with Acute Unilateral Cerebral Ischemia (A.U.C.I.). In H. Lechner and A. Aranibar (Eds.), *EEG and Clinical Neurophysiology,* Excerpta Medica, Amsterdam–Oxford–Princeton, pp.131–137.

Van Huffelen, A.C., Poortvliet, D.C.J. and Van der Wulp, C.J.M. (1980d) Quantitative EEG in cerebral ischemia. C. The significance of photic stimulation (PS) in patients with Acute Unilateral Cerebral Ischemia (A.U.C.I.). In H. Lechner and A. Aranibar (Eds.), *EEG and Clinical Neurophysiology*, Excerpta Medica, Amsterdam–Oxford–Princeton, pp.138–142.

Van Huffelen, A.C., De Weerd, A.W., Mosmans, P.C.M. and Jonkman, E.J. (1981) Quantitative EEG and cerebral blood flow in patients with minor cerebral ischemia. *Electroenceph. clin. Neurophysiol.*, 52: 143.

Van Huffelen, A.C., Veering, M.M., De Weerd, A.W., Mosmans, P.C.M. and Jonkman, E.J. (1982) Evaluation of non-invasive techniques (qEEG, rCBF, CT) in minor cerebral ischemia. *Clin. Neurol. Neurosurg.*, 84: 204–205.

Wieneke, G.H., Deinema, C.H.A., Spoelstra, P., Storm van Leeuwen, W. and Versteeg, H. (1980) Normative spectral data on alpha rhythm in male adults. *Electroenceph. clin. Neurophysiol.*, 49: 636–645.

Yanagihara, T., Houser, O.W. and Klass, D.W. (1981) Computed tomography and EEG in cerebrovascular disease. *Arch. Neurol.*, 38: 597–600.

*Brain Ischemia: Quantitative EEG and Imaging Techniques, Progress in Brain Research, Vol. 62, edited by
G. Pfurtscheller, E.J. Jonkman and F.H. Lopes da Silva
©1984 Elsevier Science Publishers B.V.*

Quantitative EEG in Normals and in Patients with Cerebral Ischemia

V. KÖPRUNER[1], G. PFURTSCHELLER[1,*] and L. M. AUER[2]

[1]*Department of Computing, Institute of Biomedical Engineering, Technical University of Graz, A-8010 Graz and*
[2]*Department of Neurosurgery, University of Graz, A-8036 Graz (Austria)*

INTRODUCTION

The EEG represents the bioelectrical activity generated in cortical tissue that is controlled by subcortical structures. Disturbances in cerebral perfusion caused by occlusion and/or stenosis of cerebral vessels result in a reduced cell metabolism and this can affect the generation of the EEG. Obrist et al. (1963), Ingvar et al. (1976) and Sulg et al. (1981) are among those who have emphasized this close coupling between brain electrical activity, blood flow and the metabolic activity of the brain. The EEG is, therefore, a valuable tool for estimating global or regional brain dysfunction in cerebrovascular insufficiency.

In patients with extensive cortical infarctions and severe neurological deficits, the EEG shows clear patterns of abnormality (Ladurner and Lechner, 1971); in patients with absent or mild deficits, however, the EEG often shows no abnormalities, if visually assessed (Strauss and Greenstein, 1948; Paddison and Ferriss, 1961; Enge et al., 1980).

The technique of computer-based EEG analysis or quantified EEG (qEEG) provides us with objective data and parameters (for reviews see Barlow, 1979; Lopes da Silva, 1981) more suitable for detecting mild forms of brain dysfunction than visual EEG assessment (Gotman et al., 1973; Pfurtscheller et al., 1981). In a recent study, Van Huffelen et al. (1980) found an abnormal qEEG in about half of a group of 20 patients with acute unilateral ischemia who had "normal" EEGs according to the visual assessment. This example demonstrates the ability of qEEG to detect brain dysfunction related to minor ischemia.

Provocative methods, such as hypoxia (Gastaut et al., 1961) or physical exercise (Kamp and Troost, 1978), may be applied to provoke EEG abnormalities in patients with minor or no abnormal EEG signs during rest. Another type of provocation is the voluntary fist clenching of a rubber ball, where sensorimotor regions are activated and the central mu rhythm is blocked (Jasper and Penfield, 1949; Pfurtscheller and Aranibar, 1979).

EEG changes in centro-temporal regions may appear if the cerebral blood flow and/or the oxygen metabolism in the territory of the middle cerebral artery (MCA) is affected. Assuming that a strong correlation exists between EEG, cerebral blood flow and metabolism, it should be possible to find abnormalities in qEEG from bipolar

---

*To whom correspondence should be addressed

[29]

centro-temporal derivations in most of the patients with minor cerebral insufficiency in the supply territory of the MCA. Furthermore, it should even be possible to discriminate between patients with and without cortical ischemia. In order to test this hypothesis, the qEEG was studied in a group of 32 patients with cerebral insufficiency, most of them candidates for extra-intracranial arterial bypass (EIAB) surgery, before and after which the EEG was recorded from the centro-temporal region during rest and motor activity. In order to discriminate this group of patients suffering from chronic ischemia from a group of 50 neurologically normal subjects, univariate, bivariate and multivariate statistical analyses of the qEEG data were used, and the parameters showing the largest discrimination power were evaluated.

METHOD – DATA ACQUISITION

Subjects

Normals

Two groups of neurologically normal subjects were investigated in these experiments. The first group consisted of 31 students aged between 20 and 32 years, and the second group of 19 subjects, aged between 35 and 80 years. The average age of all normals was 37 years. There were 32 men and 18 women. For statistical analysis, both groups were either pooled together or, in case age was considered of interest, they were treated separately. All subjects were paid.

Patients

EEGs were recorded in a group of 32 patients varying in age between 29 and 72 years, 22 males and 10 females. All patients had cerebrovascular insufficiencies and were admitted to the Department of Neurosurgery of the University of Graz for revascularization surgery; 30 had an EIAB and two a carotid endarterectomy. For the statistical analyses, two measurements from each patient were used, one before operation and the other 7 days thereafter. The perfusion and therefore the brain activity as well can be assumed to have been altered by the time the second EEG recording was made, owing to the surgical intervention. This was reflected in the fact that a certain degree of independence between both EEGs, although obtained from the same patient, was found. The time interval between the cerebrovascular event and the EEG recordings used for computerized analysis lay between 3 weeks and 2 years.

Neurological deficits. Six patients suffered from transitory ischemic attacks (TIA) and 26 from completed stroke. At the time of the EEG recording, 6 were without neurological symptoms, in 20 there were mild to moderate neurological deficits and in 6 these were severe. All were able to perform the task of squeezing a rubber ball at least with the hand on the nonaffected side. Twenty-four patients were able to use both hands. One patient could only squeeze with the right hand, and seven could only use the left hand.

Computerized tomography. Cortical infarction was reported in 17 patients and subcortical infarction in 6 (9 patients had cortical and subcortical infarction as well). One patient had severe one-sided atrophy and eight had a normal CT scan with some atrophy mainly associated with age.

Angiography. All but three patients had occlusion either of the internal carotid artery (ICA) or of the MCA. One had high cervical stenosis of the ICA and two had stenosis of the common carotid artery. The latter two were candidates for endarterectomy. Of the 32 patients, 17 had a single lesion, 11 patients had two and 4 had multiple lesions.

EEG – data acquisition

Six EEG channels were recorded, using a bipolar transverse montage involving a coronal row along the central areas and across the vertex. The positions of the electrodes and their numbering can be seen in Fig. 1.

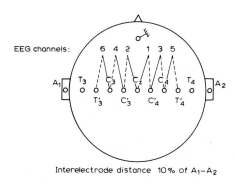

Fig. 1. Electrode positions.

Two experimental conditions were used: recording during rest and recording during voluntary, self-paced squeezing of a rubber ball. If possible, the squeezing was performed first with the right and then with the left hand, but when a patient's affected hand was too weak, only the nonaffected hand was used. The subjects sat in a comfortable chair and were instructed to keep their eyes closed during the whole experiment.

During each test condition (control or hand movement), 60 EEG epochs were recorded, each of 6-sec duration. In the movement condition the interstimulus intervals were a minimum of 10 sec, and each epoch consisted of 4 sec preceding the onset of the movement and 2 sec following it.

Recordings were made with a time constant of 0.3 sec and an upper cutoff frequency of 30 Hz (-3 dB). The analog-to-digital conversion was done at a rate of 64/sec.

EEG – data processing

Artifacts

Each EEG epoch was checked for distortions by an automatic procedure prior to the calculation of the parameters. If artifacts were found within an epoch, it was rejected, and only undistorted epochs were taken for parameter extraction. The following criteria for artifact recognition were applied:

(i)   Overload of the A/D converter;
(ii)   Short lasting transient artifacts of less than 1-sec duration (e.g. caused by switching impulses or eye blinks);

(iii)   High-frequency distortions (e.g. EMG);
(iv)   Low-frequency distortions (mostly caused by movement of the subject).
The artifact recognition and rejection were done online during sampling of the EEG. Figure 2 shows a terminal printout of this phase.

39	–	–	–	–	–	–	39
40	–	–	–	–	–	–	40
41	–	–	–	B	–	–	41
42	–	–	–	–	–	–	42
43	–	–	–	B	–	A	43
44	O	–	O	–	–	–	44
45	–	–	–	–	–	–	45
46	–	–	–	–	–	–	46
47	–	–	–	–	–	S	47
48	–	–	–	–	–	–	48
49	–	–	–	B	–	–	49
50	–	–	–	–	–	–	50
51	–	–	–	–	–	–	51
52	S	S	–	–	–	S	52

Fig. 2. Terminal printout during sampling (extract). From left to right: Number of epoch, then for channel 1–6 indication of type of distortion: - no distortion, O overload of the A/D-converter; S transient distortion, A low-frequency distortion, B high-frequency distortion.

Parameters

For the test under the control condition, the whole 6-sec epochs were taken to calculate the parameters. For the test during ball squeezing, two intervals, each of 2-sec duration, were considered for parameter extractions. The first 2 sec of the pre-movement period were taken as a reference and therefore called the "reference interval", while the interval including the moment of the occurrence of the trigger, which marked the onset of the movement, was considered as the "action interval".

The parameters that were calculated can be classified into three groups:
(i)   Power parameters (total power, absolute and relative band powers);
(ii)   Peak parameters (peak frequency and peak power);
(iii)   ERD parameters (event-related desynchronization in the alpha and beta bands).

Ad (i): The whole 6-sec epoch during the control condition and the 2-sec reference interval during movement conditions were taken for calculating the power spectra by applying an FFT algorithm. From these power spectra, absolute and relative delta (0–4 Hz), theta (4–8 Hz), alpha (6–14 Hz) and beta (14–24 Hz) powers were calculated.

Ad (ii): These parameters are difficult to obtain from the discrete FFT spectrum, because of its large variance and the limited frequency resolution (0.5 Hz corresponding to the 2-sec interval). Therefore, an autoregressive approach was chosen by approximating the spectrum by a polynomial of high order (Box and Jenkins, 1970). The frequency resolution was chosen to be 0.1 Hz.

Ad (iii): The ERD parameters were calculated according to a procedure developed in our laboratory (Pfurtscheller and Aranibar, 1980). The averaged band power was calculated for the alpha and beta bands as a function of time. The ERD parameters were then obtained as the percentage of the power decrease in the action interval with respect to the average power in the reference interval.

The peak parameters were often not reliable, because the automatic procedure simply considered the highest peak in the alpha band as the right one. As a matter of fact, some of our subjects had no peak at all or two or more peaks in that frequency band. In our investigation, the so-called "mu" rhythm was the one that was of interest, and therefore had to be determined by visual comparison of spectral plots with the values given by the peak detection procedure.

The reason for choosing a very wide alpha range was that the peaks sometimes were at lower frequencies than 7 Hz in patients with severe ischemia; in contrast, in some subjects a movement-reactive peak (mu) was found above 13 Hz.

Each parameter was available from each of the six channels and from each of the different testing conditions (except the ERD parameters, which were only calculated from the movement conditions). For example, in the case of a complete series of test sequences in a normal (control condition, right-hand squeezing, left-hand squeezing), 150 parameters were obtained. In addition, the age of the subjects was taken into consideration.

METHOD – STATISTICAL ANALYSIS

The aim of our investigation was the development of a procedure that would allow clear discrimination of normals and patients with cerebral ischemia on the basis of multiple EEG data recorded during rest and voluntary movement.

For our analysis, the method of multivariate linear discriminant analysis (MLDA) was chosen because of its simplicity and its robustness against non-normally distributed data.

In the literature there are two major approaches to MLDA, both of them leading to the same solution, known as "Fisher's linear discriminant function".

The first approach assumes that the data of the groups have multivariate normal distributions. Moreover, the covariance matrices of the groups have to be equal. This approach was described in detail by Anderson (1958) and by other authors, including Rao (1973), Morrison (1976) and Chatfield and Collins (1980).

Another approach is followed by Schuchard-Ficher et al. (1980). Here the linear discriminant function is yielded by maximizing the ratio of the "departures between the groups" to the "mean departure within the groups". No assumptions have to be made concerning the distributions or the covariance structures.

Statistical tests concerning differences between group means, like Student's t-test and Hotelling's T^2, or analyses concerning the probabilities of misclassification, however, are only meaningful if the assumptions of normality and equal covariances hold.

RESULTS

Initial analyses

These analyses were performed in order to describe the properties of different parameter combinations and the properties of the groups with respect to these combinations.

Averaged parameters

In a first step, the mean of each parameter was calculated by averaging over all six channels (A-parameters). Only the central and mid-central channels, however, were used for parameters concerning the beta band (the centro-temporal channels 5 and 6 were often affected by muscle activity, which showed its main effect in this frequency band).

Correlation analysis of the normal group. A correlation analysis of the A-parameters was performed in order to test whether certain parameters are correlated with age and with each other. The result was as follows:

The peak frequency within the alpha band is highly negatively correlated with age ($r = -0.7$); that means that frequency decreases with increasing age. This correlation has also been found by Matejcek (1980). The power parameters are moderately positively correlated with age (0.4–0.5), whereas the ERD parameters show no significant correlation.

The correlation between the other parameters formed five clusters:

1st Cluster: total power, theta and alpha power are highly positively correlated with each other (0.75–0.9).

2nd Cluster: peak frequency is negatively correlated with the parameters of the first cluster (-0.3–-0.4).

3rd Cluster: beta power is moderately correlated with the first cluster (0.65–0.7).

4th Cluster: delta power is very weakly correlated with the other power parameters.

5th Cluster: the ERD parameters show no significant correlation with all other parameters.

Comparison of normals and patients. The A-parameters obtained from both groups were tested for equal means by t- and T^2-tests. The result is shown in Table I. Here the parameters' names are given. A preceding "A" indicates "average", the character following the dot indicates control (C) or movement (M) condition. The second character stands for the EEG parameter: P = total power, D = delta, T = theta, A = alpha, B = beta power, F = peak frequency, H = peak power, EA = ERD in the alpha band, EB = ERD in the beta band. The corresponding group means for the first (normal) and the second (patient) group and the pooled standard deviation (S.D.) are displayed. An asterisk (*) at the side of the t-value indicates significance at the level of 5%. Apparently, the low frequency parameters (delta and theta power) are higher in the patient group (negative t-values). All other parameters seem to be higher for the normals. Above all, the peak frequencies are significantly different as indicated by the t-test.

We tested whether this frequency decrease in the patient group was caused by the different age distribution or by another effect.

A regression analysis in the normal group resulted in the following dependence of the "age-specific" frequency (ASF) and age:

$$ASF = 11.95 - 0.053 \times age$$

Hence, a measure of an "age-normalized" frequency (ANF) can be obtained as follows:

TABLE I

TABLE I

AVERAGE PARAMETERS: COMPARISON OF NORMAL (1) AND PATIENT (2)
GROUPS WITH t-TESTS

Group 1: 47 cases, group 2: 49 cases (for explanation see text, p. 34.)

Name	Mean 1	Mean 2	S.D.	t-Value (1.99)
AP.C	15.58	15.85	11.13	−0.12
AD.C	5.88	6.54	4.43	−0.72
AT.C	2.14	3.38	2.94	−2.07*
AA.C	6.78	6.22	6.59	0.42
AB.C	1.51	1.28	1.75	0.66
AF.C	9.95	8.58	1.06	6.40*
AH.C	3.12	2.03	3.55	1.50
AP.M	15.63	15.16	11.19	0.20
AD.M	4.70	5.83	4.44	−1.24
AT.M	2.24	3.26	2.92	−1.71
AA.M	7.56	6.09	6.76	1.06
AB.M	1.61	1.26	1.79	0.96
AF.M	9.82	8.48	1.01	6.45*
AH.M	3.14	2.04	3.44	1.58
AEA.M	0.30	0.21	0.16	2.69*
AEB.M	0.30	0.24	0.19	1.79

$$ANF = F + 0.053 \times age$$

ANF is independent of age. Figure 3 displays ANF on the x-axis and the averaged ERD from the alpha band on the y-axis for both groups. The values of the normal group are displayed as squares, and the patients' data are marked by triangles. The confidence regions (assuming normal distributions) are plotted, together with the corresponding confidence regions for the group means (level 80%). The empirical (shaded for the normal group) and theoretical marginal distributions show whether the assumption of normality is fulfilled or not. The straight line in the plot is the discrimination line. The result of MLDA was about 63% of correct classifications. Since the two most significantly different parameters were used (frequency and ERD in the alpha band, see Table I), a better classification result would not be possible with the A-parameters.

Normalized differences

Unilateral ischemia affects the generation of the EEG mainly in one hemisphere and therefore can result in an interhemispheric asymmetry of certain parameters. Analyses of differences between homologous electrode positions can be used to measure such asymmetries. Since many parameters show a very large interindividual variance, it appeared that it was better to use normalized parameters: $(R - L)/(R + L)$. If the parameters have a positive sign, this expression yields values between 0 and +1 or −1. All parameters used in this study have positive signs since powers and frequencies can never be zero or negative, except the ERD parameters. The latter therefore are not normalized. An expression for the overall normalized difference (D-parameters) was obtained by summing the normalized differences of the three pairs of homologous derivations.

36

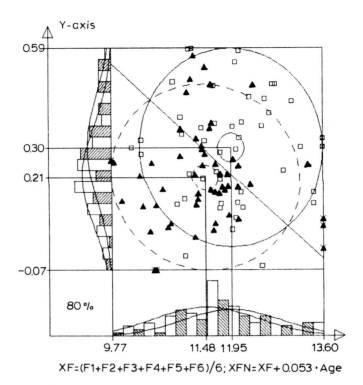

Fig. 3. Bivariate scatter plot with discriminant line. Normal and patient group. *X*-axis: average of age-normalized frequency during control situation; *y*-axis: average of blocking response in the alpha band. Further explanations in text, p. 35.

Again, only the inner two pairs were used for parameters concerning the beta band.

D-parameters in the normal group. A correlation analysis of the D-parameters including age showed that none of these parameters is significantly correlated with age. The other correlations behave similarly to those described in the preceding subsection.

The means of all D-parameters are negative, indicating that in the normal group the parameters in the left hemisphere are larger than those in the right. These differences are not significant by the *t*-test, although a trend seems to exist (an overall T^2-test yielded significance at a level of 5%)

Comparison of normal group and patients. No significant difference could be found between the group means. The overall T^2-test also gave no reason for rejecting the hypothesis of equal means.

This result is easy to explain, because the patients in our investigation were suffering from different forms of unilateral ischemia, and nearly the same number were affected in the right as in the left hemisphere.

Figure 4 shows a bivariate example. The D-parameters are the frequency on the *x*-axis and the ratio theta to beta on the *y*-axis, both of them measured during control conditions. It can be seen that the data from the normals are clustered close around the mean, which is almost zero. The data from the patient group have about the same mean, but a substantially larger confidence region. The application of MLDA is, therefore, not meaningful.

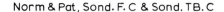

Norm & Pat, Sond. F. C & Sond. TB. C

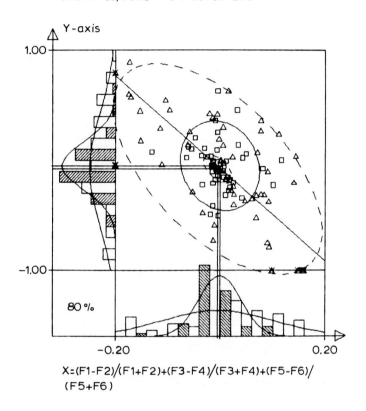

$$X=(F1-F2)/(F1+F2)+(F3-F4)/(F3+F4)+(F5-F6)/(F5+F6)$$

Fig. 4. Normal and patient group. *X*-axis: sum of normalized differences (SOND) between homologous derivations of peak frequency, *y*-axis: SOND of ratio theta/beta, both during control situation.

A special asymmetry measurement

Figure 5 presents a technique that allows the separation of the groups. The picture marked with "A" is just the same as Fig. 4. The full circle represents the confidence region of the normal group. Most of the patient data lie outside the circle. The mean was subtracted in order to shift the data toward the origin (this step can be omitted in our case, because the means of all D-parameters can be assumed to be zero). Then the absolute value of the parameters is taken, leading to the result shown under "B". The effect is a "folding" of the whole data into the first quadrant of the system of coordinates. Such a transformation will cause a non-normal distribution (Chi-square-like). A logarithmic transformation (Fig. 5C), however, is a suitable way of transforming the distribution into an approximately normal one.

38

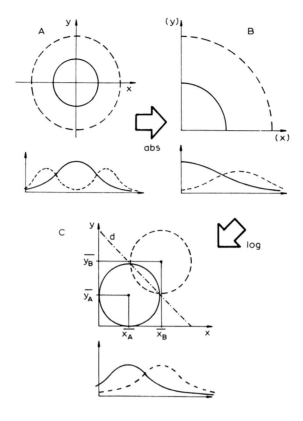

Fig. 5. Separation of overlapping groups with same means, but different confidence regions. For explanation see text, p. 37.

There are two ways of taking the absolute value. First, the absolute value can be taken of the sum of normalized differences, obtaining:

$$S_1 = \left| \sum_{i=1}^{3} \frac{R_i - L_i}{R_i + L_i} \right|$$

The second method is to take the absolute value of each of the three normalized differences, corresponding to the homologous pairs, and then sum them:

$$S_2 = \sum_{i=1}^{3} \left| \frac{R_i - L_i}{R_i + L_i} \right|$$

Apparently, the second method yields a more rigid criterion for symmetry, because S_2 can be zero if and only if perfect symmetry exists between all pairs of positions. Thus this measurement was used in the further considerations.

In Figs. 6 and 7 the effect of taking the absolute value and of transforming it is shown using the data of Fig. 4. It can be seen that the group means are clearly separated now, but the marginal distributions depart from normal (Fig. 6). An MLDA yielded about 80% correct classifications. Adding a small constant to the symmetry measurement of Fig. 6 and taking the logarithm leads to a result shown in Fig. 7. Here the data can be assumed to be (at least approximately) normally distributed. Furthermore, the confidence regions, displaying the covariance structures of the groups, look rather similar. Thus, any statistical technique can be applied to the data without restrictions. The quality of the classification by MLDA is again about 80%. This symmetry measurement will be abbreviated to "S" in the following.

S-parameters in the normal group. The correlation analysis revealed that none of the S-parameters shows a significant correlation with age. Most correlations between the parameters are relatively weak (less than 0.4), but there is one cluster containing theta, alpha and beta power with higher correlations (less than 0.7).

Comparison of normal group and patients. A comparison between both group means by *t*-test gave the following results:

(1) All the S-parameters are less negative for the patient group, thus indicating that the patients in general have more asymmetric data.

(2) The largest differences appear with frequency, absolute theta/beta, delta, theta and relative beta power.

(3) There are only small differences (without any significance) between both groups in the alpha-band parameters.

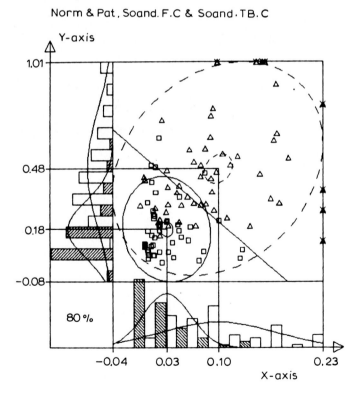

Fig. 6. Same as Fig. 4, but sums of absolute normalized differences (SOAND).

40

(4) There is no difference between the parameters measured in the control condition and those obtained during hand movement. That means that movement does not yield a better discrimination. (Note: in this analysis, the average of the parameters for right- and left-hand squeezing was taken.)

(5) The overall T^2-test yields a very high significance. Since the parameters are approximately normally distributed (see Fig. 7), this test will be valid.

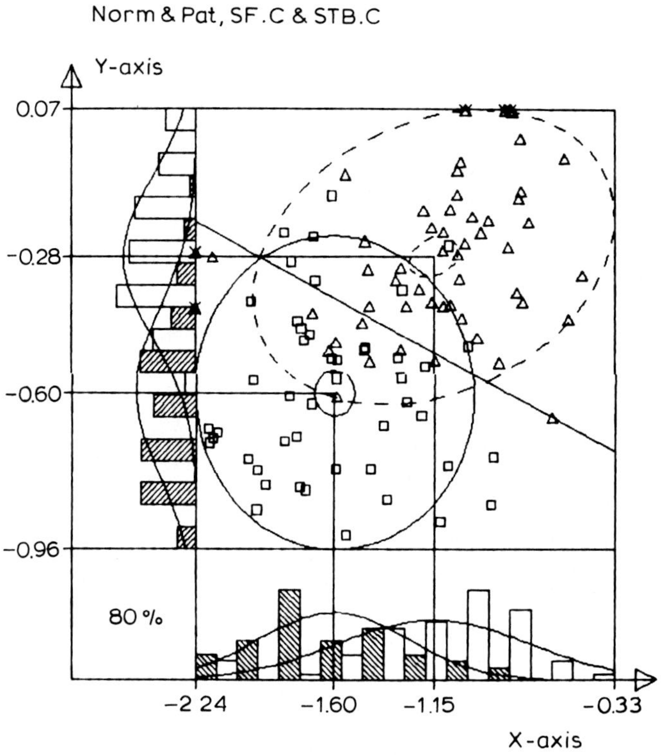

Fig. 7. Same as Fig. 6, but with logarithmic transformation.

These results demonstrate that the S-parameters are in fact a good basis for starting an MLDA, of which the following features are:
(1) No dependence on age;
(2) Large differences between data from normals and from patients;
(3) Small correlations with each other;
(4) Roughly normal distributions with the same covariances for both groups.

Multiparametric asymmetry score (MAS)

Criteria for optimal subsets

The aim of MLDA is to derive an optimal set of parameters and to determine the corresponding coefficients in the linear discriminant function. Let us consider some criteria necessary for optimal subsets. An example is shown in Table II. Here an

TABLE II

MLDA (EXTRACT) BETWEEN NORMAL (47 CASES) AND
PATIENT GROUP (49 CASES);
20 S-PARAMETERS

No.	Name	Coefficient	Power(%)
1	SF.C	−4.885	13.3
2	SA.M	10.196	13.0
3	ST.M	−9.124	12.6
4	SEA.M	−8.530	10.4
5	STB.C	−6.445	10.0
6	SHA.C	−4.376	5.5
.	.	.	.
.		.	.
20	SHA.M	−0.268	0.3

MLDA was performed on the S-parameters described in the preceding subsection. The names of the parameters are shown, together with their discriminant coefficient and their relative discrimination power in percent. The quality of the classification was about 92%.

This example was chosen to demonstrate a typically unstable result. The parameter SA.M (alpha power during movement), for example, has the second largest discrimination power, although it was stated above that the S-parameters concerning the alpha band were the weakest discriminators. Thus here a contradiction results. Moreover, SA.M has a positive discriminant coefficient, meaning that a positive value of this parameter for a certain case (indicating a high degree of asymmetry) might result in a positive value of the whole discriminant function (this case will then be classified as "normal"); this is also a contradiction to the above finding that patients are more asymmetric than normals.

What is the explanation for these phenomena? First, as seen in the previous section, the parameters concerning the alpha band have no significant differences between the normal and the patient group. Second, these parameters are relatively highly correlated with the theta and beta powers, and third, the group sizes of about 50 individuals are relatively small, compared with the number of parameters (20). These three effects cause the described unstable and invalid behavior.

Regarding stable subsets we must formulate a few general rules: first, the order of the parameters, according to their discriminative power, should be roughly the same as in the univariate consideration. Second, the coefficients must be negative (this is not a general rule for MLDA; it only holds for our special data). Third, it would seem to be better to remove very weak parameters (e.g. SHA.M in Table II), because of their uncertainty. Fourth, if a subset of parameters is highly correlated, only one of them should be used. Fifth, the number of parameters should be as small as possible, but as large as necessary.

The greatest problem in MLDA is the choice of the optimal set. If N-parameters are given originally, and one has to determine an optimal subset, 2^N analyses will be used to find it (all possible subsets of size 1 plus all subsets of size 2, etc.). In the above example, 20 parameters are given, so that we would have had to try out about one

42

million analyses. This is, of course, impossible.

In practice, another approach is used, called "stepwise" MLDA. Here, in a stepwise manner, by including and removing parameters in the analysis, more or less
optimal sets can be found, though there is no guarantee that the global optimum will
be reached (Dixon, 1979; Schuchard-Ficher et al., 1980).

We used a similar approach in our investigation, starting with all parameters and
then, according to the above criteria, removing invalid ones. In addition, some a
priori knowledge, stemming from previous analyses, was also taken into consideration.
In this way, optimal subsets could be established relatively fast.

Different movement conditions

In the last subsection it was stated that the S-parameters, measured during right-
and left-hand squeezing and then averaged, do not allow a better discrimination
between normals and patients than the control parameters. An exact analysis had to
be tried out in order to test whether or not certain movement conditions bring more
information. The six most powerful parameters were used: SF (frequency), SD (delta), ST (theta), STB (theta/beta power), SEA (ERD in the alpha band), SEB (ERD
in the beta band).

The following conditions were considered: C (control), M (movement averaged), R
(movement right), L (movement left), A (movement with affected hand), U (movement with unaffected hand).

The results for the univariate parameters are shown in Table III. As a measure of
discrimination power, Wilks' Lambda was applied. Its maximum value can be 1,
meaning no discrimination at all. The smaller the Lambda value, the better the
discrimination.

TABLE III

WILKS' LAMBDA FOR S-PARAMETERS, DIFFERENT TEST
CONDITIONS

(C = control, M = movement averaged, R = right hand, L = left hand, A =
affected hand, U = unaffected hand)

Name	C	M	R	L	A	U
SF	0.678	0.761	0.818	0.807	0.845	0.701
SD	0.748	0.778	0.723	0.862	0.744	0.844
ST	0.791	0.783	0.769	0.822	0.782	0.807
STB	0.572	0.557	0.679	0.511	0.653	0.542
SEA	–	0.913	0.948	0.904	0.940	0.913
SEB	–	0.941	0.964	0.954	0.954	0.964

Table III shows the following points:
(i)   The parameter SF is best in the control condition.
(ii)   SD and ST are best during movement of the right hand.
(iii) STB shows a very clear minimum for left-hand movement.
(iv)   SEA is also best for left-hand movement.
(v)   SEB shows no clear minimum.
(vi)   Squeezing of the affected and unaffected hand, respectively, shows no clear

pattern. The values of Lambda generally lie between those for C, R and L.

A multivariate analysis has established these statements. Above all, it seems that squeezing of the affected hand will not give good discrimination, as we had previously assumed.

Optimal sets

Several optimal sets had to be established because of the fact that not all of the subjects were able to perform hand squeezing with both hands. Therefore, four combinations of testing sequences had to be considered:

(i)   Control test alone (C);
(ii) Control and right hand (C–R);
(iii) Control and left hand (C–L);
(iv) Control, right and left hand (C–R–L).

In addition, the peak frequencies often could not be determined, either because no peak was found in the spectrum or it could not be clearly assigned. Thus eight optimal discriminant functions had to be derived.

The starting set was constructed according to Table III. The parameters SF, SD, ST, STB and SEA were taken from the two best conditions, i.e. for a certain parameter, the condition for which it had the weakest discrimination power was omitted. Thus 10 parameters were in the starting set: SF.C and SF.L, SD.C and SD.R, ST.C and ST.R, STB.C and STB.L and SEA.R and SEA.L. Now, in a stepwise manner, the optimal sets for the various combinations of conditions were sought, according to our previously discussed criteria. Only complete cases (i.e. cases where the complete C–R–L sequence was performed) were used for establishing the discrimination functions.

The optimal sets were (in order of discrimination power):

(C):   STB.C, SF.C, ST.C, SD.C;
(C–R):   STB.C, SF.C, SD.R, ST.R, SEA.R;
(C–L):   STB.L, SF.C, STB.C, SEA.L, ST.C, SD.C;
(C–R–L): STB.L, SF.C, STB.C, SEA.L, ST.R, SD.R.

Based on these optimal subsets, a classification procedure was constructed; the aim was to classify every case. For this, the computer program has to look for the tests given for a certain case, see whether peak frequencies are available or not, and then to compute the corresponding discriminant function. If the score (multiparametric asymmetry score – MAS) is positive, the case is classified as "normal", otherwise as "abnormal". For analysis purposes, however, all possible scores have been computed for each case. The results, based on 50 normals and 64 patient cases, are shown in the following tables.

Table IV shows the numbers of missing and false classifications. It is seen that, with only one discriminant function, there would have been many cases that could not be classified at all, because of missing peak frequencies or missing test sequences.

In Table V the resulting quantities of specificity (i.e. the percentage of correctly classified normals), sensitivity (percentage of correctly classified patients) and the overall percentage of correct classifications are given, together with the theoretical percentage of correct classifications (calculated from Mahalanobis' D^2) and the value of Wilks' Lambda. The last column of the table presents the percentages when the best discrimination function has been applied.

44

TABLE IV

CLASSIFICATION RESULT, FALSE AND MISSING
CLASSIFICATIONS

Normals: 50 cases, patients: 64 cases

	With peak frequency				Without peak frequency			
	C	C–R	C–L	C–R–L	C	C–R	C–L	C–R–L
Normals (n = 50)								
false	6	6	3	3	10	7	4	3
missing	3	3	3	3	0	0	0	0
Patients (n = 64)								
false	8	7	4	4	11	8	5	4
missing	7	19	10	22	0	14	3	17
Overall (n = 114)								
false	14	13	7	7	21	15	9	7
missing	10	22	13	25	0	14	3	17

TABLE V

CLASSIFICATION RESULT, PERCENTAGES AND WILKS' LAMBDA

Normals: 50 cases, patients: 64 cases

	With peak frequency				Without peak frequency				
	C	C–R	C–L	C–R–L	C	C–R	C–L	C–R–L	Opt.
Specificity	87.2	87.2	93.6	93.6	80.0	86.0	92.0	94.0	94.0
Sensitivity	86.0	84.4	92.6	90.5	82.8	84.0	91.8	91.5	92.2
Overall	86.5	85.9	93.1	92.1	81.6	85.0	91.9	92.8	93.0
Theoretical	85.7	87.5	91.3	92.6	82.2	84.6	90.1	91.3	
Lambda	0.46	0.43	0.35	0.32	0.54	0.49	0.37	0.35	

These results appear very clear cut. An overall quality of 93% correct classifications, however, may raise the question whether there is not a systematic error in the analysis (in MLDA, there is such a systematic error if the same data are used for establishing the discriminant function and for classifying them according to this function). But there are several reasons that let us assume that the results are in fact valid. First, only 47 of the 64 patients who performed the movement task with both hands were used to determine the discriminant functions, but all the cases were classified. Second, the results have been proved by cross-validation and the "jackknife" and the "bootstrap" methods (Efron, 1982). These techniques confirmed the stability of the results. And third, the values of Lambda and the theoretical percentage of correct

45

classifications show a very similar behavior to the real percentages.

Table V shows that the additional information of hand squeezing is much higher for the left than for the right hand, and that the additional information of the frequency is highest when a control test alone was performed. In the authors' opinions, the information from the left-hand test was higher because most of our subjects were right-handed, so that the left hand was nondominant in most cases. But a further study should be made in order to establish this statement or to reject it.

Relationship between MAS and neurological deficits

The patients were divided into three groups according to their neurological deficits. In the first group there were those patients without neurological deficits (TIA, PRIND), in the second those with mild or moderate and in the third group those with severe neurological deficits. The mean MAS (± S.D.) was calculated for each group (Fig. 8). In addition, the mean MAS for the reference group of neurologically normal subjects was also calculated. The diagram in Fig. 8 clearly demonstrates that the MAS fits very well with the severity of the neurological impairment and allows a relatively clear separation even between normals and patients with TIA. A MAS of −1, for example, can be interpreted as result of minor brain dysfunction, a MAS of −8, however, as result of widespread cerebral ischemia and severe dysfunction.

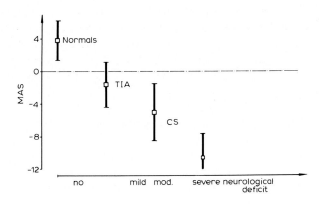

Fig. 8. MAS and severity of neurological deficits. CS = completed stroke.

Relationship between MAS and CT scan

Here the patients were grouped according to their CT scan: no lesion, small and large lesions in the CT scan. Figure 9 shows the MAS of these three groups of patients, together with that of the normal group. Again, a clear dependence can be seen between the MAS and the size of the lesion. Above all, even the patients with a normal CT scan are clearly separated from the normal group.

46

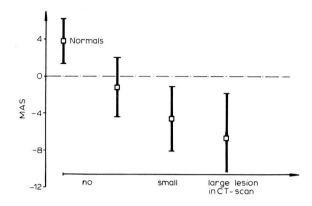

Fig. 9. MAS and size of lesion in the CT scans.

Differences between cortical and noncortical infarction

For this study, only the patient group was considered and divided into two subgroups: the patients who had cortical infarction in the CT scan and those with all other types of lesions shown by the CT scan, including a normal scan. Each group contained 32 cases.

It was found that again the S-parameters were the best discriminators, especially SF (frequency), STB (theta/beta power) and ST (theta power). The parameters obtained from the control condition were slightly better than those from the movement tests.

As a result, the data from the group with cortical infarction are much more asymmetric than those from the other group. An MLDA including the peak frequency yielded about 70% correct classifications; without frequency, the quality of the classification was reduced to 67%.

Differences between affected and nonaffected hemispheres

Two subgroups of the patients were considered, the first containing the patients with the lesion in the right hemisphere (28 cases), the second with those whose left hemisphere was affected (36 cases). For obvious reasons the S-parameters could not be used for this discrimination (absolute value!); therefore, the D-parameters were taken. The results were as follows:

(1) The band powers from the lower frequency bands (delta, theta) were higher from the affected hemisphere. Alpha power also showed this behavior, but without significance (*t*-test).

(2) The peak frequencies were significantly lower from the affected side. ERD in the alpha band was also lower there than from the nonaffected hemisphere.

(3) The other parameters (beta power, ERD in the beta band) showed no differences between the hemispheres.

(4) In general, the parameters from the movement test were more significant than those from the control condition.

(5) There were very high correlations between the alpha and the theta parameters, and also between the corresponding parameters from control and movement test (greater than 0.75).

An MLDA, using DTB.C, DEA.M, DT.M and DF.C (order according to discrimination power) yielded an overall of 73% correct classifications. Without frequency, the result was 71%.

DISCUSSION

One of the most remarkable results of this study was that the quotient theta/beta power showed the highest contribution to the overall discriminative power of the MAS. In addition, the symmetry measurements especially of delta power (SD) and theta power (ST) showed highly significant differences between the normal and the patient group. The peak frequency (SF) also demonstrated a very clear dissimilarity between the groups, but this parameter suffers from the great disadvantage that it cannot be determined in subjects without a clear peak or unclear double peaks in the power spectra. The parameter concerning the blocking in the alpha band (SEA) showed only a moderate discriminative power, but it was completely independent from the other parameters, so that its inclusion into the discriminant function resulted in a considerably increased percentage of correct classifications. All the relative powers showed a very poor behavior in comparison with the absolute band powers.

Regarding the influence of the hand movement on the quality of the discrimination, it was found that the parameters SD and ST were best during right-hand squeezing, whereas STB and SEA were more significant in the left-hand test. It can hardly be said whether these results are valid or may originate from special characteristics of the data, but it was apparent that squeezing of the left hand gave much more discrimination power than right-hand movement (see Table V). Since most of our subjects were right-handed it seems that movement of the nondominant hand will be more powerful for discrimination than movement of the dominant hand, but further studies with a control group of left-handed subjects should be made in order to confirm this hypothesis.

An analysis of the behavior of the parameters with respect to the side of the ischemic lesion demonstrated that the delta and theta powers and the quotient theta/beta were significantly increased in the affected hemisphere, whereas the peak frequency and the blocking response were reduced there. The increase of delta and theta power and the decrease of frequency were also found in visually scored EEGs (Birchfield et al., 1959) and confirmed by other qEEG studies (Van Huffelen et al., 1980).

In general, it can be said that the MAS (multiparametric asymmetry score) provides a very sensitive indicator for discriminating between neurologically normal subjects and patients with cerebral ischemia. Two points, however, should receive special emphasis:

First, the MAS is only a weighted sum of certain symmetry (S-)parameters, and these S-parameters are logarithmically transformed sums of absolute normalized differences between homologous positions. Thus, the MAS is simply a measurement for the degree of symmetry or asymmetry, respectively, between the hemispheres. The logarithmic transformation is only done in order to obtain approximately normally distributed data.

Second, it was found that the members of the normal group on the average show a very high degree of symmetry in all parameters (peak frequency, band powers, ERD responses), whereas the patients are more asymmetric in all these parameters. In the authors' opinions, this asymmetric behavior of qEEG parameters will not only be restricted to patients with unilateral ischemia but will also be valid for other diseases of the brain (such as expansive processes or an epileptic focus) with more or less clear lateralization. The weights of the parameters in the MAS might be changed, however, when considering other forms of brain dysfunction or brain lesions.

SUMMARY

Computer-aided EEG analysis and multivariate statistics are valuable in the study of minor brain dysfunction due to cerebral ischemia. EEG recordings using a bipolar montage, as a coronal chain along the central areas and across the vertex, were made from 50 neurologically normal subjects and from a group of 32 patients with transitory ischemic attacks (TIAs) or completed strokes, most of them with minor neurological deficits; nine of the patients had a normal EEG scored visually. Two test conditions were used:

(i)   Recording during rest and
(ii) recording during voluntary, repetitive, self-paced squeezing of a rubber ball using first the right and then the left hand.

The following EEG parameters were calculated: total power, absolute and relative band powers in the delta, theta, alpha and beta bands, peak frequency within the alpha band, peak power and the movement-related blocking in the alpha and beta bands. The age of the subjects was also taken into consideration. Using all three experimental tests, 151 parameters were obtained for each subject.

The application of multivariate linear discriminant analysis (MLDA) showed that in general symmetry measurements between homologous regions yield the most powerful discrimination between normals and patients.

The expression $[(R - L)/(R + L)]$ is a normalized symmetry measurement between two homologous regions. A measurement of the overall symmetry can be obtained by summing the absolute normalized differences from the three pairs of homologous derivations.

The parameters showing the best discrimination between the normal and the patient group were the peak frequency in the alpha band, the ratio theta/beta power, delta and theta power and the blocking response in the alpha band. For example, an MLDA using the above parameters yielded an overall of 93% correct classifications. Bivariate scatter plots, cross-validation and the jackknife and bootstrap procedures confirmed the power of these symmetry measurements.

ACKNOWLEDGEMENT

The authors wish to thank G. Lindinger, W. Reczek and Mrs. E. Mandl for the EEG recordings, Dr. H. Schneider for doing the CT reports and Dr. R. Oberbauer for clinical examinations. The investigation was supported by the "Fonds zur Förderung der wissenschaftlichen Forschung", Projekt Nr. 4593.

REFERENCES

Anderson, T. W. (1958) *An Introduction to Multivariate Statistical Analysis*, John Wiley & Sons, New York.

Barlow, J. S. (1979) Computerized clinical electroencephalography in perspective. *IEEE Trans. Biomed. Eng.*, 26: 377–391.

Birchfield, R. I., Wilson, W. P. and Heyman, A. (1959) An evaluation of electroencephalography in cerebral infarction and ischemia due to arteriosclerosis. *Neurology*, 9: 859–870.

Box, G. E. P. and Jenkins, G. M. (1970) *Time Series Analysis, Forecasting and Control*, Holden-Day, San Francisco.

Chatfield, C. and Collins, A. J. (1980) *Introduction to Multivariate Analysis*, Chapman and Hall, London–New York.

Dixon, W. J. (1979) *BMDP – Biomedical Computer Programs*, University of California Press, Berkeley.

Efron, B. (1982) *The Jackknife, the Bootstrap and other Resampling Plans*, Society for Industrial and Applied Mathematics, Philadelphia.

Enge, S., Lechner, H., Logar, Ch. and Ladurner, G. (1980) Clinical value of EEG in transient ischemic attacks. In H. Lechner and A. Aranibar (Eds.), *EEG and Clinical Neurophysiology*, Excerpta Medica, Amsterdam–Oxford–Princeton, pp. 173–180.

Gastaut, H., Fischgold, H. and Meyer, J. S. (1961) Conclusions of the international colloquium on anoxia and the EEG. In H. Gastaut and J. S. Meyer (Eds.), *Cerebral Anoxia and the Electroencephalogram*, Thomas, Springfield, Il., pp. 599–617.

Gotman, J., Skuce, D. R., Thompson, C. J., Gloor, P., Ives, J. R. and Ray, W. F. (1973) Clinical applications of spectral analysis and extraction of features from electroencephalograms with slow waves in adult patients. *Electroenceph. clin. Neurophysiol.*, 35: 225–235.

Ingvar, D. H., Sjölund, B. and Ardö, A. (1976) Correlation between dominant EEG frequency, cerebral oxygen uptake and blood flow. *Electroenceph. clin. Neurophysiol.*, 41: 268–276.

Jasper, H. and Penfield, W. (1949) Electrocorticograms in man: Effect of voluntary movement upon the electrical activity of the precentral gyrus. *Arch. Psychiat. Z. Neurol.*, 183: 163–174.

Kamp, A. and Troost, J. (1978) EEG signs of cerebrovascular disorder, using physical exercise as a provocative method. *Electroenceph. clin. Neurophysiol.*, 45: 295–298.

Ladurner, G. and Lechner, H. (1971) EEG-Veränderungen bei Verschlüssen im Strömungsgebiet der Arteria carotis und ihre klinische Wertung. *Wien. Z. Nervenheilkd.*, 29: 295–309.

Lopes da Silva, F. H. (1981) Analysis of EEG ongoing activity: Rhythms and nonstationarities. In N. Yamaguchi and K. Fujisawa (Eds.), *Recent Advances in EEG and EMG Data Processing*, Elsevier/North-Holland Biomedical Press, Amsterdam–New York–Oxford, pp. 95–115.

Matejcek, M. (1980) Cortical correlates of the aging process as revealed by quantitative EEG, the value of quantitative EEG in evaluating the effects of treatment. *Proc. Int. Cerebrovascular Diseases*, SIR, 55–66.

Morrison, D. F. (1976) *Multivariate Statistical Methods*, 2nd Edn., McGraw-Hill Kogakusha, Tokyo.

Obrist, W. D., Sokoloff, L., Lassen, N. A., Lane, M. H., Butler, R. N. and Feinberg, I. (1963) Relation of EEG to cerebral blood flow and metabolism in old age. *Electroenceph. clin. Neurophysiol.*, 15: 610–619.

Paddison, R. M. and Ferriss, G. S. (1961) The electroencephalogram in cerebrovascular disease. *Electroenceph. clin. Neurophysiol.*, 13: 99–110.

Pfurtscheller, G. and Aranibar, A. (1979) Evaluation of event-related desynchronization (ERD) preceding and following voluntary self-paced movement. *Electroenceph. clin. Neurophysiol.*, 46: 138–146.

Pfurtscheller, G. and Aranibar, A. (1980) Voluntary movement ERD: normative studies. In G. Pfurtscheller, P. Buser, F. H. Lopes da Silva and H. Petsche (Eds.), *Rhythmic EEG Activities and Cortical Functioning*, Elsevier, Amsterdam, pp. 151–177.

Pfurtscheller, G., Sager, D. and Wege, W. (1981) Correlations between CT scan and sensimotor EEG rhythms in patients with cerebrovascular disorders. *Electroenceph. clin. Neurophysiol.*, 52: 473–485.

Rao, C. R. (1973) *Linear Statistical Inference and its Applications*, 2nd Edn., John Wiley & Sons, New York–London–Sydney–Toronto.

Schuchard-Ficher, C., Backhaus, K., Humme, U., Lohrberg, W., Plinke, W. and Schreiner, W. (1980) *Multivariate Analysemethoden*, Springer-Verlag, Berlin–Heidelberg–New York.

Strauss, H. and Greenstein, L. (1948) The electroencephalogram in cerebrovascular disease. *Arch. Neurol. Psychiat.*, 59: 395–403.

Sulg, I. A., Sotaniemi, K. A., Tolonen, U. and Hokkanen, E. (1981) Dependence between cerebral metabolism and blood flow as reflected in the quantitative EEG. *Advanc. biol. Psychiat.*, 6: 102–108.

Van Huffelen, A. C., Poortvliet, D. C. J. and Van der Wulp, C. J. M. (1980) Quantitative EEG in cerebral ischemia. A. Parameters for the detection of abnormalities in "normal" EEGs in patients with acute unilateral cerebral ischemia. In H. Lechner and A. Aranibar (Eds.), *EEG and Clinical Neurophysiology*, Excerpta Medica, Amsterdam–Oxford–Princeton, pp. 125–130.

Brain Ischemia: Quantitative EEG and Imaging Techniques, Progress in Brain Research, Vol. 62, edited by
G. Pfurtscheller, E.J. Jonkman and F.H. Lopes da Silva
©1984 Elsevier Science Publishers B.V.

Parametric Relationships Between Four Different Quantitative EEG Methods in Cerebral Infarction

UOLEVI TOLONEN

Department of Clinical Neurophysiology, University of Oulu, SF-90220 Oulu 22 (Finland)

INTRODUCTION

A variety of approaches has been used for quantification of the EEG and extensive reviews of the various analyses have been published (Matoušek, 1973; Barlow 1979). Only a few studies, however, concern the interrelationships between these quantification techniques.

A fairly high degree of statistical equivalence has been shown between some EEG quantification methods (Beatty and Figueroa, 1974; Pigeau et al., 1981), but in cerebral ischemia there is some evidence of a certain superiority of spectral parameters (Binnie et al., 1978; Sotaniemi et al., 1980; Tolonen and Sulg, 1981). Furthermore, in different brain conditions (e.g. in cerebral ischemia and migraine) somewhat different single quantitative EEG (qEEG) parameters seem to be more appropriate for revealing abnormalities (Van Huffelen et al., 1980; Jonkman and Lelieveld, 1981). In cerebral ischemia the parameters reflecting changes in the delta and alpha bands or mean frequency index are often used as qEEG indexes (Mies et al., 1976; Cohen et al., 1977; Van Huffelen et al., 1980). The combined intensity of slow wave activity (delta and theta bands) or the ratios of slow wave activity/alpha and beta bands can also be used successfully as parameters for the evaluation of EEG changes caused by ischemia (Gotman et al., 1973; Herrschaft et al., 1977). Quantification of the EEG response to photic stimulation has also been shown to be significant (Van Huffelen et al., 1980).

The present work evaluates the relative value and reciprocal dependence of four different EEG quantification techniques (combined period and amplitude analysis, normalized slope descriptor technique, a zero-line crossing variant analysis and Fast Fourier Transform (FFT) for power density spectrum (PDS) analysis), the EEGs being recorded from three different brain areas (frontocentral, temporal and parieto-occipital regions) in patients with cerebral infarction. The value of single qEEG parameters in different brain areas is also examined.

PATIENTS

Eighty-two EEGs of 48 patients with supratentorial cerebral infarction were recorded and processed. Patients with TIA or PRIND were not included in the series. The group consisted of 18 females and 30 males, aged 19–76 (mean 50) years. The diagnosis of infarction was made by a neurologist on the basis of clinical signs, brain scans, EEGs, and, in a few cases, angiograms. The infarction was most often situated in the area supplied by the middle cerebral artery; the lesion was on the right side in 23 patients and on the left side in 25 patients. At the moment of EEG recording, the time elapsed since infarction varied from one day to several years (mean 2 months), but half of the examinations were carried out within the first 3 weeks after the infarction. In the visual scoring, 67 out of all 82 EEGs (82%) showed more or less clear disturbances and thus one fifth of the EEGs appeared as normal by visual estimate.

METHODS

The EEGs were recorded with a 16-channel electroencephalograph. During recording the patients lay awake with their eyes closed. The low frequencies were reduced using a time constant of 0.30 sec, and the high frequency cutoff point was set at 70 Hz. Six channels were selected for quantification: F_4–C_4, F_3–C_3, T_4–T_6, T_3–T_5, P_4–O_2 and P_3–O_1. The analysis of three representative artifact-free epochs of 10 sec from each channel was performed off line (from an analogue 7 channel tape recorder) by means of an HP 2100S microprogrammable 32 kiloword minicomputer. The analogue signal was low-pass filtered (KEMO VBF17J, −3 dB point at 31.5 Hz, slope −36dB/oct) and then digitized at the sampling frequency of 100 Hz using a HP 2313B A/D converter (12-bit resolution, full-scale input ±10.24 V).

The EEG quantification was performed using four different quantification techniques: (1) combined period and amplitude analysis; (2) the normalized slope descriptor technique of Hjorth (1973); (3) a modified zero-line crossing variant analysis, and (4) power spectral density (PDS) with Fast Fourier Transform (FFT). The parameters yielded by these methods are seen in Table I. The method is described in more detail in Tolonen and Sulg (1981). In the combined period and amplitude analysis, the EEG wave period and the EEG wave amplitude were calculated as described by Stigsby et al. (1973). In this method not only baseline crossings but also superimposed waves are determined, and the method thus deviates from the pure zero-line crossing estimation. The superimposed waves were included, when their root mean square value exceeded that of sine wave of 3 μV. The mean frequency parameter of the period analysis, the averaged frequency, was obtained by dividing the total number of waves by the analysis time. In the present zero-line crossing variant analysis, four level crossing parameters were calculated: the parameter zero-line crossing 0 indicates the number of upcrossings of zero; zero-line crossing +u is the number of upcrossings at the level 2/3 standard deviation above the zero level; zero-line crossing −u is correspondingly the number of upcrossings of the level of 2/3 standard deviation below the zero level; and the zero-line crossing mean is the combination of the first three as follows:

$$f_{\mathrm{m}} = 1/3(f_0 + f_{+\mathrm{u}} + f_{-\mathrm{u}}).$$

In this study the values of zero-line crossing 0 and mean are presented. In the spectral density analysis the mean frequency was obtained by weighting the averaged frequency by power density according to the formula:

TABLE I

MEAN VALUES (±S.D.) OF THE CALCULATED qEEG PARAMETERS IN BOTH HEMISPHERES FROM ALL BRAIN AREAS STUDIED

1 = period and amplitude analysis, 2 = Hjorth's parameters, 3 = zero-line crossing variant analysis and 4 = power spectrum with Fast Fourier Transform.

Parameter	F_4-C_4, F_3-C_3 (N=45)		P_4-O_2, P_3-O_1 (N=82)		T_4-T_6, T_3-T_5 (N=41)	
	Lesion side	Control side	Lesion side	Control side	Lesion side	Control side
1. Averaged frequency (Hz)	9.6±2.0	10.1±1.7	9.2±1.7	9.7±1.8	9.2±1.7	9.9±1.6
Mean voltage (µV)	5.7±2.7	5.8±3.0	6.4±3.2	6.2±3.1	7.6±3.3	6.8±2.6
Mean energy	4.7±6.6	4.8±8.9	5.9±7.5	5.3±6.9	8.1±9.0	6.0±5.5
2. Activity (µV)	5.7±2.7	5.8±3.1	6.4±3.3	6.2±3.1	7.6±3.4	6.9±2.6
Mobility (Hz)	9.1±2.7	9.7±2.1	8.8±2.1	9.4±2.0	8.6±2.1	9.4±1.9
Complexity (Hz)	14.1±2.1	14.1±1.9	11.1±2.5	10.9±2.4	12.0±2.8	12.0±2.3
3. Zero-line crossing 0 (Hz)	9.2±2.6	9.8±2.2	8.9±2.2	9.5±2.2	8.7±2.3	9.6±2.0
Zero-line crossing mean (Hz)	9.0±2.6	9.6±2.2	8.7±2.1	9.3±2.1	8.6±2.2	9.4±1.9
4. Mean frequency (Hz)	7.5±2.8	7.9±2.3	7.7±2.4	8.4±2.3	7.4±2.4	8.3±2.0
Peak frequency (Hz)	5.2±4.6	5.9±2.3	6.9±4.1	7.4±4.0	6.5±4.1	7.5±3.6
50th percentile (Hz)	6.1±3.4	6.4±3.2	7.4±3.1	8.2±2.8	6.8±3.0	8.1±2.0
75th percentile (Hz)	10.7±4.6	11.3±3.9	10.0±3.1	10.8±3.1	9.7±3.0	10.6±2.6
Alpha mean frequency (Hz)	9.7±0.6	9.7±0.5	9.5±0.7	9.6±0.7	9.3±0.8	9.5±0.9
Delta activity (%)	37±18	32±15	27±18	22±15	29±18	23±12
Theta activity (%)	19±9	17±7	16±9	14±7	16±7	14±9
Alpha activity (%)	30±14	35±15	49±21	52±20	49±19	51±14
Skewness	1.7±0.9	1.5±0.7	1.9±0.9	1.4±0.9	1.8±0.7	1.5±0.7
Kurtosis	8.1±5.5	6.8±4.3	10.3±5.7	9.8±8.8	10.6±4.5	8.9±4.9

$$f_\mathrm{m} = \frac{\displaystyle\int_{O}^{F} f \cdot P(f) \cdot \mathrm{d}f}{\displaystyle\int_{O}^{F} P(f) \cdot \mathrm{d}f}.$$ The frequency resolution was 0.1 Hz.

The alpha mean frequency was calculated according to the same formula as the spectral mean frequency but now only for the alpha range (7.5–13.5 Hz). The spectral peak frequency indicated the frequency of maximum power density above 3.5 Hz. The percentiles 50 and 75 indicated the frequency below which 50% (or 75%) of the whole power density of the signal was situated. The frequency bands used for calculations of the percentages for alpha, theta and delta were 7.5–13.5 Hz for alpha, 3.5–7.5 Hz for theta and 0.5−3.5 Hz for delta.

RESULTS

Parameter values of both hemispheres

The mean values of the calculated qEEG parameters from all three brain areas studied of both hemispheres are presented in Table I. The mean frequency values of the combined period and amplitude analysis (averaged frequency), Hjorth's technique (mobility) and zero-line crossing were broadly similar, but the spectral mean frequency was slower.

Interrelationships between the four EEG quantification techniques studied

All four quantification techniques produced a mean frequency parameter. Linear correlation coefficients between these mean frequency values showed an overall high interdependence between the methods: all correlations were significant at p-level <0.001 in both hemispheres from all three brain areas examined. The correlation coefficients ranged parieto-occipitally from 0.89 to 0.99, frontocentrally from 0.84 to 0.99 and temporally from 0.90 to 1.0. In spite of this high equivalence between these methods, significant differences (even at p-level <0.001) in these correlations could, however, be seen. The lowest correlation coefficients appeared between the period and amplitude and spectral mean frequencies.

Of the three spectral frequency band parameters (percentages of delta, theta and alpha), the delta activity was the only one which showed significant correlations with all four calculated mean frequencies in both hemispheres (Table II). The highest correlation of the delta activity was with spectral mean frequency and the lowest with period and amplitude mean frequency (averaged frequency). The spectral alpha activity also showed a tendency to a higher correlation with spectral mean frequency than with the other three mean frequencies. The averaged frequency did not show any correlation with the amplitude parameter mean voltage in any brain areas studied, though especially in the infarction hemisphere the other three mean frequency

TABLE II

THE LINEAR CORRELATION COEFFICIENTS (r) BETWEEN ALL FOUR MEAN FREQUENCY
VALUES (AVERAGED FREQUENCY FROM PERIOD AND AMPLITUDE ANALYSIS,
MOBILITY (HJORTH'S METHOD), ZERO-LINE CROSSING MEAN FREQUENCY FROM A
ZERO-LINE CROSSING ANALYSIS AND SPECTRAL MEAN FREQUENCY FROM FFT POWER
DENSITY SPECTRUM) AND SOME OTHER QUANTITATIVE EEG PARAMETERS IN BOTH
HEMISPHERES FROM ALL BRAIN AREAS

(N = 45 frontocentrally, 82 parieto-occipitally and 41 temporally)

F_4-C_4, F_3-C_3

	Lesion side				Control side			
	Averaged frequency	Mobility	Zero-line crossing mean	Spectral mean frequency	Averaged frequency	Mobility	Zero-line crossing mean	Spectral mean frequency
Delta activity	−0.63	−0.75	−0.74	−0.81	−0.55	−0.60	−0.61	−0.72
Alpha activity	0.17	0.31	0.27	0.40	0.05	0.12	0.12	0.27
Theta activity	−0.30	−0.28	−0.29	−0.22	−0.24	−0.27	−0.24	−0.20
Mean voltage	−0.25	−0.55	−0.52	−0.51	−0.23	−0.51	−0.51	−0.42
Skewness	−0.83	−0.89	−0.90	−0.88	−0.87	−0.90	−0.91	−0.87
Kurtosis	−0.76	−0.83	−0.83	−0.79	−0.78	−0.82	−0.83	−0.72
Alpha mean frequency	0.50	0.48	0.52	0.40	0.42	0.43	0.41	0.32

p<0.05 when r is 0.29–0.38, p<0.01 when r is 0.38–0.47, p<0.001 when r is >0.47

P_4-O_2, P_3-O_1

Delta activity	−0.51	−0.67	−0.67	−0.79	−0.53	−0.61	−0.62	−0.74
Alpha activity	0.09	0.26	0.27	0.42	0.02	0.10	0.11	0.11
Theta activity	−0.46	−0.48	−0.48	−0.50	−0.48	−0.46	−0.48	−0.48
Mean voltage	−0.15	−0.41	−0.41	−0.33	−0.14	−0.34	−0.32	−0.23
Skewness	−0.62	−0.63	−0.67	−0.61	−0.71	−0.73	−0.73	−0.70
Kurtosis	−0.57	−0.58	−0.59	−0.48	−0.56	−0.60	−0.58	−0.51
Alpha mean frequency	0.70	0.65	0.62	0.57	0.69	0.67	0.65	0.60

p<0.05 when r is 0.22–0.28, p<0.01 when r is 0.28–0.35, p<0.001 when r is >0.35

T_4-T_6, T_3-T_5

Delta activity	−0.56	−0.68	−0.68	−0.81	−0.44	−0.56	−0.55	−0.69
Alpha activity	0.21	0.36	0.35	0.52	0.14	0.21	0.20	0.34
Theta activity	−0.60	−0.66	−0.68	−0.66	−0.66	−0.61	−0.60	−0.56
Mean voltage	−0.18	−0.37	−0.33	−0.29	−0.26	−0.40	−0.38	−0.32
Skewness	−0.76	−0.79	−0.79	−0.81	−0.51	−0.53	−0.51	−0.54
Kurtosis	−0.76	−0.72	−0.71	−0.61	−0.63	−0.67	−0.66	−0.63
Alpha mean frequency	0.67	0.61	0.62	0.52	0.69	0.60	0.57	0.52

p<0.05 when r is 0.30–0.39, p<0.01 when r is 0.39–0.49, p<0.001 when r is >0.49

parameters often correlated significantly with mean voltage, as seen in Table II. In all examined areas, spectral skewness and kurtosis showed significant correlations with all the four mean frequency values.

Interhemispheric EEG differences

Many of the calculated qEEG parameters showed significant differences between the infarcted hemisphere and the control hemisphere (Tables III, IV and V). Not all the parameters showing significant asymmetry of the EEG are listed in these tables, but in each group the parameters of the highest *p*-values are shown.

$$P_4\text{--}O_2; P_3\text{--}O_1$$

TABLE III

QUANTITATIVE INTERHEMISPHERIC PARAMETRIC EEG DIFFERENCES ±S.D. LISTED ACCORDING TO p-VALUES (PAIRED t-TEST) PARIETO-OCCIPITALLY IN THE WHOLE MATERIAL (1), AND IN FAST (2), SLOW (3), HIGH AMPLITUDE (4) AND LOW AMPLITUDE (5) EEG GROUPS

1. Whole material (N=82)

Averaged frequency	-0.5 ± 0.8 Hz	$p<0.0001$
Mobility	-0.6 ± 1.0 Hz	$p<0.0001$
Zero-line crossing mean	-0.6 ± 1.0 Hz	$p<0.0001$
Zero-line crossing 0	-0.6 ± 1.1 Hz	$p<0.0001$
Spectral mean frequency	-0.7 ± 1.3 Hz	$p<0.0001$
Spectral 75th percentile	-0.8 ± 1.5 Hz	$p<0.0001$
Delta activity	5 ± 11 %	

2. Spectral mean frequency >7.7 Hz (N=44)

Averaged frequency	-0.3 ± 0.6 Hz	$p<0.002$
Zero-line crossing mean	-0.3 ± 0.7 Hz	$p<0.004$
Mobility	-0.3 ± 0.7 Hz	$p<0.005$

3. Spectral mean frequency ≤ 7.7 Hz (=38)

Mobility	-1.0 ± 1.2 Hz	$p<0.0001$
Zero-line crossing mean	-1.0 ± 1.2 Hz	$p<0.0001$
Spectral mean frequency	-1.2 ± 1.5 Hz	$p<0.0001$
Delta activity	10 ± 13 %	$p<0.0001$

4. Mean voltage >6.4 µV (N=37)

Zero-line crossing 0	-1.2 ± 1.3 Hz	$p<0.0001$
Spectral mean frequency	-1.3 ± 1.5 Hz	$p<0.0001$
Mobility	-1.1 ± 1.3 Hz	$p<0.0001$
Zero-line crossing mean	-1.1 ± 1.3 Hz	$p<0.0001$
Delta activity	10 ± 13 %	$p<0.0001$

5. Mean voltage ≤6.4 µV (N=45)

Averaged frequency	-0.3 ± 0.6 Hz	$p<0.0005$
Mobility	-0.3 ± 0.7 Hz	$p<0.001$
Zero-line crossing mean	-0.4 ± 0.7 Hz	$p<0.001$

In the parieto-occipital area (the whole material) the mean frequency values of all the four quantification techniques used showed a clear asymmetry (Table III). Very clear asymmetries could also be seen in many other calculated spectral parameters.

In both the slow and fast EEGs as well as in both the high and low amplitude EEGs, all the mean frequency parameters showed clear interhemispheric asymmetry (Table III). Especially in the slow and high amplitude EEGs the spectral delta activity seemed to be of great importance. In the fast and low amplitude EEGs of the parieto-occipital area, however, the spectral density parameters did not seem to show the EEG asymmetry at so high a p-level as did some of the parameters of the other three quantification techniques used.

$$F_4–C_4; \; F_3–C_3$$

The parameters showing the interhemispheric EEG differences frontocentrally at the highest p-levels (all EEGs surveyed) were spectral theta and alpha activities (Table IV); interestingly, these were not the same as in the parieto-occipital area.

TABLE IV

QUANTITATIVE INTERHEMISPHERIC PARAMETRIC EEG DIFFERENCES ±S.D. LISTED ACCORDING TO p-VALUES (PAIRED t-TEST) FRONTOCENTRALLY IN THE WHOLE MATERIAL (1), AND IN FAST (2), SLOW (3), HIGH AMPLITUDE (4) AND LOW AMPLITUDE (5) EEG GROUPS

1. Whole material (N=45)			
Theta activity	2.3±5.2	%	$p<0.005$
Alpha activity	−4.9±12	%	$p<0.007$
Averaged frequency	−0.5±1.3	Hz	$p<0.02$
Zero-line crossing 0	−0.6±1.8	Hz	$p<0.04$
Zero-line crossing mean	−0.5±1.7	Hz	$p<0.04$
Delta activity	5±14	%	$p<0.04$
2. Spectral mean frequency >7.5 Hz (N=25)			
Theta activity	2.1±4.9	%	$p<0.04$
3. Spectral mean frequency ≤7.5 Hz (N=20)			
Mobility	−1.5±1.7	Hz	$p<0.001$
Spectral mean frequency	−1.4±1.9	Hz	$p<0.003$
Averaged frequency	−0.9±1.3	Hz	$p<0.004$
Zero-line crossing mean	−1.3±1.8	Hz	$p<0.004$
4. Mean voltage > 5.7 μV (N=17)			
Alpha activity	−10±12	%	$p<0.002$
Mobility	−1.6±1.9	Hz	$p<0.003$
Zero-line crossing mean	−1.4±1.8	Hz	$p<0.005$
Delta activity	13±16	%	$p<0.005$
Spectral mean frequency	−1.5±2.0	Hz	$p<0.005$
5. Mean voltage ≤ 5.7 μV (N=28)			
Theta activity	2.4±4.2	%	$p<0.006$
Mean voltage	−0.4±1.2	μV	$p<0.10$

58

Furthermore, in fast and low voltage EEGs of the frontocentral area the theta activity was the only one of importance in recording the EEG asymmetry, though also frontocentrally in the slow and high amplitude EEGs the mean frequency parameters (together with spectral alpha activity) showed the EEG asymmetry at a high p-level.

$$T_4–T_6;\ T_3–T_5$$

In the temporal area (Table V), the most interesting observation was that in fast EEGs the amplitude parameters (mean voltage of the period and amplitude analysis and activity of Hjorth) together with mean energy of the period and amplitude analysis, showed the EEG asymmetry at a high p-level, though in slow EEGs these parameters together with spectral theta activity and kurtosis were the only parameters that did not show significant EEG asymmetry.

TABLE V

QUANTITATIVE INTERHEMISPHERIC PARAMETRIC EEG DIFFERENCES ±S.D. LISTED ACCORDING TO p-VALUES (PAIRED t-TEST) TEMPORALLY IN THE WHOLE MATERIAL (1), AND IN FAST (2), SLOW (3), HIGH AMPLITUDE (4) AND LOW AMPLITUDE (5) EEG GROUPS

1. *Whole material (N=41)*

Spectral 50th percentile	-1.3 ± 2.2 Hz	$p<0.0004$
Zero-line crossing 0	-0.9 ± 1.6 Hz	$p<0.0005$
Mobility	-0.9 ± 1.5 Hz	$p<0.0006$
Averaged frequency	-0.7 ± 1.3 Hz	$p<0.0007$
Spectral mean frequency	-0.9 ± 1.7 Hz	$p<0.0008$

2. *Spectral mean frequency >7.4 (Hz) (N=17)*

Mean energy	$2.3-2.8$	$p<0.004$
Mean voltage	1.3 ± 1.6 μV	$p<0.004$
Activity	1.3 ± 1.6 μV	$p<0.005$

3. *Spectral mean frequency ≤ 7.4 Hz (N=24)*

Spectral 50th percentile	-2.2 ± 2.4 Hz	$p<0.0001$
Spectral mean frequency	-1.4 ± 1.6 Hz	$p<0.0002$
Zero-line crossing 0	-1.2 ± 1.4 Hz	$p<0.0005$

4. *Mean voltage >7.6 μV (N=18)*

Mobility	-1.6 ± 1.0 Hz	$p<0.0001$
Zero-line crossing 0	-1.7 ± 1.2 Hz	$p<0.0001$
Zero-line crossing mean	-1.5 ± 1.1 Hz	$p<0.001$
Spectral mean frequency	-1.8 ± 1.3 Hz	$p<0.001$

5. *Mean voltage ≤7.6 μV (N=23)*

Mean energy	-1.8 ± 4.9	$p<0.09$
Activity	-0.8 ± 2.0 μV	$p<0.09$
50th percentile	-0.7 ± 1.9 Hz	$p<0.09$

Ratio parameters

The ability of the ratios of slow wave activity to alpha activity to show the interhemispheric differences was also tested.

Parieto-occipitally in the slow and the high amplitude EEGs as well as in all the subjects (groups 1, 3 and 4 in Table III) the ratio of spectral theta plus delta activities/alpha activity [(t + d)/a] appeared at the p-level of 0.0001, at which level the ratio of spectral delta activity/alpha activity (d/a) also appeared in groups 1 and 3 of this table. In both the fast and the low amplitude EEGs these ratio parameters were of less importance: the highest p-values of these ratio parameters were shown by the ratio of spectral theta activity/alpha activity (t/a): 0.05 in the group 2 and 0.08 in group 5 of Table III.

Frontocentrally in the whole group, the ratio (t+d)/a revealed EEG asymmetry at the significance level of $p<0.003$. In the fast and the low amplitude EEGs in the frontocentral area among the three ratio parameters studied, the ratio t/a showed the highest p-values for EEG asymmetry: $p<0.05$ in group 2 of Table IV and $p<0.006$ in group 5 of Table IV.

TABLE VI

LINEAR CORRELATION COEFFICIENTS BETWEEN SPECTRAL ALPHA, THETA AND DELTA ACTIVITIES (%) IN VARIOUS BRAIN AREAS STUDIED (INFARCTION SIDE)

	P_4-O_2, P_3-O_1		F_4-C_4, F_3-C_3		T_4-C_6, T_3-T_5	
	Theta	*Delta*	*Theta*	*Delta*	*Theta*	*Delta*
Alpha	-0.34^b	-0.83^c	0.02	-0.72^c	-0.47^b	-0.88^c
Theta		0.33^b		-0.15		0.53^c

[a] $= p <0.05.$ [b] $= p <0.01.$ [c] $= p <0.001.$

Temporally in the whole material, the ratios d/a ($p<0.006$) and (t + d)/a ($p<0.003$) showed significant asymmetry, but t/a did not ($p<0.17$). Furthermore, in the slow EEGs the ratio t/a did not reveal any asymmetry ($p<0.39$), though d/a did ($p<0.0009$). However, in high amplitude EEGs both these parameters showed significant asymmetry, t/a ($p<0.0003$) and d/a ($p<0.002$).

Interrelationships of spectral band parameters

Table VI illustrates the interrelationships of the spectral parameters of delta, theta and alpha activities. It can be seen that in all the brain areas studied, the correlation was highest between the delta and alpha activities, and that frontocentrally the theta activity showed no correlation with either the delta or alpha activities.

DISCUSSION

Correlations of the EEG quantification techniques used

Only a few studies have been devoted to the degree of statistical comparability of different qEEG methods. Beatty and Figueroa (1974) showed in five volunteers (using EEGs from the occipital region) that the percent alpha as measured using standard spectral methods has a correlation of 0.79 with period and 0.82 with the period and amplitude estimates of the same percentages. Pigeau et al. (1981) compared period analysis and Fast Fourier Transform (FFT) in waking and sleeping groups, measuring the EEG in the waking group from the P_4 position and in the sleeping group from the C_4 position. A high degree of statistical equivalence was found between the period analysis and the FFTs. Linear regression revealed a high correlation (0.70–0.94) in all frequencies (beta, sigma, alpha, theta and delta) except for beta (0.54) and delta (0.41) in the waking group. Matoušek (1973) has also shown a remarkable degree of correspondence between the zero crossings and power spectrum.

In cerebral infarction a high statistical equivalence was also detected in the present work between the four qEEG methods used: the linear correlation between the mean frequencies of these four techniques varied between 0.84 and 1.0. In spite of these significant correlations between these methods, significant differences, however, existed in these correlation coefficients. The PDS mean frequency and the mean frequency of period and amplitude analysis gave the lowest correlation coefficients, neglect of the amplitude (period analysis) possibly being one cause for this. The ignoring of signal amplitude of the period analysis was also reflected in the absence of correlations between the amplitude parameter mean voltage and the mean frequency of the period analysis. According to Obrist et al. (1973), both the mean frequency and the amplitude of the EEG reflect the degree of brain hypoxia quite closely, thus suggesting that qEEG parameters useful in cerebral ischemia should contain information about both of these.

EEG asymmetries

Clear interhemispheric qEEG differences could be seen in all three brain areas studied even though many of the patients were studied late after the infarction when EEG abnormalities had declined or even totally disappeared in visually interpreted EEGs (Roseman et al., 1951; Silverman, 1960). In the visual scoring one fifth of the EEGs of this series appeared as normal. On the other hand, because it has been shown that in normal subjects significant interhemispheric differences in the peak frequencies within the alpha band occur in the central and occipital regions (Pfurt-scheller et al., 1977), perhaps not all the interhemispheric differences were solely due to ischemic changes.

Parieto-occipitally, the clearest interhemispheric differences of the present series could be seen in all four mean frequency parameters, in the PDS 75th percentile and in the PDS delta activity. In this brain area in cerebral infarction patients the delta activity, the 75th percentile and the averaged frequency were among the first four parameters obtained from the stepwise regression analysis performed among all the qEEG parameters of the present four EEG quantification techniques and CBF (Tolonen and Sulg, 1981). There is thus a good correlation in this brain area between the parameters that show the clearest interhemispheric differences and those parameters that include most of the information in relation to the CBF. This therefore supports the value of these parameters as qEEG indexes in this brain area.

Zero-line crossing counts easily underestimate the contribution of low-frequency components and/or overestimate fast frequency components (see Lopes da Silva, 1982). This fact was possibly reflected in the present results of both the fast and low amplitude EEGs of the parieto-occipital area, where PDS parameters did not show EEG asymmetry at so high a *p*-level as the zero-line crossing estimates did.

The parameters that revealed the EEG interhemispheric differences at the highest *p*-levels frontocentrally were different from those that revealed them parieto-occipitally. It was interesting that in the frontocentral area the theta activity in the fast and low amplitude EEGs was the only parameter to reveal the EEG asymmetry, though, e.g. in the occipital and temporal regions in patients with cerebrovascular accidents the greatest deviation from the controls was found by Cohen et al. (1976) in the delta band. Furthermore, in the present study the theta activity seemed frontocentrally to be an independent parameter in relation to the delta and alpha activities for it showed no correlation with these parameters. However, significant temporal and parieto-occipital correlations were seen.

Because of considerable physiological fluctuations of the theta activity, Matoušek (1968) has preferred the ratio of theta/alpha activity (t/a) for evaluation of the EEG background activity. The magnitude of the ratio t/a, especially after empirical correction, is comparable to the visual estimation of the amount of theta activity (Matoušek, 1968). However, as to the ability to reveal EEG asymmetry, the different ratio parameters of slow wave activity/alpha activity did not seem in the present work to improve essentially the results obtained by using only single parameters. Mies et al. (1976) has earlier shown that in cerebral ischemia the frequency index was a more reliable indicator for focal changes than the parameters of delta-, theta-, alpha- and beta-band intensities.

Spectral band parameters

The changes in the delta and alpha bands in infarction patients seemed to be dependent (inversely) on each other to a fairly high degree, but the information content of theta activity was especially different frontocentrally. This is in accordance with the observation of Van Huffelen et al. (1980) that in a follow-up study in a patient with an extensive frontocentral and parietal ischemia the frequencies of the theta peaks for the occipital, parietal and posterior temporal regions remained stable, though the alpha peak frequencies changed.

Sainio et al. (1983) have shown that in recent infarctions a high proportion of delta or a low proportion of alpha power is a reliable indicator of a poor outcome, but theta power changes are not. The different role of the delta and theta band in cerebral infarction patients also supports the observation that occipital delta activity correlates well with CBF of the same hemiphere, but that theta activity does not (Tolonen and Sulg, 1981). For further evaluation of the significance of the theta activity parameter in infarction patients, the local CBF and also clinical correlations with the theta changes should be studied frontocentrally. It would be interesting to do the same estimate for the amplitude and mean energy parameters of the temporal regions, where these parameters in certain EEG profiles were the only ones to show significant EEG asymmetry.

Conclusions

Beatty and Figueroa (1974) and Pigeau et al. (1981) have concluded that period analysis and FFT analysis show similar types of information, and hence a faster period analysis method can be used more often in EEG research. While they studied healthy volunteers, the present work investigated cerebral infarction patients and a high statistical equivalence was still found between all the four methods used (combined period and amplitude analysis, normalized slope descriptors, zero-line crossing variants and FFT power density spectrum). This suggests that these methods are close alternatives for each other. In spite of this high correlation between these four methods, however, significant differences could be seen, especially between the period analysis and the power density spectral analysis. Moreover, some data published earlier suggest a certain advantage of spectral parameters in cerebral ischemia: (1) Binnie et al. (1978) obtained more accurate data from the power spectrum method than from normalized slope descriptors; moreover, according to Denoth (1975), Hjorth's parameters are of limited applicability; (2) Sotaniemi et al. (1980) showed that in open-heart surgery, patients' spectral parameters provided a higher correlation between clinical disturbances and the EEG than combined period and amplitude analysis or normalized slope descriptors; (3) Tolonen and Sulg (1981) found that in cerebral infarction patients the spectral density parameters showed a tendency to a higher correlation with CBF than the parameters from combined period and amplitude analysis, normalized slope descriptors or a zero-line crossing variant analysis did. Altogether, therefore, in cerebral ischemia there is evidence for some independence and superiority of the power density spectral analysis in the quantification of the EEG.

At the parametric level it seems that in cerebral infarction patients different qEEG parameters may be more useful in different brain areas, in slow versus fast EEGs, and in high voltage versus flat EEGs. The present results support the applicability of the often used qEEG parameters of mean frequency, delta band and alpha band intensities in cerebral ischemia. The theta band may also be of importance as an EEG index frontocentrally while the amplitude parameters may be so temporally, at least as far as the ability to show EEG asymmetry is concerned.

SUMMARY

In the present study four different EEG quantification techniques are compared in patients with cerebral infarction.

The 82 EEGs of 48 patients with unilateral cerebral infarction were recorded and processed. The EEG analysis was performed using four different quantification techniques: (1) period and amplitude analysis, (2) normalized slope descriptors of Hjorth, (3) a zero-line crossing variant analysis and (4) spectral density analysis with Fast Fourier Transform.

The linear correlation coefficients (r) between the mean frequency values of these four quantification techniques showed an overall high interdependence between the methods: the r value ranged from 0.84 to 1.0 (in all $p<0.001$). However, in spite of this high equivalence between these methods significant differences could be seen, especially between the period and amplitude and spectral analyses.

The parameters which showed significant interhemispheric EEG differences were not the same in the three brain areas studied. For example, frontocentrally the theta activity was the only parameter indicating significant EEG asymmetry in fast and low amplitude EEGs; temporally, amplitude parameters showed the clearest EEG asymmetries in fast EEGs. However, in all three brain areas studied the mean frequency and delta activity parameters were the most useful indicators in the majority of EEG groups.

Although these four EEG quantification techniques seem to correlate well with each other, there are some differences between them. At the parametric level somewhat different EEG parameters appear to be more useful in different brain areas as well as in different EEG profiles, at least as far as the ability to display EEG asymmetry is concerned.

REFERENCES

Barlow, J. S. (1979) Computerized clinical electroendephalography in perspective. *IEEE Trans. Biomed. Eng.* BME-26,377–391.

Beatty, J. and Figueroa, C. (1974) Period analytic algorithms for the estimation of selected spectral properties of short segments of EEG data. *Behav. Res. Meth. Instrum.*, 6: 293–295.

Binnie, C. D., Batchelor, B. G., Bowring, P. A., Darby, C. E., Herbert L., Lloyd, D. S. L., Smith, D. M., Smith, G. F. and Smith M. (1978) Computer-assisted interpretation of clinical EEGs. *Electroenceph. clin. Neurophysiol.*, 44: 575–585.

Cohen, B. A., Bravo-Fernandez, E. J. and Sanches, Jr., A. (1976) Quantification of computer analyzed serial EEGs from stroke patients. *Electroenceph. clin. Neurophysiol.* 41: 379–386.

Cohen, B. A., Bravo-Fernandez, E. J. and Sanches, Jr., A. (1977) Automated electroencephalographic analysis as a prognostic indicator in stroke. *Med. Biol. Eng. Comput.*, 15: 431–437.

Denoth, F. (1975) Some general remarks on Hjorth's parameters used in EEG analysis. In G. Dolce and H. Künkel (Eds.), *CEAN-Computerized EEG Analysis*, Fischer, Stuttgart, pp. 9-18.

Gotman, J., Skuce, D. R., Thompson, C. J., Gloor, P., Ives, J. R. and Ray, W. F. (1973) Clinical applications of spectral analysis and extraction of features from electroencephalograms with slow waves in adult patients. *Electroenceph. clin. Neurophysiol.*, 35: 225–235.

Herrschaft, H., Hossman, K.-A., Mies, G. and Zülch, K. J. (1977) Relationship between cerebral blood flow and EEG frequency content in patients with acute brain ischaemia. *Acta Neurol. Scand.* 56, (Suppl. 64): 414–415.

Hjorth, B. (1973) The physical significance of time domain descriptors in EEG analysis. *Electroenceph. clin. Neurophysiol.*, 34: 321–325.

Jonkman, E. J. and Lelieveld, M. H. J. (1981) EEG computer analysis in patients with migraine. *Electroenceph. clin. Neurophysiol.*, 52: 652–655.

Lopes da Silva, F. (1982) EEG analysis: Theory and practice. In E. Niedermaeyer and F. Lopes da Silva (Eds.), *Electroencephalography. Basic Principles, Clinical Applications and Related Fields*, Urban & Schwarzenberg, Baltimore–Munich, pp. 685–711.

Matoušek, M. (1968) Frequency analysis in routine electroencephalography. *Electroenceph. clin. Neurophysiol.*, 24: 365–373.

Matoušek, M. (Ed.) (1973) Frequency and correlation analysis. In A. Remond (Editor-in-Chief), *Handbook of Electroencephalography and Clinical Neurophysiology, Vol 5 (Part A)*, Elsevier, Amsterdam, pp. 5A1–5A137.

Mies, G., Hossman, K.-A. and Zülch, K. J. (1976) *EEG analysis in patients with cerebrovascular disorders*, Proceedings DECUS Symposium, Munich September 1976 3, 411–414.

Obrist, W. D., Saltzman, H. A., Sulg, I. A., Thompson, L. W. and Townsed, R. E. (1973) The quantitated EEG in hypoxic and hyperbaric conditions. *Swed. J. Defence Med.*, 9: 466–471.

Pfurtscheller, G., Maresch, H. and Schuy, S. (1977) Inter- and intrahemispheric differences in the peak frequency of rhythmic activity within the alpha band. *Electroenceph. clin. Neurophysiol.*, 42: 77–83.

Pigeau, R. A., Hoffman, R. F. and Moffitt, A. R. (1981) A multivariate comparison between two EEG analysis techniques: period analysis and Fast Fourier Transform. *Electroenceph. clin. Neurophysiol.*, 52: 656–658.

Roseman, E., Schmidt, R. P. and Foltz, E. L. (1951) Serial electroencephalography in vascular lesions of the brain. *Neurology*, 2: 311–331.

Sainio, K., Stenberg, D., Keskimäki, I., Muuronen A. and Kaste, M. (1983) Visual and spectral EEG analysis in the evaluation of the outcome in patients with ischemic brain infarction. *Electroenceph. clin. Neurophysiol.*, 56: 117–124.

Silverman, D. (1960) Serial electroencephalography in brain tumors and cerebrovascular accidents. *Arch.*

Neurol. Psychiat. 2: 122–129.

Sotaniemi, K. A., Sulg, I. A. and Hokkanen, E. (1980) Quantitative EEG as a measure of cerebral dysfunction before and after open-heart surgery. *Electroenceph. clin. Neurophysiol.*, 50: 81–95.

Stigsby, B., Obrist, W. D. and Sulg, I. A. (1973) Automatic data acquisition and period-amplitude analysis of the electroencephalogram. *Comput. Progr. Biomed.*, 3: 93–104.

Tolonen, U. and Sulg, I. A. (1981) Comparison of quantitative EEG parameters from four different analysis techniques in evaluation of relationships between EEG and CBF in brain infarction. *Electroenceph. clin. Neurophysiol.*, 51: 177–185.

Van Huffelen, A. C., Poortvliet, D. C. J., Van der Wulp, C. J. M. and Magnus, O. (1980) Quantitative EEG in cerebral ischaemia. In H. Lechner and A. Aranibar (Eds.), *EEG and Clinical Neurophysiology*, Excerpta Medica Int. Congr. Ser. 526, Excerpta Medica, Amsterdam, pp. 115–143.

Brain Ischemia: Quantitative EEG and Imaging Techniques, Progress in Brain Research, Vol. 62, edited by
G. Pfurtscheller, E.J. Jonkman and F.H. Lopes da Silva
©*1984 Elsevier Science Publishers B.V.*

Quantitative EEG as a Measure of Brain Dysfunction

ILMAR SULG

University Hospital, Department of Clinical Neurophysiology, Trondheim (Norway)

INTRODUCTION

Since the EEG was discovered and developed into a valuable tool for studies on brain activity, evidence has accumulated on a close but complex coupling between the electrical activity of the brain, cerebral blood flow and metabolism. This evidence was first deduced from the fact that impairment of brain function, e.g. in hypoxia, hypoglycemia, coma etc., is usually accompanied by a slowing of the EEG. Also, most metabolic diseases and dysmetabolic encephalopathies are more or less reflected in the EEG.

On the basis of many experimental and clinical studies, it seems justified to conclude that the EEG has to be seen as a paraphenomenon of integrated metabolic brain activity.

With the advent of quantitative techniques for measurement of blood flow and oxygen uptake (Kety and Schmidt, 1948; Lassen and Munck, 1955) it became possible to correlate the EEG to these parameters, globally as well as regionally. The invasive method for measurement of the regional cerebral blood flow (rCBF) by means of intracarotid injection of isotopes (Lassen and Ingvar, 1961), was later supplemented by such noninvasive techniques as inhalation and intravenous injection of isotopes (Mallett and Veall, 1965; Obrist et al., 1975; Kuikka et al., 1977). However, these nontraumatic methods are lower in resolution and reliability. This deficit is more or less compensated by the fact that the noninvasive CBF measurements can be repeated without any harm to the patient.

During the last 20 years the quantitative analysis of the EEG has been improved with a variety of highly effective and sophisticated techniques (Blackman and Tukey, 1958; Kaiser and Petersén, 1966; Dumermuth and Flühler, 1967; Walter and Brazier, 1968; Zetterberg, 1969; Hjorth, 1973; Pfurtscheller and Haring, 1972). Combined quantitative studies on metabolic, hemodynamic and electrical activities, have produced new information about the brain in health as well as in different pathological states and the future seems to be even more promising. By combining quantitative EEG with single-photon-emission computerized tomography, highly interesting results have been obtained (Henriksen et al., this volume; Buchsbaum et al., this volume). The era of nuclear magnetic resonance techniques is just beginning, offering in the near future a still closer look into the metabolic events within the brain than ever before. Because the EEG is directly dependent on cerebral metabolism, these new methods will certainly contribute to better understanding of this dependence. By studying relationships between EEG, CBF and cerebral metabolism, we can learn how to utilize the EEG more effectively and how to extract as much relevant information as possible from the complex EEG pattern.

[65]

The main goal of the present study, which began about 10 years ago, was primarily a comprehensive statistical evaluation of the relationship between different qEEG parameters and the CBF as well as cerebral metabolism. The secondary goal was, especially regarding clinical requirements, to find out which analysis technique could offer a meaningful data reduction, because this is an imperative prerequisite for reliable and clinically acceptable monitoring of the brain in high-risk conditions.

QUANTITATIVE ANALYSIS OF THE EEG

The EEG, a continuous and complex flow of bioelectric events, offers several objective measures of brain activity. Although there is as yet no exhaustive explanation for the neurophysiological basis of the EEG, it has proved possible to identify abnormal frequency and wave patterns indicative of different pathological conditions in the brain. These empirical findings have led to the general use of the EEG as a diagnostic tool with many clinical and experimental applications. Both in the past and at present, most clinical EEGs have been evaluated visually: the actual recording has to be compared with known EEG patterns. The interpretation is thus based on this comparison. When gross changes are present, this method is adequate, but if minor deviations or differences have to be detected and evaluated, a set of quantitative standards is necessary, especially when statistical relationships are sought between electrical and other parameters of brain activity.

Various attempts have been made to supplement descriptive EEG interpretation with quantitative techniques. Modern computers offer several very effective methods for transformation of the EEG into digital data. At present, however, only a few laboratories have fully developed programs for computerized analysis of the EEG at their disposal.

When an instrumental analysis is not available or applicable, the manual analysis or, alternatively, a semi-automatic digitalization of the EEG trace is still a useful alternative (Sulg, 1969a). This approach is time consuming, but compared to instrumental techniques offers some essential advantages, such as immediate availability and optimal selectivity of a multi-channel record and further, the quantification can be made from any EEG sample of any length. Using this method, it is also possible to minimize the influence of artifacts, because every single graphic component not originating from the brain can easily be excluded. The fact that visual descriptive interpretation of wave patterns has made a basic contribution to the clinical EEG diagnosis is the main reason for the present method of EEG quantification. The most rewarding aspect of this method, however, is the fact that the very subject of analysis is the same as that for routine EEG interpretation in clinical applications. Even when the laboratory equipment has advanced to computer technology, one still has to check and compare the computer output with the traditional EEG recording.

Manual Period and Amplitude Analysis

The graphic wave phenomenon, more or less aberrant from the sine wave, is the main feature in the EEG trace. Any individual wave can be quantitatively described when its duration or period, amplitude and pattern are determined. Of these parameters, only the first two can be conveniently measured manually. The present technique (Sulg, 1969a) is similar to the so-called period analysis, presented in a mathematical approach by Burch et al. (1964). It is called manual period and amplitude analysis (MPAA). Using a specially designed transparent, multiscaled ruler, all EEG activity in the 1–20 Hz frequency band was measured with the resolution for successive frequency classes of 1 Hz (e.g. frequency class 1 Hz included all waves between 0.5 and 1.5 Hz).

Frequency index

The activity time (accumulated waves present) in every frequency class is added over all frequency classes. The ratio of all counted waves to the corresponding total activity time in seconds gives the frequency index (F. I.), also called mean frequency:

$$\frac{\text{total number of waves}}{\text{total activity time}} = \text{F. I.}$$

Energy index

In order to calculate a parameter, which could approximately correspond to the power density achieved with Fourier analysis, an "energy index" was calculated from wave amplitudes and duration.

Assuming that a single wave is sinusoidal, the energy E is proportional to A/8f, when A is the peak-to-peak amplitude and f the frequency. The sums of the energy of all consecutive waves in one frequency class will be denoted by Ef. By adding the Ef values throughout the frequency spectrum (1–20 Hz), the total energy and the energy index (E. I.) can be calculated:

$$\frac{\text{total energy}}{\text{total number of waves}} = \text{E. I.}$$

Computer aid in manual analysis

In the MPAA only the measurement and classification of EEG waves required manual performance. The resulting data were then computer processed for the following values: wave counts (n) in alpha, beta, theta and delta frequency bands; total number of waves (N), activity time (AT) profile, total activity time (TAT), percent activity time (%AT) profile including plotted polygon, total energy, energy index, statistical parameters (mode, mean, median, S.D., variance, skewness and kurtosis of quantitative polygons).

Computerized EEG analysis

Period and amplitude analysis

An IBM 1800 computer was programmed for automatic frequency analysis using zero-crossing detection, combined with integrated amplitude measurements (Stigsby et al., 1973).

Multivariable analysis

A combined multivariable analysis of the EEG was performed using four computer techniques: power density analysis using Fast Fourier Transformation (FFT), period and amplitude analysis, computing of normalized slope descriptors (Hjorth, 1973) and averaged frequency from a modified zero-crossing analysis (Sulg et al., 1977a).

With this computer program it is possible to compare different analysis techniques on the same EEG sample. FFT and combined period-amplitude analysis are computed for frequencies of 1 to 25 Hz and also separately for conventional EEG frequency bands. The mean frequency and other central tendencies (such as peakedness and skewness) are also computed.

MEASUREMENT OF CEREBRAL BLOOD FLOW

There have been two main research projects on relationship between qEEG and CBF: the first one was done in cooperation with D. H. Ingvar, S. Cronquist and J. Risberg at the University Hospital in Lund, Sweden (Sulg and Ingvar, 1968; Ingvar and Sulg, 1969; Sulg, 1969b). The second was also a team project done at the University Hospital of Oulu, Finland (Ahonen et al., 1979; Tolonen and Sulg, 1981). In Lund the rCBF measurements were made with the intracarotid 133-Xenon clearance technique. In the second study the CBF was measured by gamma camera, after intravenous injection of 133-Xenon. In Lund, data from manual EEG analysis were used for statistical evaluation of relationships between EEG and cortical cerebral blood flow. In Oulu, the extensive package of computer subroutines as described above was used. Both projects resulted in academic theses (Sulg, 1969b; Tolonen, 1981).

QUANTITATIVE EEG AS A MEASURE OF CEREBRAL DYSFUNCTION

qEEG and CBF in ischemic brain

qEEG/CBF relationships were studied in a large neurological patient group (144 patients, most of them suffering from ischemic brain lesions), compared to six healthy controls, all examined by means of the intra-carotid isotope clearance method. The age range of the patients was 14–79 years (mean 51 years). Nearly all patients were studied in the subacute or chronic stage of their disease with relatively stable neurological symptomatology in order to avoid interference from major acute sequelae of ischemic brain lesions, such as focal hyperfusion and brain edema. In nearly all of them, the CBF measurements and the qEEG studies were done within 24 h. Although noncompartmental as well as "grey" and "white" flow were measured, only the flow values within the rapidly perfused tissue compartment were used in the present study, since the EEG is very probably generated in the grey matter of the brain. The CBF measurements were usually combined with cerebral arteriography; blood pressure, hemoglobin concentration, as well as the arterial pCO_2 were also measured. The qEEG samples were taken from the parieto-occipital and temporo-occipital regions.

CBF and frequency content of the EEG

The relation between mean hemisphere grey rCBF and amount of measured percent activity time (%AT) in patients as well as in healthy controls is displayed in Figure 1. It can be seen that all quantitative EEG profiles derived from patients deviate clearly from the reference polygon of healthy individuals, although one of the patient groups shows a mean grey CBF not differing from the normal level. Here the EEG seems to be more sensitive for the actual brain disease than the CBF. It can be further seen that parallel to decreasing flow levels, there was a bimodal shift in EEG activity toward the lower frequencies, i.e. a decrease in the alpha range and an increase in slower activity. This trend is surprisingly clearcut for all flow levels, except in the patient group with the highest flow, also exceeding the normal level. The corresponding qEEG profile shows the most abnormal distribution of brain activity, even more abnormal than patients with the lowest CBF. The physiological coupling between EEG and CBF seems to persist within a wide range of progressing impairment in brain function, but only to a certain limit. The group of patients with the highest CBF in combination with the most abnormal qEEG profile illustrates impressively the so-called luxury-perfusion syndrome (Lassen, 1966), although this syndrome has been described mainly as a decoupling between CBF and cerebral metabolism.

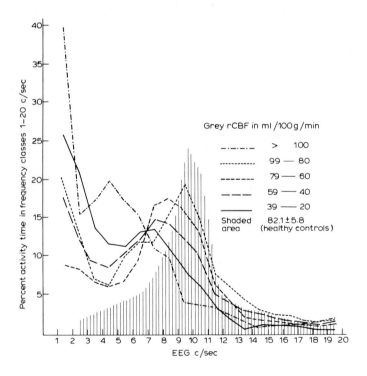

Fig. 1. Graphic display of relationships between the qEEG (i.e. percent activity derived from manual period analysis) and the rCBF (i.e. the hemispheric mean fast compartment flow, or "cortical" flow). Different polygon profiles represent group mean values of EEG activity distribution in five groups of neurological patients with pathological EEGs. Grouping has been made according to the CBF level. Group mean values differ from each other by about 20 ml/100 g brain weight per min. Shaded area: the mean profile representing the distribution of EEG activity in a group of healthy controls with a hemispheric mean rCBF of 82.1 ml (S.D. = 5.8) per 100 g brain weight per min. (From Sulg et al., 1981, with permission of Karger, Basel).

The profound EEG abnormality is to be considered as the third sign in the triad of the luxury-perfusion syndrome. Thus it is important to realize that in this situation as well, the EEG still reflects the pathological state of the brain, because it is primarily dependent on neuronal metabolism. Figure 1 shows further that EEG profiles in groups with different mean CBF values differ most clearly in the alpha and delta activity ranges, whereas the visible difference nearly disappears within theta frequencies, as well as in higher frequencies beyond the alpha range. Similar trends can be seen in Figure 2, which shows Spearman rank order correlation coefficients for actual frequency classes in relation to the CBF in a limited group of patients that excluded all cases with an apparent or suspected luxury-perfusion syndrome. There appears to be a negative correlation (most pronounced within the delta range) for slow frequencies, and a positive correlation for activity within the alpha range. There are no abrupt changes at the margins between "classical" frequency bands, a fact that demonstrates that these frequency bands are more or less artificial.

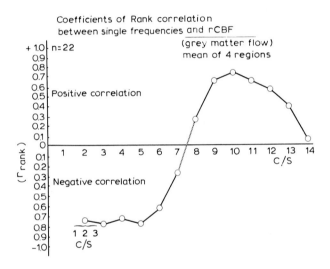

Fig. 2. Spearman rank correlation coefficients for EEG activity in single frequency classes in relation to the mean hemisphere noncompartmental rCBF in 22 neurological patients with a pathological EEG. (From Sulg et al., 1981, with permission of Karger, Basel).

qEEG, CBF and age

Stepwise regression analyses of correlations between qEEG parameters, CBF and the age of the patients were performed. Twenty-five qEEG variables were included, such as data from every frequency class and band, total area of profile polygons (primary EEG variables) and furthermore, all meaningful statistical parameters of the polygons (secondary EEG variables), such as mean, median, skewness, peakedness etc. Because a certain influence from the age factor was expected, this factor was also included in some of the analysis steps.

Single frequency classes and CBF. Here the CBF is the dependent variable and the computer was programmed to seek among the other available variables the one with the highest multiple correlation coefficient (MCC), because this variable would offer the best prediction of the CBF. Activity in the frequency class 11 Hz was given the first place (MCC = 0.32, regression coefficient 0.43, F-value 13.2, significant at the 0.1% level). The next place was given to 15 Hz, but with considerably weaker significance (deduced from the F-value) than for the 11 Hz. The program then stopped, because the F-value became insufficient.

Single frequency classes, rCBF and age. When the age factor was included in the regression analysis according to single frequency classes and CBF, it was given the first place with a high significance (MCC = 0.35), i.e. as the best predictor for the CBF. The age was followed by 2 Hz and then by 4 Hz. The age factor seems thus to have a peculiar effect on the order of entry of the frequency classes, where the entering order is dependent on the value of the variable for the prediction of the CBF.

EEG frequency bands, CBF and age. The age factor was again given the first place, followed by the alpha, beta and delta frequency bands.

Secondary qEEG variables and CBF. The mean frequency was entered with high significance into the first place (MCC = 0.36), followed by the skewness of the polygon.

Secondary qEEG variables, CBF and age. When the age factor was included, the highest correlation was achieved for the combination EEG mean frequency and age (MCC = 0.52, F-value 14.86 corresponding to significance at 0.01%); the significance was even higher than what was obtained from all primary variables with sufficient F-values. When all secondary variables with sufficient F-values were utilized, a MCC as high as 0.56 (significance at the 0.01% level) was obtained.

Discriminant analysis

Using this statistical method, patients included in the study are classified into an arbitrary number of groups according to the estimated CBF values (see Figure 1). Then the coefficients for the discriminant functions of EEG variables are calculated from the CBF/qEEG correlations. The EEG profiles included in the analysis are reclassified, using these so-called function coefficients. In the present study more than half of the EEG profiles (54%) were reclassified correctly.

Polygon–profile clustering analysis

This is a quite different approach to the analysis of relationships between two variables, such as qEEG and CBF. The analysis is built on a profile similarity measure. The distance function (D-measure) was used for this purpose. In computation, quantitative profiles will be "aggregated" into "clusters" by the power of the D-measure. The profile pattern alone is thus the basis for classification. The material consisted of qEEG profiles from 100 patients. The analysis produced four different clusters: the corresponding average profiles are displayed in Figure 3. These clustered groups also showed interesting relationships to the clinical diagnoses. In clusters I and III, cerebrovascular lesions dominated; the ischemic lesions, however, were found in all clusters in the following order: 20% in cluster II, 18.7% in clusters I and IV, and 14% in cluster III; tumor cerebri dominated in clusters II (47%) and IV (25%).

Clustering analysis seems to offer a new way of obtaining information about relationships between EEG and other brain functions. The quantitative EEG profile is a bioelectrical "finger-print" of an individual. Clustering of EEG profiles from a large population could open new vistas for psychology and behavioral science. This method could also be of some advantage if neither descriptive EEG analysis nor quantitative

72

EEG estimates are sufficient to differentiate brain dysfunction syndromes of miscellaneous genesis.

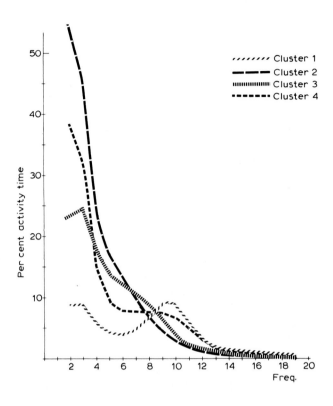

Fig. 3. Mean profiles as result of cluster analysis. For explanation see text, p. 71.

Prediction of the CBF from the qEEG

Linear regression analysis has been used to predict the CBF from a given set of qEEG parameters.

Figure 4 shows the polynomial plotting of the prediction error (residuals) against estimated rCBF values when the blood flow was predicted from the EEG mean frequency. It is seen that most of the predicted values differed by less than 20 ml/100 g/min from the estimated ones.

Regional relationships between qEEG and rCBF

Correlations between mean hemispheric CBF and qEEG from parieto-occipital regions were analyzed and described in previous chapters. In the present study the EEG mean frequency and the rCBF were measured in six additional patients with an occlusion of the middle cerebral artery: rCBF values were correlated to corresponding regional qEEG variables for the same hemisphere. One patient underwent five consecutive rCBF and qEEG examinations during the first 43 days of illness. The overall correlations between the mean hemispheric blood flow and the mean hemispheric

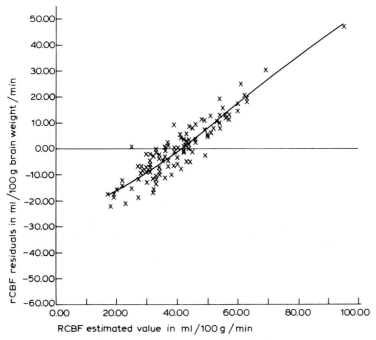

Fig. 4. Relationship between estimated rCBF values and rCBF residuals when the mean frequency was used (see text, p. 72).

frequency were also significant in this study; the product-moment correlation coefficient was 0.5 (significant at the 0.01% level).

Exceptions, however, were found when qEEG and rCBF values were correlated regionally; low frequency EEG coincided with an unexpected high flow, probably due to luxury perfusion. As seen in Figure 5, in the acute stage there was a lack of co-variation between the EEG mean frequency and the rCBF, especially within the center of the lesion. Follow-ups 22 and 44 days later showed a striking co-variation of these two variables outside the infarcted area and a trend in the same direction within the lesion. This case demonstrates convincingly that in the human brain a focal ischemic injury may "uncouple" the physiological coupling between brain activity (as reflected in the EEG) and the regional CBF.

Effect of cardiac pacemaker on CBF and qEEG

It is a well-known clinical fact that cardiac arrhythmia may have a profound effect on systemic circulation and that more pronounced arrhythmias may also induce cerebral symptoms such as syncopal-convulsive attacks. The result is a transitory brain ischemia. Treatment by implantation of an artificial pacemaker has proved to be successful in relieving such syncopal symptoms. It is also common experience that patients with a total heart block, when treated with artificial pacing, show progressive somatic as well as mental improvement (Lagergren, 1975).

The purpose of this study was to establish whether changes in CBF could explain the effect of pacing, and if such a beneficial effect would also be reflected in the qEEG.

74

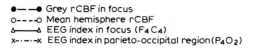

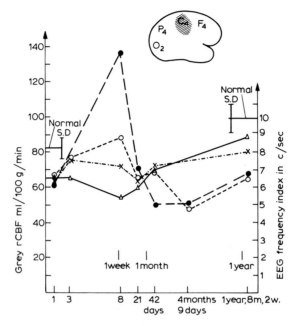

Fig. 5. Focal and perifocal relationships between qEEG and rCBF. Trends of EEG mean frequency as well as fast compartment flow (grey rCBF) are shown within the focus of an ischemic lesion and outside of it. Seven examinations were performed within 22 months.

Six male patients with a complete atrioventricular (AV) block and Adams–Stokes syndrome were subjected to rCBF and qEEG studies. The methods were the same as in previous studies. Heart volume was measured in five patients pre- and postoperatively; no significant differences were found. Signs of more pronounced cardiac decompensation were noted in only one patient, who also had an enlargement of the heart. In four other patients the cardiac decompensation was only slight; the main symptom was stress dyspnea. None of the patients showed any focal neurological signs. However, in all of them a slight to moderate reduction of physical well-being and mental capacity was noted, but there was no evidence of pronounced dementia or signs of psychosis. The heart rate varied preoperatively between 30 and 48 per min. With the pacemaker the heart rate was fixed to a frequency of 72 per min in all cases.

In all six patients the mean hemispheric noncompartmental rCBF was found to be significantly below normal values as measured in the previously described healthy controls. The mean of all six patients was 40 (S.D. = 3.9) ml/100 g/min upon the first examination; this represents a 21.5% decrease from the normal 51.1 ml/100 g/min. The mean hemispheric fast flow was found to be 60.4 (S.D. = 5.1) ml/100 g/min, which was 25.9% below the normal level (82.1, S.D. = 5.8). Upon follow-up 6 months later all six patients showed an increase in hemispheric rCBF, 5.6 ml for cortical flow (9.3%) and 3.7 ml for the mean hemispheric rCBF (9.2%).

Preoperatively, the quantitative average profile for the total group showed a clear-cut deviation from the normal. Re-examination 6 months later showed a shift toward the normal pattern in all cases, i.e. a decrease of slow wave content and increase in activity in the alpha range. The EEG frequency index (F. I) increased in four and decreased in two patients. One of these, however, showed a regional slow wave abnormality in the preoperative EEG which disappeared post-operatively. In the third EEG examination about 2 years later, the F. I. had risen considerably above the preoperative level. The increase of the group mean value, however, did not reach the level of statistical significance. If, however, the areas of EEG profile polygons were calculated and the difference between pre- and postoperative profiles tested with a χ^2-test, the result turned out to be highly significant ($p < 0.001$).

The correlation between rCBF and the frequency index (calculated for differences between pre- and postoperative values) showed higher coefficients (up to 0.57) for rCBF values corrected for arterial CO_2 than for noncorrected values. The correlation between F. I. and the fast flow was shown to be higher ($r = 0.57$) than correlation between noncompartmental rCBF and F. I. ($r = 0.46$).

There was also a general improvement, pronounced in one patient, substantial in three and slight in two. All patients had subjective relief and an increased sense of well-being after the initiation of pacemaker therapy. Syncopal symptoms did not occur after the start of artificial pacing. It should be pointed out, however, that in spite of the relative improvement observed, the rCBF values still remained subnormal postoperatively.

Obrist and Henry (1958) have shown that the alpha rhythm was significantly slower and the incidence of delta activity was greater in elderly patients (mean age 69 years) with cardiovascular diseases than in healthy subjects of the same age. One possibility would be that the insufficient circulation in the elderly patients had also damaged other organs such as the kidneys to some extent, and that the brain suffered secondarily because of metabolic disorders. A second and more probable explanation would be that the decrease of CBF and slowing of EEG was due to ischemic episodes during Adams–Stokes attacks. The third possibility, also quite real, is that the low perfusion pressure of the brain during extreme bradycardia could have caused the decreased CBF. Also a combination of different causative factors, including those mentioned above could have been responsible for the development of a chronic encephalopathy. Frequent Adam–Stokes attacks could have caused prolonged sequences of cerebral hypoxia with long-lasting effects on neuronal metabolism.

Following artificial pacing, an increase in heart rate and an improvement in cerebral hemodynamics probably takes place. At the same time, hypoxic attacks are avoided. The result is a successive improvement in CBF and neuronal metabolism, as well as in the EEG (Sulg et al., 1969; Lagergren, 1975).

qEEG in open-heart surgery

This study, initiated by the author (Sulg et al., 1977b) was performed at the University Hospital of Oulu (Finland). The risk of brain disorders arising during open-heart surgery has been established in a number of clinical and electroencephalographic studies. Despite recent advances in surgical techniques and devices for extracorporeal circulation, brain disorders are still reported to occur quite frequently. Attempts have been made to find some preoperative signs and tests of prognostic value, unfortunately without sufficient results. Guided by our previous neurological and neuropsycholog-ical studies (Sotaniemi et al., 1980), we considered it worthwhile to investigate the predictive usefulness of the EEG.

Sixty-five consecutive cardiac valvular replacement cases were investigated (age 15–65 years). An aortic valve operation was performed in 44 cases, mitral valve in 16 and multiple valve replacement was carried out in 5 cases. The patients were grouped according to their neurological outcome postoperatively: the cases showing no cere-bral complications ($N = 37$) and patients displaying cerebral complications ($N = 28$). The patients were investigated twice within the preoperative week and 5 times (10 days, 2,5,8 and 12 months) after surgery. All investigations included neurological examination and qEEG analysis was carried out using the previously described multi-variable analysis (Sulg, 1975). The EEG was recorded from the parieto-occipital and fronto-central regions. The preoperative incidence of an abnormal EEG was 49%. The presence of such a normal conventionally interpreted EEG was prognostically highly favorable.

The qEEG amplitude parameters did not show any statistically significant meaning for the prognosis. The frequency parameters had a greater prognostic weight, espe-cially the mean frequency derived from the FFT analysis. When this parameter (spec-tral mean frequency) was abnormally low (7 Hz) the incidence of postoperative clini-cal complications was doubled (60%) compared to cases with higher mean frequency values.

The combination of a low mean frequency (<8.5 Hz) together with a low alpha mean frequency (<9 Hz) was also unfavorable: hemispheric complications were observed in all the six such cases.

Presence of slow wave activity in the first postoperative EEG (recorded 10 days postoperatively) correlated clearly with the clinical findings: cerebral disorders were observed in nearly 80% of the corresponding 18 cases. The following postoperative qEEG changes proved to have the most significant correlation to a poor clinical outcome:

(1) Slowing of the FFT mean frequency by 2 Hz or more;
(2) Slowing of the alpha mean frequency by 1 Hz or more, and
(3) fall in percentage alpha activity by 30% or more.

The present results show that the EEG carries some prognostically predictive information. The observations indicate that both conventional and quantitative EEG can provide warning of impaired tolerance to exceptional stress as occurs during extracorporeal circulation, and that these prognostic signs should not be overlooked in preoperative patient evaluation.

qEEG in brain infarction

This study was performed in cooperation with U. Tolonen and E. Hokkanen, University Hospital, Oulu, Finland. The multiparameter EEG analysis program (Sulg et al., 1977a) was used for EEG quantification. The rCBF was measured by gamma camera immediately after intravenous injection of 133-Xenon (Kuikka et al., 1977). Twenty-two patients with unilateral supratentorial infarction were investigated.

The EEG mean frequency was determined by all four computer-techniques (com-pare section on Regional relationships between qEEG and rCBF, p. 72) and corres-ponding values showed significant or nearly significant correlations with the mean rCBF in the infarcted hemisphere; the highest correlation was found between the amount of delta activity and hemispheric mean flow (CBF_m): $r = 0.75$, $p < 0.001$. When using stepwise regression analysis, the first three qEEG variables with maximum preditive value for CBF were all from the power spectral density analysis. The correlation coefficients between the qEEG and regional fast compartmental flow were lower than those between the qEEG variables and the mean hemispheric CBF (Tolonen and Sulg, 1981).

qEEG in monitoring of anesthesia

The first part of this study was performed in cooperation with A. Hollmen, P. Eskelinen and E. Hokkanen at the University Hospital in Oulu. The project was later extended to involve university hospitals in Helsinki (Finland) and in Trondheim (Norway).

In general anesthesia there are potential risks for cerebral complications, especially in such complicated procedures as open-heart surgery. The anesthesio-surgical team has to keep the patient at an optimal level between sufficient analgesia/relaxation and deep anesthesia to minimize the stress for the patient and risk of cerebral hypoxia. Continuous monitoring of well-chosen vital variables is an invaluable help here. The outcome depends ultimately on the postoperative state of the brain.

In a pilot study, 20 patients were monitored during open-heart surgery for cardiac valve defects. The perfusion pressure was monitored parallel to mean frequency and mean amplitude of the EEG (Sulg et al., 1977b; Sotaniemi, 1980). These studies resulted in the following conclusions: signs of slight as well as profound hypoxia (as a result of falling blood pressure or insufficient oxygenation) are readily detectable by means of these two qEEG parameters (Figure 6). As long as there is a reciprocity between the trends of mean frequency and mean amplitude, there is no risk for the patient. A successive decrease in both trends, however, is a sign of dangerous progressive cerebral hypoxia. Because the effects of corrective measures and compensative treatment (e.g. increasing of perfusion pressure, etc.) are also reflected in the qEEG trends, these measures can be optimally guided. The work described above has led to the development of a new computerized device to monitor anesthesia and brain activity (Anesthesia and Brain Monitor, ABM) in high-risk anesthesia and intensive care situations (Sulg et al., 1982). This easily transportable device calculates at regular intervals two qEEG variables (mean frequency and mean amplitude). Because cerebral vessels and blood flow are influenced by pCO_2, and because this variable is of great importance during anesthesia, the end-tidal pCO_2 is also monitored parallel to the EEG. In addition, the EMG is monitored in one channel as the mean amplitude of spontaneous muscle activity (from any scalp muscle) and in another channel in terms of responses to serial stimuli to a peripheral nerve in order to check the effect of neuromuscular blocking agents. The reactivity and awareness of the patient are well reflected in spontaneous frontal muscle tension.

GENERAL DISCUSSION

The bulk of the information presented here concerns the physiological relationships between the EEG, CBF and cerebral metabolism. Although qEEG variables have not

78

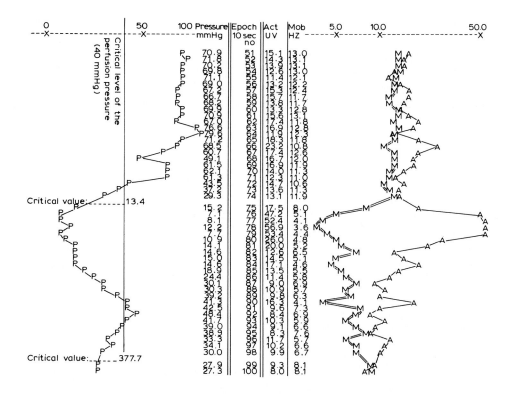

Fig. 6. Multiparameter monitoring during open-heart surgery. The computer delivers from consecutive 10-sec analysis epochs the following data, displayed on the line-printer along appropriate scales: (A) mean amplitude of the EEG, (M) mean frequency of the EEG (calculated as the mobility according to Hjorth), (P) mean perfusion pressure (= arterial blood pressure in a. subclavia minus pressure in vena cava superior), cumulative value of critical hypotension, i.e. the total time of perfusion pressure beneath 40 mm Hg, and consecutive numbers of analysis epochs. Within the actual sequence of monitoring a typical EEG reaction to hypotonic hypoxia is seen.

been correlated directly to cerebral metabolism, the qEEG parameters have shown significant correlations to other laboratory findings in uremic encephalopathy (Hagstam, 1971) and in hepatoportal encephalopathy (Rorsman and Sulg, 1970; Kardel and Stigsby, 1975). In 1976, Ingvar et al. showed that in a group of neurological patients, the mean frequency of manually analyzed EEGs had a highly significant correlation ($r = 0.78$, $p < 0.001$) to cerebral oxygen consumption.

Because the relationships between the EEG and CBF are complex, it was necessary to analyze these correlations with several statistical methods allowing different approaches to the task. The studies thus included advanced regression and correlation methods, as e.g. discriminative analysis for prediction of the CBF from the qEEG. The analysis of quantititative EEG profiles included a profile-clustering program especially designed for the present study.

Despite the heterogeneity of the patient material, we were able to demonstrate statistically highly significant correlations between qEEG and CBF except in conditions comparable to the luxury-perfusion syndrome. One of the main findings was the highly significant correlation between hemispheric mean averages of the EEG and

CBF for the fast flow component as well as for the noncompartmental flow. The discrepancy between high correlations for these mean values and the markedly lower significance levels in regional correlations may hypothetically be explained by the following consideration: the EEG generators in the brain, as well as the mechanisms controlling the hemispheric CBF, are more or less affected both in diffuse and in regional cerebral disorders. The brain generally tends to react as a whole to miscellaneous pathological noxae. There seem to be differences mainly in the degree but not in the mode of the reaction, i.e. a focal lesion in one part of the brain may cause similar although less pronounced distant effects within the same hemisphere, and often in the contralateral hemisphere as well. Very probably there are also quite close trends in EEG and CBF regionally, especially in early stage of lesions, but in the present studies this local interdependence was difficult to evaluate because of methodological limitations. Investigations were also performed at different stages of disease and on the basis of the present results we now know that the EEG/CBF interrelationships may vary, e.g. during an ischemic infarction. In a follow-up study of a patient with a focal ischemic hemispheric lesion, seven examinations in 20 months showed a profound dissociation of the EEG and CBF estimates in the subacute phase. In the chronic stage, however, there was a gradual return to covariance of the EEG mean frequency and rCBF within the focus. This usually is demonstrable 2–4 weeks after the onset of illness. It is essential to note that during a dissociation phase, caused by a posthypoxic tissue lactate acidosis combined with paralytic vasodilation, the severely disturbed tissue metabolism is also adequately reflected in the abnormal EEG pattern, whereas the autoregulative coupling of the CBF to tissue metabolism is lost. The present study thus confirms that in man the EEG/CBF dissociation is an essential phenomenon of the abnormal superperfusion or luxury-perfusion syndrome (Lassen, 1966; Freeman and Ingvar, 1968). Furthermore, because such an abnormal condition of the brain, especially when focal, cannot be diagnosed with a CBF measurement alone, the EEG/CBF dissociation by an abnormal EEG and "normal" or increased CBF indicates the presence of severe tissue damage. In clinical routine, the same conclusion can also be drawn from coexistence of a profound EEG abnormality and regionally increased flow, visualized by angiography. Does the EEG/CBF dissociation, when demonstrated, always indicate pathological changes in the brain tissue? The answer seems positive as far as conditions with the luxury-perfusion syndrome are concerned. There are, however, also some hemodynamic disturbances, where regional EEG/CBF covariance may not exist, e.g. in malformations of cerebral vessels, in arteriovenous shunts and in reactive cerebral hyperemia in an inflammatory process (e.g. encephalitis). There are also conditions where the EEG improves without any demonstrable increase in CBF, e.g. in postinfarction stages. Here the reversed dissociation of EEG/CBF is due to reparative, reconstructive and regenerative events in the recovering neuronal tissue, perhaps parallel to adaptation to a lower perfusion than before the infarction. In encephalitis, the initially protective EEG/CBF dissociation may as the disease progresses turn into a hypoxic decoupling between tissue metabolism and the CBF; but here as well the EEG still reflects in its progressive abnormal pattern the abnormal state of the brain. It has also been shown (by means of manual EEG analysis) that the autoregulation of the CBF can be eliminated by experimentally induced profound hypoxia (Freeman and Ingvar, 1968). The question then arises that if there are infarcted areas with entirely dissociated EEG/CBF, how can the overall correlation between corresponding estimates achieve such a high level of significance for hemispheric mean values, as we have demonstrated? The answer probably lies at least partly in the averaging effect of multi-regional CBF measurements, and partly in the remoteness of cerebral structures controlling the basic EEG frequency. In rCBF measurements with multiple extracranial detectors, usually only one or few of them will pick up the abnormal superflow around a focus, while the rest or most of other detectors record the distant flow decrease. Hemispheric mean values will thus be influenced to a limited degree by dissociative values, while most of the measured regions reflect the indirect reaction of the hemisphere involved. This reaction is usually also reflected in the background activity of the EEG.

There are probably subcortical structures that control rhythmic cortical activity. Several experimental studies have established the presence of these structures in the thalamus and reticular formation of the upper brain stem, which might influence intrinsic cortical rhythms. Furthermore, Garoutte and Aird (1958) have found evidence that both normal and abnormal EEG rhythms have a high degree of bilaterally homologous synchrony, except in focal abnormalities. This phenomenon has been explained by a central regulating pacemaker, which utilizes the diffuse and bilateral projection systems (Jasper 1949). This assumption appears to fit to some extent with the inhibitory phasing theory proposed by Andersen and Sears (1964). According to this theory, the basic EEG rhythm is generated by reverberating thalamocortical circuits that produce synchronized postsynaptic potentials in the cortical neurons.

Our main task, the statistical analysis of correlations between EEG and CBF, offered a unique opportunity to "rank" different qEEG estimates according to the degree to their relationship to the CBF. This was done mainly with stepwise regression analysis. Beginning with the primary data it was found, surprisingly, that the regression coefficients of EEG activity in single frequency classes varied considerably between nonsignificant and highly significant values within the frequency range of 1 to 20 Hz. In the material including focal lesions, the activity in the delta band, and especially the 2-Hz class, had the highest partial and multiple correlation coefficients. On the other hand, in cases without focal EEG abnormalities in the parieto-occipital regions, the higher frequencies in the alpha, theta and beta bands turned out to have the closest relationship to the mean CBF. This varying covariance throughout the EEG spectrum explains the strange finding that the qEEG/rCBF correlation coefficients produced the lowest values when the whole spectrum was taken into account. This conclusion, however, is valid at the present only for the frequency content derived from manual period analysis. Here the secondary polygon statistics, such as the mean, the median, and the skewness were found to have the highest correlation to the CBF. The mode frequency (corresponding to the peak or dominant frequency) also obtained statistically significant although somewhat lower values. The fact that the results from computerized analyses performed later (Tolonen and Sulg, 1981) resulted in somewhat different conclusions, points to the difference in the content of quantitative profiles: in the former, there are only summed periods of EEG waves, whereas in FFT spectra, the power density forms the profile. Interestingly, the mean or averaged frequency tends to keep its prime position as the "best" predictor of CBF even in data derived from FFT techniques as well as from computerized period and amplitude analysis. Its use, together with mean amplitude, for brain monitoring in high-risk conditions therefore seems to be justified.

The significance of the age of our patients stands out clearly in all statistical relationships. In evaluation of qEEG/CBF/age relationships, applying the stepwise regression model, the age factor was given the first rank of significance. The age factor also had some unexpected influence on the "ranking" order of other qEEG estimates when this procedure was performed with or without the age factor within the regression equation.

In patients with ischemic or other focal lesions, EEG and CBF measurements more or less reflect the regional changes on the tissue level. In patients with atrioventricular block and/or valvular defects, other etiological factors are involved, such as hemodynamic events in systemic circulation. In heart-block patients, the main finding was the fact that the CBF decreased and EEG slowed without any significant decrease in blood pressure or in cardiac output. Here the question arises: what is the real cause and order of causative pathological events in the brain? Could the primary etiology be the slowness and irregularity in the pulse flow? This affects not only the blood flow, but also pulse-synchronous neuronal impulses from the baroreceptors into the brainstem structures. Could this nonphysiological irregularity of neuronal inflow via vasomotoric centers in the medulla oblongata have secondary influences not only on wakefulness, but also diffusely within the brain, mediated possibly by the reticular formation? This question cannot in any case be more than a vague hypothesis. More realistic, however, is the assumption that a combination of different causative factors is responsible for the encephalopathy.

Frequent syncopal-convulsive attacks could cause prolonged brain hypoxia, accompanied by stepwise disintegration and exhaustion of physiological autoregulation. If this vicious circle is then broken by artificial pacing, the hemodynamic abnormalities and other secondary symptoms including encephalopathy will decline and perhaps disappear slowly in the reverse order. This study also confirmed the observation by others that a certain adaptation time may be needed for cerebral circulation and metabolism, before the brain achieves the full benefit of the normalized hemodynamic conditions.

CONCLUSIONS

We have learned from this work that the EEG is really a paraphenomenon of cerebral metabolism. It cannot, however, be used to measure the metabolic rate of the brain, although this is more or less directly reflected in the EEG. Thus the EEG as well as the CBF are physiologically coupled to brain metabolism, but there is no direct coupling between flow and EEG. The CBF is indirectly reflected in the EEG as long as there is physiological autoregulation of the CBF. In pathological hyperperfusion (the luxury-perfusion syndrome), the EEG and flow are dissociated, but even then the pathological state of the brain is still reflected in the EEG. There is, however, also an EEG/CBF dissociation in physiological conditions, i.e. the EEG does not reflect closely those shifts in the CBF that are the result of activation of higher cortical functions (Stigsby et al., 1977). Therefore the EEG is not a perfect tool for measurement of normal functions, but it is an excellent measure, especially when quantified, of brain dysfunction.

SUMMARY

This study has once again confirmed the existence of close relationships between the EEG, cerebral blood flow and metabolism. Furthermore, the results of elaborate statistical analysis of these relationships have uncovered the important fact that the primary qEEG data do not always represent the best possible prediction of the CBF. By means of some few secondary statistical measures, such as the mean frequency, the skewness of the spectral distribution, etc., more reliable predictions of the CBF can be obtained from EEG parameters. This fact has been demonstrated in several studies in which the author was involved. Although there are within certain limits significant correlations between the EEG and the CBF, the coupling between EEG and cerebral metabolism is closer than between EEG and CBF. The EEG as well as the CBF are coupled to brain metabolism, but there is no direct coupling between flow and EEG. In ischemic conditions the EEG and CBF can be dissociated, but even then the pathological state of the brain is reflected in the EEG. There is also an EEG/CBF dissociation in physiological conditions: the EEG does not reflect closely the increase of CBF by activation of higher cortical functions. Therefore the EEG is not a perfect tool for measurement of normal brain function, but it is an excellent measure (especially when quantified) of brain dysfunction. The remarkably high statistical age-rCBF correlations demonstrated in the present study indicate that aging may have a complex influence on the cerebral state. Age seems to be an important factor in the interdependence of the EEG, rCBF and probably also in the cerebral oxygen uptake. Thus the results of the present study confirm earlier findings regarding the essential role of age when evaluating EEG in senescence.

REFERENCES

Ahonen, A., Tolonen, U., and Kuikka, J. (1979) Cerebral blood flow, transfer time and volume in patients with cerebral hemispheric infarction. *Acta neurol. scand.* 60, (Suppl. 72): 60–61.

Andersen, P. and Sears, W. (1964) Inhibitory phasing theory. *J. Physiol.*, 1973: 459–480.

Blackman, R. B. and Tukey, J. W. (1958) *The Measurement of Power Spectra from the Point of View of Communications Engineering*, Power Publications, Inc., New York.

Burch, N. R., Nettleton, W. J., Sweeney, J. and Edwards, R. J. (1964) Period analysis of the electroencephalogram on a general purpose digital computer. *Ann. N. Y. acad. Sci.*, 115: 827–843.

Dumermuth, G. and Fluehler, H. (1967) Some modern aspects in numerical spectrum analysis of multichannel electroencephalographic data. *Med. biol. Eng.*, 5: 319–331.

Freeman, J. and Ingvar, D. H. (1968) Elimination by hypoxia of cerebral blood flow autoregulation and EEG relationship. *Exp. Brain Res.*, 5: 61–71.

Garoutte, B. and Aird, R. B. (1958) Studies on the cortical pacemaker: Synchrony and asynchrony of bilaterally recorded alpha and beta activity. *Electroenceph. clin. Neurophysiol.*, 10: 259–268.

Hagstam, K. E. (1971) EEG frequency content related to chemical blood parameters in chronic uremia. *Scand. J. Urol. Nephrol.*, Suppl. 7: 1–56.

Hjorth, B. (1973) The physical significance of time domain descriptors in EEG analysis. *Electroenceph. clin. Neurophysiol.*, 34: 321–325.

Ingvar, D. H. and Sulg, I. A. (1969) Regional cerebral blood flow and EEG frequency content in man. *Scand. J. clin. Invest.*, 23, Suppl. 109: 47–66.

Ingvar, D. H., Sjölund, B. and Ardö, A. (1976) Correlation between dominant EEG-frequency, cerebral oxygen uptake and blood flow. *Electroenceph. clin. Neurophysiol.*, 41: 268–276.

Jasper, H. H. (1949) Diffuse projection systems: the integrative action of the thalamic reticular system. *Electroenceph. clin. Neurophysiol.*, 1: 405–420.

Kaiser, E. and Petersén, I. (1966) Automatic analysis in EEG. 1. Tape computer system for special analysis. 2. Reverse correlation. *Acta neurol. scand.*, 42, Suppl. 22: 1–38.

Kardel, T. and Stigsby, B. (1975) Period-amplitude analysis of the electroencephalogram correlated with liver function in patients with cirrhosis of the liver. *Electroenceph. clin. Neurophysiol.*, 38: 605–609.

Kety, S. S. and Schmidt, C. F. (1948) The nitrous oxide method for the quantitative determination of cerebral blood flow in man; theory, procedure and normal values. *J. clin. Invest.*, 27: 476–481.

Kuikka, J., Ahonen, A., Koivula, A., Kallanranta, T. and Laitinen, J. (1977) An intravenous isotope method for measuring regional cerebral blood flow and volume. *Phys. in Med. Biol.*, 22: 958–970.

Lagergren, K. (1975) *Perceptual and psychomotor performance in pacemaker patients: Influences of heart rate, posture and 2-oxi-pyrrolidinone-1-acetamide (Piracetam)*, Dept of Psychiatry, Karolinska Hospital, Stockholm (thesis).

Lassen, N. A. (1966) The luxury perfusion syndrome and its possible relation to acute metabolic acidosis localised within the brain. *Lancet*, 11: 1113–1115.

Lassen, N. A. and Munck, O. (1955) The cerebral blood flow in man determined by the use of radioactive Krypton. *Acta physiol. scand.*, 33: 30–49.

Lassen, N. A. and Ingvar, D. H. (1961) The blood flow of the cerebral cortex determined by radioactive [85] Krypton. *Experientia (Basel)*, 17: 42–43.

Mallet, B. L. and Veall, N. (1965) The measurement of regional cerebral clearance rates in man using Xenon-133 inhalation and extracranial recording. *Clin. Sci.*, 29: 179–191.

Obrist, W. D. and Henry, C. E. (1958) Electroencephalographic frequency analysis of aged psychiatric patients. *Electroenceph. clin. Neurophysiol.*, 10, 4: 621–632.

Obrist, W. D., Thompson, H. K., Wang, H. S. and Wilkinson, W. E. (1975) Regional cerebral blood flow estimated by [133]Xenon inhalation. *Stroke*, 6: 245–256.

Pfurtscheller, G. and Haring G. (1972) The use of an EEG autoregressive model for the time-saving calculation of spectral power density distribution with a digital computer. *Electroenceph. clin. Neurophysiol.*, 33: 113–115.

Rorsman, G. and Sulg, I. A. (1970) Lactulose treatment of chronic hepatoportal encephalopathy. *Acta med. Scand.*, 187: 337–346.

Sotaniemi, K. A. (1980) Cerebral disorders in open-heart surgery patients. A neurological, electroencephalographical and neuropsychological follow-up study. Thesis. *Acta Universit. Oulu (Finland) Serie D, No 56*.

Sotaniemi, K. A., Sulg, I. A. and Hokkanen, T. E. (1980) Quantitative EEG as a measure of cerebral dysfunction before and after open-heart surgery. *Electroenceph. clin. Neurophysiol.*, 50: 81–95.

Stigsby, B., Obrist, W. D. and Sulg, I. A. (1973) Automatic data acquisition and period-amplitude analysis of the EEG. *Computer Progr. Biomed.*, 3: 93–104.

Stigsby, B., Risberg, J. and Ingvar, D. H. (1977) EEG changes in the dominant hemisphere during memorizing and reasoning. *Electroenceph. clin. Neurophysiol.*, 42: 665–675.

Sulg, I. A. (1969a) Manual EEG analysis. *Acta neurol. scand.*, 45: 431–458.

Sulg, I. A. (1969b) The quantitated EEG as a measure of brain dysfunction. *Scand. J. clin. Invest.*, 23, Suppl. 109: 110.

Sulg, I. A. and Ingvar, D. H. (1968) Regional cerebral blood flow and EEG in occlusion of the middle cerebral artery. *Scand. J. clin. Lab. Invest.*, Suppl. 102: 16:d.

Sulg I. A. (1975) The quantitated EEG as a measure of brain dysfunction. In M. Matejcek and G. Schenk (Eds.), *Quantitative Analysis of the EEG*, AEG Telefunken, Konstanz, pp. 509–520.

Sulg, I. A., Cronqvist, S., Schüller, H. and Ingvar, D. H. (1969) The effect of intracardiac pacemaker therapy on cerebral blood flow and electroencephalogram in patients with complete atrioventricular block. *Circulation*, 39: 487–494.

Sulg, I. A., Hokkanen, T. E., von Post, B. and Reunanen, M. (1977a) Computerized quantitative multiparameter analysis of the EEG. In F. Sicuteri (Ed.), *Headache: New Vistas*, Biomedical Press, Florence, pp. 213–224.

Sulg, I. A., Hokkanen, T. E. and Hollmén, A. I. (1977b) Simultaneous monitoring of perfusion pressure and quantitative EEG in anesthesia and in other conditions with risk for hypoxia. In W. A. den Hartog-Jager, G. W. Bruyn and A. P. J. Heystee (Eds.), *11th World Congress of Neurology*, Excerpta Medica, Amsterdam, p. 152.

Sulg, I. A., Sotaniemi, K. A., Tolonen, U. and Hokkanen, E. (1981) Dependence between cerebral metabolism and blood flow as reflected in the quantitative EEG. In J. Mendlewicz and H. M. van Praag (Eds.), *Advanc. biol. Psychiat. Vol. 6*, Karger, Basel, pp. 102–108.

Sulg, I. A., Hollmén, A. I., Tammisto, T. and Hokkanen, E. T. (1982) Quantitative neuro-monitoring in intensive care and in anesthesia. *Internat. Congress Series No 612, Advances in Neurotraumatology*, Excerpta Medica: 235–237.

Tolonen, U. (1981) Cerebral infarction in man, studied by quantitative isotope and EEG methods. Thesis. Acta Universit. Oulu (Finland) serie D, No 68.

Tolonen, U. and Sulg, I. A. (1981) Comparison of quantitative EEG parameters from four different analysis techniques in evaluation of relationships between EEG and CBF in brain infarction. *EEG clin. Neurophysiol.*, 51: 177–185.

Walter, D. O. and Brazier, A. B. (1968) Advances in EEG analysis. *Electroenceph. clin. Neurophysiol.*, Suppl. 27: 105–109.

Zetterberg, L. H. (1969) Estimation of parameters for a linear difference equation with application to EEG analysis. *Math. Biosci.*, 5: 227–275.

Brain Ischemia: Quantitative EEG and Imaging Techniques, Progress in Brain Research, Vol. 62, edited by
G. Pfurtscheller, E.J. Jonkman and F.H. Lopes da Silva

Limitations of EEG Frequency Analysis in the Diagnosis of Intracerebral Diseases

G. MIES, G. HOPPE and K.-A. HOSSMANN

Max-Planck-Institut für Neurologische Forschung, Ostmerheimer Str. 200, D-5000 Köln 91 (F.R.G.)

INTRODUCTION

With the discovery by Berger (1934) of electrical brain activity in man and the subsequent technical improvement of recording devices, visual EEG evaluation has become a valuable clinical tool in the detection of EEG abnormalities. Traditionally, such abnormalities are deviations in voltage and frequency from normal electrical brain activity. When the electrodes are distributed topographically (10–20 system) over the skull, localization of pathological EEG abnormalities is possible. Computer-supported quantitative EEG (qEEG) frequency analysis has been developed in parallel with visual EEG evaluation, providing a more objective approach in the assessment of EEG alterations. The criteria chosen as signs of such alterations are changes in the total intensity of the signal or in the percentage decreases/increases in the conventional frequency bands (Gotman et al., 1973). The topography of the EEG focus can be presented with the 10–20 system familiar to most encephalographers.

This study was intended to determine whether abnormal EEG findings obtained by qEEG frequency analysis are necessarily related to the pathology of brain lesions. Quantitative EEG frequency analyses were made under experimental conditions of acute focal ischemia and experimentally induced brain tumors in various animals. In order to characterize significant features of the pathological EEG, other parameters such as blood flow, electrolyte homeostasis and water content of the brain were also measured in the same animals. Should a specific relationship between EEG alterations and such parameters exist, this may well prove to be applicable to the pathognomonic differentiation of human cerebral brain lesions. To this end, we have also examined EEG using qEEG analysis in patients suffering from cerebrovascular disease, brain tumors, intracerebral hemorrhage and head trauma.

MATERIAL AND METHODS

Experimental studies

The following models of focal ischemia and experimentally induced brain tumors were investigated.

Graded focal ischemia of the gerbil brain

The Mongolian gerbil (*Meriones unguiculatus*) possesses the unique feature of an incomplete circle of Willis. The occlusion of the common carotid artery on one side reduces arterial blood supply to the brain to such an extent that severe neurological deficits (hemiparesis, rolling seizures) are observed in one-third of the animals (symptom–positive gerbils), indicating brain infarction (Levine and Payan, 1966; Kahn, 1972). In the remaining two-thirds of the gerbils no neurological symptoms are detectable (symptom–negative gerbils).

Experimental procedures. In 124 gerbils, the left common carotid artery was exposed under 1.2% halothane (O_2:N_2/30% : 70%) anesthesia. Animals were placed in a stereotaxic frame, the skull was exposed and two pairs of silver-ball EEG electrodes were positioned to record the bipolar EEG from both hemispheres throughout the total period of investigation. The EEG was stored in an Ampex recorder for subsequent offline EEG frequency analysis (see below). After 90 min, anesthesia was discontinued in one group of animals, which was allowed to recover in order to assess any neurological symptoms. After a further 30 min, animals were sacrificed and the brains removed to determine the electrolyte and water content. In the other group of gerbils, polyethylene catheters were inserted into both femoral arteries and veins to monitor blood pressure and permit the administration of drugs or tracers and the withdrawal of arterial blood. All animals respired spontaneously. The body temperature was maintained at 37° with an infrared lamp. In this group of gerbils, cerebral blood flow was measured 30, 60, 90 and 120 min following carotid artery occlusion as described by Reivich et al. (1969). Sham-operated controls were maintained under identical experimental conditions.

Experimental qEEG frequency analysis. EEG amplifiers and the tape recorder were calibrated by applying sinus-wave signals to each channel and performing subsequent EEG frequency analysis. The EEG was digitalized off-line at 64 Hz using a Fast Fourier Transform for 4-sec epochs that were averaged four times (PDP 12, Digital, Maynard, U.S.A.). Possible changes in EEG amplitude can be linearized by calculating the square roots of the spectral power Fourier coefficients. The intensity of each frequency band was expressed as the percentage of total power with the following frequency ranges: delta band 1–3.75 Hz, theta band 4–7.5 Hz, alpha band 7.75–12.75 Hz and beta band 13–20 Hz. In addition, the frequency index was calculated by dividing the alpha plus beta by delta plus theta power.

Measurement of brain electrolyte and water content. The brains were dissected into hemispheres. After determination of the wet weight, the tissue was dried to constant weight at 105°C. Each hemisphere was then homogenized in a mortar and electrolytes were wet-extracted with 0.75 M HNO_3. Sodium and potassium concentrations in the supernatant were measured by flame photometry (Zimmermann and Hossmann, 1975).

Determination of cerebral blood flow. 30 μCi [^{14}C]antipyrine dissolved in 0.5 ml Ringer solution were infused intravenously over a period of 1 min. Simultaneously, arterial blood was sampled into preweighed vials every 10 sec. Systemic circulation was arrested by i.v. injection of saturated KCl solution; the brains were removed rapidly and frozen in methyl butane at -70°C for subsequent cryostat brain sectioning. The reweighed arterial blood samples were bleached with 0.3 ml 30% H_2O_2 and ^{14}C-radioactivity was measured after adding 10 ml scintillator (Quickszint, Zinser, Frankfurt, F.R.G.). After correcting for quenching and converting blood weight to blood volume (taking the density $p = 1.06$), the ^{14}C-concentration was expressed as nCi/ml of arterial blood.

Quantitative autoradiography. Quantitative autoradiography was used to measure the ^{14}C-concentration in brain tissue. Brains were cut into 20-μm slices at $-20°$C using a cryostat; the slices were then placed in an X-ray cassette together with ^{14}C-standards of known ^{14}C-concentration and exposed to a Kodak SB film for 4 days. Autoradiographic images were obtained from each slice together with the different ^{14}C-standards. A calibration curve of optical density and ^{14}C-concentration was plotted for the standards; thereafter, measurements of extinction of each brain slice autoradiogram permitted the corresponding ^{14}C-concentration to be determined.

Calculation of cerebral blood flow. Local cerebral blood flow was calculated according to the equation given by Reivich et al. (1969):

$$C_B = \lambda \cdot K \cdot \int_O^T C_a \cdot e^{-K\,(T-t)}\, dt\,,$$

where C_B is the local [^{14}C]antipyrine concentration in the tissue (determined by quantitative autoradiography); C_a is the arterial blood ^{14}C-concentration; λ is the blood-brain partition coefficient (for [^{14}C]antipyrine: $\lambda = 1$). K represents the blood flow per unit tissue mass weighted for λ.

Graded focal ischemia of the cat brain

A well-established method of studying focal ischemia is to occlude the middle cerebral artery (MCA) via the transorbital approach (Hudgins and Garcia, 1970) using the modification described by O'Brien and Waltz (1979) for cats.

Experimental procedure. Forty-eight cats were anesthetized by intraperitoneal injection of 30 mg/kg pentobarbital. After insertion of polyethylene catheters into both femoral arteries and veins, the animals were tracheotomized, immobilized with gallamine triethiodide and mechanically ventilated with room air to give an arterial pCO_2 of about 30 mm Hg. The EEG was recorded from both hemispheres using silver-ball electrodes positioned parietally over the territories of the MCA. Recording and evaluation of the EEG were performed as described above.

To expose the left MCA, the eyeball was removed and the optical foramen enlarged. After separation of dura and arachnoid membranes, the MCA was occluded with a Mayfield aneurysm clip.

Measurement of cerebral blood flow. Repeated blood-flow measurements were performed by the intracardiac microsphere injection technique (Rudolph and Heymann, 1967), usually 15 min before and 15 min after onset of ischemia and 1, 2 or 4 h following MCA occlusion. The diameter of the microspheres injected was 15 ± 5 micron; these were labeled with ^{141}Ce, ^{113}Zn or ^{46}Sc. At the time of injection, an arterial reference sample was withdrawn at a known constant speed. Blood and tissue radioactivity was measured using a three-channel gamma counter (Biogamma II, Beckman, Fullerton, U.S.A.).

Calculation of cerebral blood flow. Regional cerebral blood flow using the radioactive microsphere injection method was calculated according to the formula

$$\text{rCBF} = \frac{R_t \times F_b \times 100}{W_t \times R_b} \qquad \text{ml/100 g/min,}$$

where R_t is the tissue radioactivity, W_t the tissue weight, R_b the radioactivity in blood and F_b the flow rate of the reference blood sample (Rudolph and Heymann, 1967).

Experimentally induced brain tumors in cats

Details of this cat tumor model have been described elsewhere (Hossmann et al., 1979). Briefly, intracerebral tumors were produced by stereotaxic xenotransplantation of 4×10^6 cloned rat glioma cells (RG2) into the right internal capsule of the brain. Brain tumors with a diameter of 0.5 to 1 cm developed within 1 to 3 weeks.

The experimental procedure, blood flow measurements, qEEG frequency analysis and determination of electrolyte and water content were as described above.

Clinical studies

Clinical qEEG frequency analysis

qEEG frequency analysis was performed on routine EEGs to allow a direct comparison between computer-assisted parametric description of the EEG and visual EEG evaluation. The bipolar EEG was recorded with the conventional 10–20 electrode set-up. Nine different montages of eight channels were hard-copied on an electroencephalograph (Schwarzer, München, F.R.G.) and the EEG was stored simultaneously on magnetic tape (Meditape, Siemens, Erlangen, F.R.G.). In order to restrict EEG computer analysis to artifact-free EEG sections of 16 sec duration, the start of such periods was marked on tape with a trigger signal; this enabled the computer program to identify the beginning of frequency analysis recorded from each derivation. EEG frequency analysis was performed off-line on eight channels simultaneously for each of the nine montages. EEG data was reduced as described in the experimental section.

The EEG was presented topographically, achieved by referring each measured parameter to one of the corresponding 19 EEG electrodes involved in the nine different derivations. The average value of the various EEG parameters for each electrode was used to calculate the interhemispheric difference. The computer printout of regional side deviations for the percentage changes in delta, theta, alpha, and beta bands as well as the frequency index was adapted to the 10–20 electrode system and represents the average hemispheric differences on EEG recordings over a period of 2.4 min. The conventional display of the computer-assessed EEG parameters permitted adequate comparison with visual EEG evaluation as regards the localization and the main frequency of the EEG focus (Hossmann et al., 1980).

The criteria taken for the identification of an EEG focus were a unilateral decrease in the frequency index of more than 10% and, in addition, a 10% interhemispheric difference for any one of the conventional frequency bands. The EEG records obtained using qEEG computer frequency analysis were grouped as follows for each class of cerebral disease:
- according to the maximum of slow wave activity, regardless of alterations in the fast frequency bands;
- according to the pattern of intensity changes in all four frequency bands.

Clinical diagnosis of patients with cerebral disease

Quantitative EEG analysis was evaluated in patients with focal ischemia ($n = 67$; mean age $\pm$ S.D.: 65.5 $\pm$ 7.1), intracerebral hemorrhage ($n = 9$; 60.4 $\pm$ 13.2), brain tumors ($n = 46$; 49.8 ± 13.7) and head trauma ($n = 10$; 55.2 ± 17.0). Ischemic disorders were examined in the Neurological Department (by courtesy of Prof. Heiss) within 48 h after onset of stroke. Cerebral angiography revealed that focal ischemia was due to stenosis or occlusion of one internal carotid ($n = 30$; 61.0 ± 10.3) or an intracranial artery ($n = 34$; 60.0 ± 13.1) or of cardiac orgin ($n = 3$; 74.7 ± 5.1). Morphological changes were later verified by computer tomography. Cases of intracranial hemorrhage consisted of patients with subarachnoidal and mass bleeding, which was visualized in CT scan. Brain scintigraphy, angiography and CT scans were employed to confirm the diagnosis of an intracranial brain tumor.

RESULTS

Experimental studies

Graded focal ischemia of the gerbil brain

The results obtained by qEEG frequency analysis are summarized in Fig. 1. In animals exhibiting neurological signs of brain infarction, the total intensity decreased by about 80% in the corresponding hemisphere. The frequency index was reduced by more than 41% and revealed a drastic elevation of slow-wave components and additional loss of alpha and beta intensities. In contrast, a gradual increase in total power

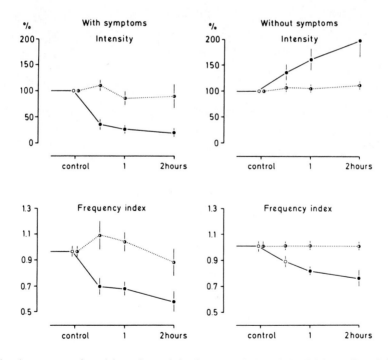

Fig. 1. The time course of total intensity and the frequency index of the EEG in affected (o—o) and unaffected (●....●) hemisphere is shown after common carotid artery occlusion in gerbils. Animals with symptoms showed a drastic reduction in EEG amplitude and frequency index. In gerbils exhibiting no symptoms, 2 h after carotid artery occlusion EEG amplitude doubled concomitant with a significant decrease in the frequency index.

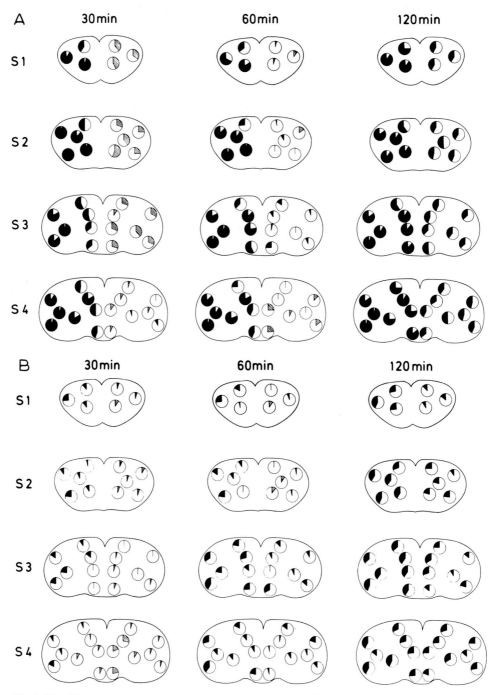

Fig. 2. Blood flow changes as percentage of controls are summarized 30, 60 and 120 min after left common carotid artery occlusion in gerbils for four different coronal levels (S1–S4). A: In symptom–positive gerbils, blood flow is drastically reduced in the affected hemisphere. The area of hypoperfusion enlarges throughout the experimental period. B: In symptom–negative gerbils, blood flow gradually declines over a period of 2 h to about 50% of control. In both experimental groups, perfusion in the contralateral hemisphere was affected to a varying extent. Symbols: ◐ 25% blood flow decrease; ◑ 25% blood flow increase.

was observed in symptom–negative gerbils over a period of 2 h following common carotid artery occlusion. One and two hours later, there was a significant and consistent slowing of the ipsilateral EEG as indicated by the frequency index.

The blood flow changes as percentage of control flow are illustrated in four different coronal brain sections (Fig. 2A, B). In symptom–positive animals, cerebral perfusion in the left hemisphere was drastically reduced in the parieto-temporal cortex, caudate putamen and thalamus (Fig. 2A). The area of hypoperfusion progressed toward the midline within 2 h and the initial hyperemia in the contralateral hemisphere was followed by a 50% reduction in blood flow. In symptom–negative gerbils (Fig. 2B), there was only a slight reduction in blood flow in the left hemisphere 30 min after carotid artery occlusion but thereafter it decreased gradually to about 50% of the control value at 2 h ($p<0.05$). Interestingly, at this time cerebral blood flow in the contralateral hemisphere was significantly reduced by about 25%.

The results for brain tissue electrolyte and water content are summarized in Table I. No changes in sodium, potassium or water content as compared to control values in symptom–negative animals could be detected. In symptom–positive gerbils, however, ipsilateral focal ischemia was severe enough to produce a significant rise in sodium and water content at 2 h concomitant with tissue potassium loss; this was also evident from the rise in the Na/K quotient.

TABLE I

ELECTROLYTE DISTURBANCES OF GERBIL BRAIN 2 H AFTER LEFT COMMON CAROTID ARTERY OCCLUSION

	Left hemisphere				Right hemisphere			
	Na^+	K^+	H_2O	Na/K	Na^+	K^+	H_2O	Na/K
	(mEq/kg d.w.)		(%)		(mEq/kg d.w.)		(%)	
Control	202.9	484.7	78.4	0.42	209.1	484.8	78.5	0.42
(n = 9)	± 1.3	± 3.4	± 0.1	± 0.01	± 1.3	− 3.3	± 0.1	± 0.01
Without symptoms	211.6	478.0	78.6	0.44	208.2	477.9	78.5	0.44
(n = 15)	± 3.8	± 9.6	± 0.1	± 0.11	± 2.2	± 14.6	± 0.1	− 0.02
With symptoms	263.9***	443.9***	79.7***	0.59***	200.9	502.4*	78.5	0.40
(n = 11)	± 4.2	± 7.4	± 0.2	± 0.01	± 3.4	± 3.7	± 0.2	± 0.01

All values are given as mean ± S.E.M., statistical differences between experimental control groups are marked with *$p < 0.01$, ***$p < 0.001$; n is the number of animals in each group; d.w. is the dry weight of brain tissue.

A significant linear correlation was found between cortical blood flow and the percentage of delta plus theta activity taken from all animals after occlusion of the common carotid artery (Fig. 3; $r = -0.6484$; $p<0.001$). However, both groups of animals differed in their changes in total power after onset of graded focal ischemia; whereas in symptom–negative gerbils the total intensity gradually increased as cortical perfusion declined, symptom–positive animals showed suppression of EEG amplitude with reduced blood flow (Fig. 4).

92

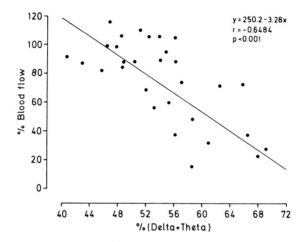

Fig. 3. Relationship between delta plus theta activity as the percentage of total power and blood flow (% of control) following common carotid artery occlusion in gerbils; this reveals a significant correlation between the increase in low-frequency activity and reduction in blood flow

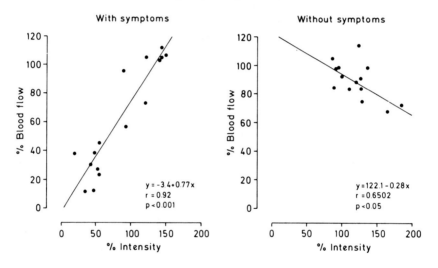

Fig. 4. Total EEG intensity in relation to blood flow (% of control) following common carotid artery occlusion in gerbils. In animals with symptoms, a suppression of EEG amplitude is observed together with a decrease in blood flow; symptom–negative animals showed a rise in EEG intensity at reduced blood flow values.

Correlation between EEG changes and changes in water and ion content were more difficult to establish; there was no significant relationship between either EEG intensity or EEG frequency index and any of the measured parameters. Only the calculated idiogenic osmotic activity of brain tissue appeared to influence the intensity in the delta band of the EEG (Fig. 5). This activity was calculated from the relative loss of tissue cations observed under conditions of focal ischemia assuming that total tissue osmolality did not change. Since idiogenic osmols are generated in part by catabolic waste products, slowing of the EEG presumably correlated with the metabolic disturbance rather than with changes in ion content.

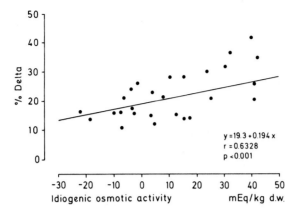

Fig. 5. Idiogenic osmotic activity (sodium deficit or cation surplus) was plotted against percentage of delta activity after common carotid artery occlusion in gerbils. Replacement of sodium cations by unknown osmoactive compounds is associated with metabolic disturbance of brain tissue and a tendency to slow-wave generation.

Graded focal ischemia of the cat brain

In cats, transorbital occlusion of the middle cerebral artery resulted in different degrees of ischemia. As shown in Figure 6, a wide range of flow values was recorded in the center of the MCA territory; this led to differences in the alterations of ion and water homeostasis. When flow remained above 15 ml/100 g/min, the sodium/potassium ratio in the cerebral cortex did not change (non-critical ischemia) but below 15 ml/100 g/min there was a severe disturbance of ion homeostatis (critical ischemia).

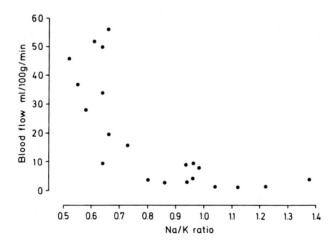

Fig. 6. Relationship between the Na/K ratio and blood flow in cerebral cortex of the cat after MCA occlusion. Electrolyte homeostasis was not disturbed above a flow value of about 15 ml/100 g/min (noncritical ischemia). Below that flow threshold, however, derangement of tissue electrolyte content was evident as indicated by the increase in Na/K ratios. (Modified from Hossmann and Schuier, 1980.)

94

EEG changes in cases of critical and non-critical ischemia also differed, although to a lesser extent than in gerbils both with and without neurological symptoms. In both critical and non-critical ischemia, EEG intensity initially decreased but there was a gradual normalization within 2 h in those animals with higher blood flow (Fig. 7). Interestingly, the EEG frequency index decreased only in animals with non-critical ischemia. If this change is an electrophysiological symptom of a partial ischemia, the absence of slow-wave activity in the animals with critical ischemia could be explained by total electrical silence in the more severely affected brain. This interpretation is also supported by the fact that blood flow correlated with EEG intensity but not with the EEG frequency index (Fig. 8).

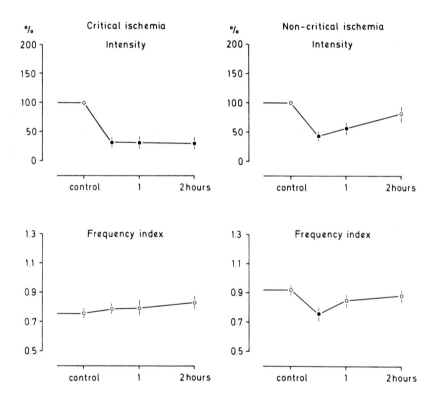

Fig. 7. Time course of EEG changes after MCA occlusion in cats. In both groups (critical or noncritical ischemia), EEG suppression is the most predominant characteristic in the case of hypoperfusion but it recovers in noncritical ischemia. The changes in frequency index are only transiently detectable, if at all. (Modified from Hossmann and Schuier, 1980.)

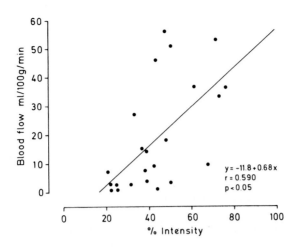

Fig. 8. Relationship between total power and blood flow in cerebral cortex after MCA occlusion in cats. In contrast to gerbils without symptoms, a reduction of blood flow in cats is accompanied by a decline in total power of the recorded EEG.

Power spectra

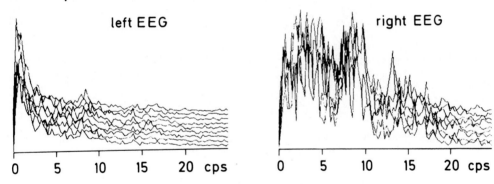

Fig. 9. EEG power spectra recorded from a tumor-bearing cat exhibiting pronounced slowing of the EEG over the affected left hemisphere. (From Hossmann et al., 1979.)

Experimental brain tumors in cats

A typical result of qEEG frequency analysis after 3 weeks of tumor growth is given in Fig. 9. In 5 out of 13 tumor-bearing animals, there was an increase in low-frequency amplitude restricted to the affected hemisphere. EEG changes were not, however, found to correlate with the electrolyte and water content of brain tissue, the size of the brain tumor or the blood flow in white and grey matter adjacent to the tumor (Fig. 10; Hossmann et al., 1979).

96

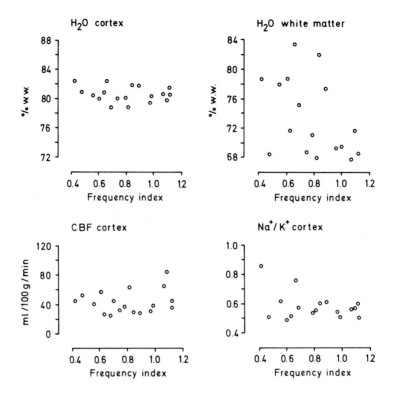

Fig. 10. No correlations were found between the frequency index of the EEG and blood flow, electrolyte or water content in experimental brain tumors in cats.

Clinical qEEG frequency analysis

A topographical display of lateral EEG differences in the conventional frequency bands and the frequency index is shown in a patient suffering from acute focal ischemia (Fig. 11). Table II demonstrates the incidence of delta and/or theta focus in various clinical conditions. The incidence is about 70% in patients with brain tumors and intracranial hemorrhage, but such foci are observed less often in brain infarcts and head trauma. To evaluate the possible contribution of other frequency band changes, EEGs were grouped according to the frequency pattern (Table III). With this classification, an EEG focus consistent with a decrease in alpha plus beta activity at elevated intensities of delta and/or theta band could be detected in 55.2% of patients suffering from brain infarction, in 70% of patients with head trauma, but only in 34.9% of brain tumor cases. On the other hand, in brain infarction only 24% of patients exhibited a concomitant increase in alpha and/or beta activity, indicating that the preferential manifestation of an EEG focus in cerebrovascular disease is represented by the increase in slow wave and the simultaneous decrease in fast wave activity.

Middle cerebral artery occlusion

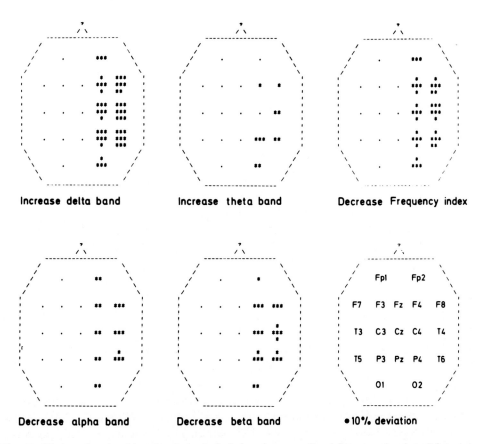

Fig. 11. Display of regional interhemispheric deviations in conventional frequency bands and frequency index obtained from clinical qEEG frequency analysis. The EEG was derived from a patient suffering from acute brain infarction. (From Hossmann et al., 1980.)

TABLE II

INCIDENCE OF DELTA AND/OR THETA FOCUS IN
PATIENTS WITH UNILATERAL HEMISPHERIC LESIONS

Disease	Incidence of slow wave focus (%)
Infarction n = 67	35.8
Hemorrhage n = 9	66.7
Tumors n = 46	71.7
Head trauma n = 10	20.0

TABLE III

PATTERN OF qEEG CHANGES IN PATIENTS WITH UNILATERAL HEMISPHERIC LESIONS

Disease	Frequency pattern						
	↑↑↓↓ (%)	↑↓↓↓ (%)	Sum (%)	↑↑↓↑ (%)	↑↑↑↓ (%)	↑↑↑↑ (%)	Sum (%)
Infarction n = 67	43.3	11.9	55.2	6.0	10.4	6.0	22.4
Hemorrhage n = 9	–	11.1	11.2	–	–	66.7	66.7
Tumors n = 46	26.1	8.8	34.9	4.3	6.5	32.6	43.4
Head trauma n = 10	60.0	10.0	70.0	–	–	–	–

Percentage of patients with respective pattern of qEEG changes on the side of brain lesion. Arrows indicate (from left to right) increases and decreases of delta, theta, alpha and beta intensities greater than 10% change as compared with the unaffected hemisphere

DISCUSSION

The objective of the present study was to clarify to what extent the pathological anatomy of brain lesions contributes to characteristic abnormalities in the EEG assessed quantitatively using computerized EEG frequency analysis. For this purpose, EEG changes were studied with respect to amplitude and frequency content of the signal under certain experimental conditions. This allowed the additional determination of possible pathophysiological characteristics related to the EEG abnormalities observed.

In focal ischemia, the derangement of electrolytes and water content occurs when cerebral blood flow decreases to a certain threshold for which the absolute value seems to be species-dependent (Branston et al., 1977; Hossmann and Schuier, 1980; Tamura et al., 1981). It is tempting to assume that the concomitant electrophysiological changes in spontaneous neuronal activity under these experimental conditions behave similarly. However, our experimental data clearly revealed that the EEG changes during the acute stage of focal ischemia differed markedly. In MCA occlusion in cats, the suppression of the EEG amplitude was related to the severity of the blood-flow reduction and this was the most striking EEG abnormality. Changes in the frequency content do not appear to be an important characteristic of pathological EEG in this infarction model. In gerbils, however, a different response to unilateral common carotid artery occlusion was apparent: here an immediate onset of stroke causes a reduction in EEG amplitude; when cerebral blood flow declines slowly but remains above a critical perfusion value, the EEG amplitude evidently increases with time. Gerbils exhibited elevated delta activity regardless of the EEG amplitude changes. Although no relationship was found between frequency content and cortical blood flow in the cat brain following MCA occlusion, in gerbils the increase of delta plus theta activity was evidently proportional to the extent of reduced perfusion.

The reason for the differing EEG behavior in both species after the onset of the same type of brain lesion remains somewhat puzzling. In general, spontaneous neuronal activity is sensitive to structural damage as well as to metabolic changes in the vicinity of, or remote from, a brain lesion. When the EEG is recorded directly from underlying transiently or chronically ischemic brain tissue, a persistent suppression of the EEG voltage is a plausible consequence. Since the gerbil brain is rather small, it cannot be excluded that a signal from subcortical hypoperfused brain areas is obtained, i.e. thalamic regions may be responsible for the presence of slow-wave activity in symptom–positive animals. On the other hand, moderately reduced blood flow in symptom–negative gerbils was found to be associated with slow-frequency activities, although subcortical tissue lesions, which induce polymorphic delta activity, can be excluded (Gloor et al., 1977). An idiogenic osmotic activity indicating the onset of metabolic disturbances is associated indirectly with this phenomenon. In the cat brain the cortico-subcortical distance is larger than in the gerbil and in critical ischemia the EEG recorded is most probably from the electrically silent cortex; during transient cerebral ischemia, the reduction in cortical activity may also be caused by subcortical inhibitory influence; another mechanism suggested is that of neurotransmitter failure (Symon et al., 1979; Strong et al., 1983).

In cerebrovascular disease in man, the most frequent EEG abnormality associated with cortical lesions was found to be slow-wave activity while deeper lesions caused minimal or no increase in delta activity (Cohn et al., 1948; Strauss and Greenstein, 1948; Roseman et al., 1952; Birchfield et al., 1959; Friedlander, 1959; McDowell et al., 1959; Silverman, 1960; Paddison and Ferriss, 1961; Van der Drift and Magnus, 1961). As mentioned above,the time elapsed from the onset of stroke has to be taken into account because shortly after brain infarction, slow-wave activity is predominant, but rapidly declines during the first 2 weeks (Roseman et al., 1952). On the other hand, there has already been reference to ipsilateral voltage reduction in the EEG (Birchfield et al., 1959; Paddison and Ferriss, 1961). It would appear that both the increase in slow-wave activity and suppression of EEG amplitude as observed using qEEG frequency analysis in the experimental brain infarction models are of importance for the interpretation of clinical EEG abnormalities in cerebrovascular disease. Commonly, both characteristics are significantly related to cerebral perfusion. In contrast to earlier reports dealing with visual EEG evaluation, the elevation of delta-wave activity as assessed using qEEG frequency analysis is not necessarily the most outstanding feature of the abnormal EEG and therefore cannot be used alone in the diagnosis of cerebrovascular disease; rather, the results obtained here demonstrate the additional significance of the frequency pattern taking all conventional frequency bands into account, and of a simultaneous decrease in alpha plus beta activity. It has been emphasized that the alpha rhythm is reduced in acute cerebrovascular lesions (Held and Lecasble, 1952; Farbrot, 1954). In our gerbil experiments, the significant decrease in the frequency index supports the validity of clinical qEEG analysis results; nonetheless, the frequency index itself could not be related to hemodynamic or metabolic parameters. The precise electrophysiological characterization of ischemic EEG disturbances in man may be complicated by the large interelectrode distances in the 10–20-electrode system. Furthermore, the inconsistency of clinical EEG frequency analysis data may also reflect the different degrees of predisposition to vascular disease, i.e. arteriosclerosis. With established cerebral collateralization, for instance, less outstanding EEG symptoms may be detectable after the onset of a vascular accident; this is due partly to the altered background activity, which does not permit either the exact localization of the EEG focus, or the area of brain infarction to be determined.

The growth of experimentally induced brain tumors in cats was accompanied by development of vasogenic brain edema restricted to the white matter (Wilmes and Hossmann, 1979). The ipsilateral volume expansion led to a shift of midline structures. These findings are similar to observations made of human brain tumors (Zülch, 1952). However, here in only 38.5% of tumor-bearing animals could a slowing of the EEG be detected over the affected hemisphere and the frequency content of the EEG was independent of blood flow, electrolyte, and water content in both gray and white matter. The spread of edema fluid in white matter did not appear to contribute to the EEG abnormalities; this is not the case for white matter lesions (Gloor et al., 1977). The high incidence of a maximum in the delta and/or theta band determined by qEEG frequency analysis in patients with brain tumors confirms earlier observations that intracranial brain tumors cause a high-voltage 'delta focus (Strauss and Greenstein, 1948); however, these results differ from our experimental findings. Similar electroencephalographic characteristics are also found in patients suffering from intracranial hemorrhage. Both types of cerebral lesions may be distinguished by classification according to the frequency pattern, whereby the simultaneous decrease of alpha plus beta activity seems to be more relevant in cases of brain tumors.

In quite a number of analyzed EEGs, an increase in the alpha and/or beta band intensity was observed over the diseased hemisphere; this should reflect either high-frequency activation within or around the brain lesion or a diaschitic loss of high-frequency voltage in the homotopic area of the opposite hemisphere. This phenomenon, however, was never detected over the affected hemisphere under the experimental conditions of focal ischemia or induced brain tumors. Occasionally, a higher alpha amplitude than on the unaffected side has been observed in small transient or chronic lesions in man (Van der Drift and Magnus, 1961). Alpha and/or beta activation may also be detected as discrete electroencephalographic signs caused by brain tumors (Niebeling, 1980). The fast component in the frequency pattern is of minor importance in brain infarctions but nonetheless detectable in 22.4% of cases. In patients with brain tumors, the frequency pattern of decreased or elevated alpha plus beta activities was also found in 34.9% and 43.4% of cases, respectively. This is not surprising, since our data on experimental brain tumors, i.e. blood flow and electrolyte homeostasis, were not related to the frequency content of the EEG.

Intracranial hemorrhage could be associated almost exclusively with a concomitant increase in fast-frequency activity. This is unlike findings from visual EEG evaluation, where voltage depression of background activity is not accompanied by any appreciable differences between the alpha activities of both hemispheres (Marquardsen and Harvald, 1964).

In summary, both experimental and clinical EEGs from the same types of pathologies have been subjected to computer-supported qEEG frequency analysis. Evidence has accumulated that some discrepancies exist between the experimental and clinical characteristics of mandatory EEG parameters. Electroencephalography during experimental focal ischemia revealed that both suppression of EEG amplitude and the slowing of the EEG as a result of increased low-frequency activities corresponded to changes in blood flow, electrolyte and water content; this relationship could not be demonstrated for these parameters in experimental brain tumors. Clinically applied qEEG frequency analysis permits the localization and documentation of EEG abnormalities but does not as yet significantly contribute to differentiation between the various brain lesions. Data were found to be more inconsistent than in experimental studies; this is most probably due to age differences, drug therapy or the individual predisposition to diseases. Nonetheless, brain infarction may be distinguished from brain tumors by comparison of the maximal deviations in the low-frequency range and the frequency pattern. Further studies are now necessary to determine whether qEEG frequency analysis in patient EEGs is of pathognomonic diagnostic value.

SUMMARY

Quantitative EEG frequency analysis was used to determine alterations of total EEG intensity, of activity in conventional slow and fast wave bands and of the ratios of delta plus theta to alpha plus beta intensity (frequency index) which were related to changes of cerebral blood flow, electrolyte homeostasis and water content in experimental brain ischemia and brain tumors. Hypoperfusion of gerbil brain led to an increase of slow-wave activity. In symptom–positive gerbils, EEG amplitude decreased immediately but increased gradually to 200% of control in symptom–negative gerbils. An increase in cerebral water content and derangement of electrolyte homeostasis was only detected in symptom–positive gerbils. After middle cerebral artery occlusion of cat brain a decline in cortical blood flow was accompanied by a reduction in total power. Changes in the frequency index were only transiently detectable. Significant alterations of electrolyte homeostasis occurred below a flow value of about 15 ml/100 g/min. In only 38.5% of cats with induced brain tumors was pronounced slowing of the EEG over the affected hemisphere recorded but the frequency index could not be related to cerebral blood flow, electrolyte and water content in the overlying cortex or white matter.

Clinical EEGs were submitted to quantitative EEG frequency analysis and grouped according to the maximum of slow-wave activity or according to the pattern of intensity changes in all frequency bands. In about 70% of brain tumors and intracranial hemorrhage cases a slow wave EEG focus was detected but only in 35.8% of patients with brain infarction. Classification of the EEG focus consistent with a decrease of alpha plus beta activity at elevated delta and/or theta band activity was found in 55.2% of patients suffering from brain infarction and in 34.9% of brain tumor cases. A concomitant increase in alpha and/or beta activity was detected in 24% of patients with brain infarction but also in 43.4% of patients with brain tumors.

Our data indicate that some discrepancies exist between the experimental and clinical characteristics of abnormal EEG from the same type of brain lesion. Clinically applied quantitative EEG frequency analysis did not contribute significantly to differentiation between the various brain lesions.

ACKNOWLEDGMENT

We wish to thank Prof. W.-D Heiss and his collaborators for their kindness in providing patient data on the clinical diagnosis.

REFERENCES

Berger, H. (1934) Über das Elektroenkephalogramm des Menschen. IX. Mitteilung. *Arch. Psychiat.*, 102: 305–318.

Birchfield, R.I., Wilson, W.P. and Heyman, A. (1959) An evaluation of electroencephalography in cerebral infarction and ischemia due to arteriosclerosis. *Neurology (Minneap.)*, 9: 859–870.

Branston, N.M., Strong, A.J. and Symon, L. (1977) Extracellular potassium activity, evoked potential and tissue blood flow. *J. Neurol. Sci.*, 32: 305–321.

Cohn, R., Raines, G.N., Mulder, D.W. and Neumann, M. (1948) Cerebral vascular lesions: electroencephalographic and neuropathologic correlations. *Arch. Psychiat. (Chic.)*, 60: 165–181.

Farbrot, O. (1954) Electroencephalographic study in case of cerebrovascular accidents. *Electroencephalogr. clin. Neurophysiol.*, 6: 678–681.

Friedlander, W.J. (1959) Electroencephalographic changes in acute brain stem vascular lesion. *Neurology (Minneap.)*, 9: 24–34.

Gloor, P., Ball, G. and Schaul, N. (1977) Brain lesions that produce delta waves in the EEG. *Neurology*, 27: 326–333.

Gotman, J., Skuce, D.R., Thompson, C.J., Gloor, P., Ives, J.R. and Ray, W.F. (1973) Clinical applications of spectral analysis and extraction of features from electroencephalograms with slow waves in adult patients. *Electroencephalogr. clin. Neurophysiol.*, 35: 225–235.

Held, J.P. and Lecasble, R. (1952) Corrélations électrocliniques à propos de 100 cas d'accidents vasculaires cérébraux. *Rev. Neurol.*, 87: 201–202.

Hossmann, K.-A. and Schuier, F.J. (1980) Experimental brain infarcts in cats. I. Pathophysiological observations. *Stroke*, 11: 583–592.

Hossmann, K.-A., Wechsler, W. and Wilmes, F. (1979) Experimental peritumorous edema. Morphological and pathophysiological observations. *Acta Neuropathol. (Berl.)*, 45: 195–203.

Hossmann, K.-A., Heiss, W.-D., Bewermeyer, H and Mies, G. (1980) EEG frequency analysis in the course of acute ischemic stroke. *Neurosurg. Rev.*, 3: 31–36.

Hudgins, W.R. and Garcia, H.J. (1970) Transorbital approach to the middle cerebral artery of the squirrel monkey: A technique for experimental cerebral infarction applicable to ultrastructural studies. *Stroke*, 1: 107–111.

Kahn, K. (1972) The natural course of experimental cerebral infarction in the gerbil. *Neurology*, 22: 510–515.

Levine, S. and Payan, H. (1966) Effects of ischemia and other procedures on the brain and retina of the gerbil (Meriones unguiculatus). *Exp. Neurol.*, 16: 255–262.

Marquardsen, J. and Harvald, B. (1964) The electroencephalogram in acute cerebrovascular lesions. *Neurology (Minneap.)*, 14: 275–282.

McDowell, F., Wells, C.E. and Ehlers, C. (1959) The electroencephalogram in internal carotid artery occlusion. *Neurology (Minneap.)*, 9: 678–681.

Niebeling, H.-G. (1980) *Einführung in die Elektroenzephalographie*, Springer-Verlag, Berlin–Heidelberg–New York.

O'Brien, M.D. and Waltz, A.G. (1973) Transorbital approach for occluding the middle cerebral artery without craniectomy. *Stroke*, 4: 201–206.

Paddison, R.M. and Ferriss, G.S. (1961) The electroencephalogram in cerebral vascular disease. *Electroencephalogr. clin. Neurophysiol.*, 13: 99–110.

Reivich, M., Jehle, J. Sokoloff, L. and Kety, S.S. (1969) Measurement of regional blood flow with antipyrine-^{14}C in awake cats. *J. Appl. Physiol.*, 27: 296–300.

Roseman, E., Schmidt, R.P. and Foltz, E.L. (1952) Serial electroencephalography in vascular lesions of the brain. *Neurology (Minneap.)*, 2: 311–331.

Rudolph, A.M. and Heymann, M.A. (1967) The circulation of the fetus in utero: Methods for studying distribution of blood flow, cardiac output and organ blood flow. *Circulat. Res.*, 21: 163–184.

Silverman, D. (1960) Serial electroencephalography in brain tumors and cerebrovascular accidents. *Arch. Neurol. (Chic.)*, 2: 122–129.

Strauss, H. and Greenstein, L. (1948) The electroencephalogram in cerebrovascular disease. *Arch. Neurol. Psychiat. (Chic.)*, 59: 395–403.

Strong, A.J., Tomlinson, B.E. Venables, G.S., Gibson, G. and Hardy, A. (1983) The cortical ischaemic penumbra associated with occlusion of the middle cerebral artery in the cat. 2. Studies of histopathology, water content, and in vitro neurotransmitter uptake. *J. Cereb. Blood Flow Metab.*, 3: 97–108.

Symon, L., Branston, N.M. and Chikovani, O. (1979) Ischemic brain edema in baboons: Relationship between regional cerebral water content and blood flow at 1 to 2 hours. *Stroke*, 10: 184–191.

Tamura, A., Graham, D.I., McCulloch, I. and Teasdale, G.M. (1981) Focal cerebral ischemia in the rat. 2. Regional cerebral blood flow determined by ^{14}C-iodoantipyrine autoradiography following middle cerebral artery occlusion. *J. Cereb. Blood Flow Metab.*, 1: 61–69.

Van der Drift, J.H. and Magnus, O. (1961) The EEG in cerebral ischemic lesions: correlations with clinical and pathological findings. In J.S. Meyer and H. Gastaut (Eds.), *Anoxia and the Electroencephalogram*, Thomas, Springfield, Il., pp.180–196.

Wilmes, F. and Hossmann, K.-A. (1979) A specific immunofluorescence technique for the demonstration of vasogenic brain edema in paraffin embedded material. *Acta Neuropathol. (Berl.)*, 45: 47–51.

Zimmermann, V and Hossmann, K.-A. (1975) Resuscitation of the monkey brain after 1 h complete ischemia. II. Brain water and electrolytes. *Brain Res.*, 85: 1–11.

Zülch, K.J. (1952) Hirnödem, Hirnschwellung, Hirndruck. *Zentralbl. Neurochir.*, 12: 174–186.

SECTION II

Quantitative EEG Follow-up Studies

Brain Ischemia: Quantitative EEG and Imaging Techniques, Progress in Brain Research, Vol. 62, edited by
G. Pfurtscheller, E.J. Jonkman and F.H. Lopes da Silva

Non-invasive Follow-up Studies of Stroke Patients with STA–MCA Anastomosis; Computerized Topography of EEG and 133-Xenon Inhalation rCBF Measurement

IWAO YAMAKAMI, AKIRA YAMAURA, TAKAO NAKAMURA and KATSUMI ISOBE

Department of Neurological Surgery, Chiba University, School of Medicine, Inohana 1-8-1, Chiba-shi, Chiba (Japan 280)

INTRODUCTION

The extra-intracranial arterial anastomosis (STA–MCA anastomosis) is a widely accepted surgical technique for the treatment of various cerebral ischemic processes, but the indication and efficiency are still controversial, in spite of many investigations dealing with clinical examination, angiography, regional cerebral blood flow (rCBF) studies and electroencephalogram (EEG). The recent development of computer technology has enabled the quantitative and objective evaluation of EEG activities, and CT–EEG can display a two-dimensional equipotential map of EEG activities. To investigate the efficiency of STA–MCA anastomosis, we adopted two objective and non-invasive methods for assessment; one was the CT–EEG, and the other was the rCBF study with the 133-xenon inhalation method.

CLINICAL MATERIAL

This study includes 32 patients who underwent STA–MCA anastomosis for their cerebral ischemic processes (24 males and 8 females, mean age 53 years, range 23–71 years). The patency of the anastomosis was confirmed by postoperative angiography in all patients. The clinical diagnosis was transient ischemic attacks (TIA) in 3 cases and completed stroke in 29 cases. Preoperative angiographic findings of these cases were as follows: occlusion of internal carotid artery (ICA) in 6 cases, stenosis of ICA in 10 cases, occlusion of middle cerebral artery (MCA) in 5 cases, stenosis of MCA in 4 cases and other disorders in 7 cases. In each case, the symptomatic side was clearly defined by the clinical symptoms, angiographic findings and/or computerized tomography. In the patients with a completed stroke the STA–MCA anastomosis was made approximately 4 weeks (30 ± 4 days) after the ischemic attack.

METHODS

Computerized topography of the EEG (CT–EEG)

Pre- and postoperative EEG recordings were made in all cases and each of these recordings was analyzed with CT–EEG (MCE-1100, Nihon Kohden, Japan). During the EEG recordings, the patients were in a state of quiet attentiveness with closed eyes. The 10–20 international system of electrode placement was employed and two ear and 16 scalp electrodes were attached.

The computerized EEG processing was as described in the flow chart (Fig. 1). An EEG segment of at least 30 sec, which should be free of artifacts, was used for spectral CT–EEG analysis. The average power of each frequency band (delta: 2.0–3.5 Hz,

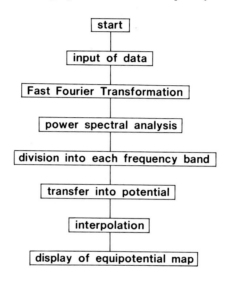

Fig. 1. Flow chart of computerized EEG analysis by CT–EEG.

theta: 4.0–7.5 Hz, alpha: 8.0–12.5 Hz, beta 1: 13.0–19.5 Hz, beta 2: 20.0–29.5 Hz) was calculated with the Fast Fourier Transformation (FFT) technique. In CT–EEG, the square root of the average power in each frequency band was defined as the equivalent potential of its frequency band. Then the average power was transformed into the equivalent potential according to this definition. The equivalent potentials were so calculated, only for the 16 points on the scalp where the scalp electrodes actually recorded the EEG potential. Potentials at the points that did not actually have a scalp electrode were interpolated (Matsuoka et al., 1978) and the CT–EEG displayed the two-dimensional map of the equivalent potential (equipotential map) of each frequency band. The equipotential maps were represented by 10 corresponding colors for color display. The more reddish an area, the higher a potential it represented and on the contrary, the more bluish areas represented the lower potentials. Figure 2 shows a conventional EEG and its equipotential maps by CT–EEG in a 50-year-old female with aphasia and moderate right hemiparesis due to the occlusion of the left internal carotid artery. On the equipotential map of the delta band, a high voltage focus is clearly visualized as a gray focus in the left hemisphere. Also in the theta band, a high

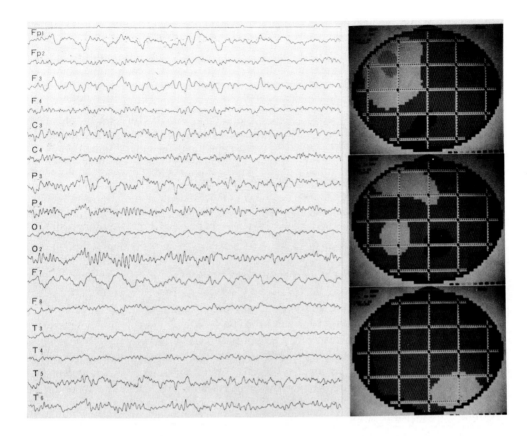

Fig. 2. A conventional EEG and its gray-display CT–EEG maps in a completed stroke patient. The conventional EEG is on the left side; the corresponding equipotential maps (CT–EEG) are on the right (top, the equipotential map of delta band; middle, that of theta band; bottom, that of alpha band). In a gray scale-display CT–EEG equipotential map, bright gray indicates the highest potential and black the lowest potential.

voltage focus is present in the symptomatic hemisphere. The authors defined a high voltage focus of delta and/or theta wave bands, clearly visualized in the symptomatic hemisphere in CT–EEG, as "high voltage slow focus:HVSF". In the alpha wave band, the amplitude in the occipital region of the symptomatic hemisphere was lower than that of the asymptomatic hemisphere. As the authors already mentioned in a previous report (Yamakami et al., 1981), there are two important parameters in CT–EEG related to cerebral function; one is HVSF and the other is alpha activity. In this communication, special attention is paid to HVSF. Changes of HVSF before and after the STA–MCA anastomosis are reported in comparison with the rCBF studies and the clinical effects of anastomosis.

Measurements of regional cerebral blood flow (rCBF)

Using the 133-xenon inhalation method (Novo Inhalation Cerebrograph, Novo Diagnostic Systems, Denmark), rCBF studies were conducted in each patient before and 3 months after STA–MCA anastomosis. The rCBF study was conducted with the

110

patients at rest; 133-xenon in a concentration of about 3.0 mCi per liter mixed with air was inhaled by the patients for one minute through a close-fitting face mask with a one-way valve. The clearance of the radioisotope from the brain was monitored for 10 min by 20 NaI collimated scintillation detectors applied over homologous regions of both hemispheres (10 over each hemisphere), perpendicular to the sagittal plane of the head. The end-tidal 133-xenon curves were used for correction of recirculation. The rCBF was calculated from the "fast" component from the desaturation curves (Fl: ml/100 g/min) derived from each head probe (Obrist et al., 1975). In this study, the hemispheric mean value of Fl (mCBF) was calculated for each hemisphere.

Cerebral angiography and computerized tomography (X-ray CT)

Pre- and postoperative cerebral angiography was performed and the patency of the anastomotic channel was confirmed in each case. The X-ray CT was frequently examined pre- and postoperatively.

Assessment of the clinical results of STA–MCA anastomosis

The clinical results of bypass surgery in each case were classified as "GOOD", "FAIR" or "POOR" according to the neurological status 3 months postoperatively. In TIA patients, "GOOD" means the cessation of TIAs after surgery, "FAIR" is a decreased frequency of TIAs and "POOR" is no change or an increased frequency of TIAs. In completed stroke patients, "GOOD" means a marked neurological improvement, "FAIR" is a moderate improvement and "POOR" is no improvement or deterioration.

Student's t-test was employed in the statistical analysis of the data.

RESULTS

"High voltage slow focus" in CT–EEG

Clinical diagnosis and preoperative HVSF in CT–EEG

Table I shows the relationship of the clinical diagnosis and preoperative HVSF in CT–EEG. Preoperatively, 11 out of 32 patients (35%) had HVSF in CT–EEG and

TABLE I

CLINICAL DIAGNOSIS AND THE PREOPERATIVE
"HIGH VOLTAGE SLOW FOCUS" IN CT–EEG

Preoperative High voltage slow focus	Clinical diagnosis	
Present (11 cases)	TIA	(0 cases)
	Completed stroke	(11 cases)
Absent (21 cases)	TIA	(3 cases)
	Completed stroke	(18 cases)

they belonged exclusively to the completed stroke group. None of TIA group showed HVSF. On the other hand, about half of the completed stroke patients (11 out of 29) showed preoperative HVSF in CT–EEG.

Changes of HVSF in serial CT–EEG studies

Table II shows the results of serial CT–EEG studies with regard to HVSF. All 11 cases with preoperative HVSF retained their HVSF throughout the postoperative course. Of the 21 patients without preoperative HVSF, 10 patients did not have HVSF throughout the postoperative course and six patients had a transient HVSF during the first postoperative week. The other five patients had HVSF at one week and at 3 months after surgery.

TABLE II

CHANGES OF "HIGH VOLTAGE SLOW FOCUS" IN
SERIAL CT–EEG STUDIES

High voltage slow focus			No. of cases
Before surgery	*Postoperative first week*	*Postoperative third month*	
(+)	(+)	(+)	11
(−)	(−)	(−)	10
	(+)	(−)	6
		(+)	5

"High voltage slow focus" in CT–EEG and the clinical results of the STA–MCA anastomosis

The clinical results of STA–MCA anastomosis in 32 patients were as follows: 8 patients were classified as "GOOD", 24 patients as "FAIR", and fortunately there was no "POOR" case. Table III shows the relationship of the clinical diagnosis and

TABLE III

CLINICAL DIAGNOSIS AND CLINICAL RESULTS OF
STA–MCA ANASTOMOSIS

Clinical diagnosis	*No. of cases*	*Clinical results of STA–MCA anastomosis*		
		GOOD	FAIR	POOR
TIA	3	3/3	0/3	0/3
Completed stroke	29	5/29	24/29	0/29
Total	32	8/32	24/32	0/32

the clinical results of bypass surgery. All the TIA patients could be classified as "GOOD". On the other hand, out of 29 completed stroke patients, 5 patients were considered as "GOOD" and 24 patients as "FAIR". The relationship of HVSF in CT–EEG and the clinical results is shown in Table IV. All 11 patients with preoperative HVSF and also sustained HVSF throughout the postoperative course could not achieve the "GOOD" classification. Out of 21 patients without the preoperative HVSF, 8 patients (40%) could be classified as "GOOD" and the other 13 patients as "FAIR". None of the 16 patients with HVSF in the postoperative third month were considered as "GOOD". Eight of the 16 patients without HVSF in the postoperative third month could be considered as "GOOD".

TABLE IV

RELATIONSHIP OF "HIGH VOLTAGE SLOW FOCUS" IN
CT–EEG AND CLINICAL RESULTS OF STA–MCA ANASTOMOSIS

High voltage slow focus			Clinical results of STA–MCA anastomosis	
Before surgery	Postoperative first week	Postoperative third month	GOOD	FAIR
(+)	(+)	(+)	0	11
	(−)	(−)	5	15
(−)	(+)	(−)	3	3
		(+)	0	5
Total			8 cases	24 cases

"High voltage slow focus" in CT–EEG and rCBF

The rCBF studies were conducted in 20 cases before and 3 months after bypass surgery. To investigate the relationship of HVSF with CT–EEG and rCBF, these 20 cases were, according to the presence or absence of the preoperative HVSF in CT–EEG, divided into two groups, a "HVSF group" that included 7 cases with the preoperative HVSF and a "non-HVSF group" with 13 cases lacking the preoperative HVSF.

Preoperative rCBF studies (Fig. 3)

The hemispheric mean value of Fl (mCBF) of all cases was 63 ml/100 g/min in the symptomatic hemisphere, and 66 ml/100 g/min in the asymptomatic hemisphere. In the symptomatic hemisphere, the mCBF of the "HVSF group" (51 ± 7 ml/100 g/min) was significantly decreased compared to that of the "non-HVSF group" (69 ± 9 ml/100 g/min) ($p<0.005$). Although the mCBF of the "HVSF group" (59 ± 9 ml/100 g/min) was significantly decreased compared to that of the "non-HVSF group" (71 ± 10 ml/100 g/min) in the asymptomatic hemisphere ($p<0.05$), the difference in mCBF between the two groups was greater in the symptomatic hemisphere than in the asymptomatic hemisphere.

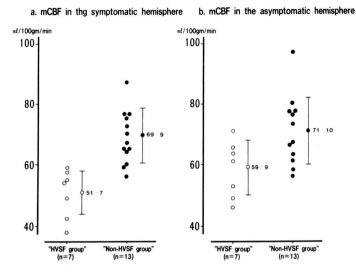

Fig. 3. Results of the preoperative rCBF study. a: Hemispheric mean value of Fl(mCBF) in the symptomatic hemisphere; b: mCBF in the asymptomatic hemisphere. The mean values and standard deviations are indicated.

rCBF studies in the third postoperative month (Fig. 4)

The mCBF of all cases was 66 ml/100 g/min in the symptomatic hemisphere and 67 ml/100 g/min in the asymptomatic hemisphere. The mCBF in the third postoperative month was slightly greater than the preoperative mCBF in both hemispheres. In the symptomatic hemisphere, the mCBF of the "HVSF group" (54 ± 11 ml/100 g/min) was significantly decreased compared to that of the "non-HVSF group" (67 ± 12 ml/100 g/min) ($p < 0.05$). Also in the asymptomatic hemisphere, the mCBF of the "HVSF group" (56 ± 9 ml/100 g/min) was significantly decreased compared to that of the "non-HVSF group" (70 ± 12 ml/100 g/min) ($p < 0.05$).

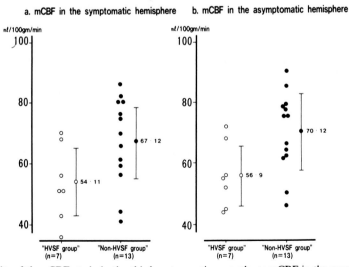

Fig. 4. Results of the rCBF study in the third postoperative month. a: mCBF in the symptomatic hemisphere, b: mCBF in the asymptomatic hemisphere.

114

"Fl symmetry index" (Fig. 5)

The authors defined the "Fl symmetry index" as follows:

$$\text{"Fl symmetry index"} = \frac{\text{Fl in the symptomatic hemisphere} \times 100}{\text{Fl in the asymptomatic hemisphere}}$$

In the preoperative rCBF study, the "Fl symmetry index" in the "HVSF group" (87 ± 6) was significantly smaller than in the "non-HVSF group" (99 ± 4) ($p < 0.005$). In the third postoperative month, there was no significant difference in "Fl symmetry index" between these two groups ("HVSF group" = 95 ± 7, "non-HVSF group" = 96 ± 5).

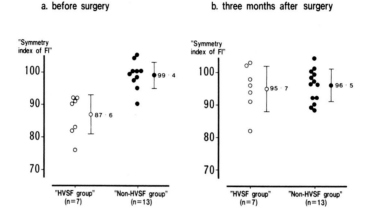

Fig. 5. "Fl symmetry index". a: before surgery, b: 3 months after surgery. For definition see text.

DISCUSSION

Since the introduction of the microsurgical technique by Yasargil in 1967, the STA–MCA anastomosis has become a widely accepted surgical technique for cerebral ischemic disease. Although there may be a general consensus that TIAs, especially in the presence of an evident morphological change, are a good indication for bypass surgery (Kletter, 1979), the effectiveness of surgery in the completed stroke patient is still controversial (Galibert and Grunewald, 1979). This is partly because there has been no objective and definite method to assess effectiveness. In this study, we adopted two noninvasive, objective methods to assess the efficiency of surgery; one was CT–EEG, in which the EEG activities were visualized topographically and semi-quantitatively, the other was the rCBF study using the 133-xenon inhalation method.

EEG study has played an important role in showing the functional influence of a cerebral lesion and many investigators have adopted the EEG as a tool for measuring cerebral function in their experimental and clinical studies of cerebral ischemia. But the visual interpretation of the conventional EEG has been mainly dependent upon the experience of the examiner and therefore it has not always been objective and quantitative. The recent introduction of computer technology in medicine has made it possible to overcome this disadvantage of the conventional EEG and to evaluate EEG activities objectively (Pfurtscheller and Wege, 1981; Tolonen et al., 1981; de Weerd et al., 1982; Nagata et al., 1982). Many attempts have been made to analyse the EEG quantitatively and CT–EEG is a computer method to display a two-dimensional map of EEG activity on the scalp semiquantitatively and topographically (Yamakami et al., 1981). In CT–EEG, the equivalent potential in each frequency band is defined as the square root of the average power spectrum of the frequency band and the equipotential maps are estimated by interpolation.

In the CT–EEG of some patients suffering from a unilateral cerebral ischemic process, there is a clearly visualized high voltage focus of delta and/or theta wave activity in the symptomatic hemisphere. The authors defined the high voltage focus of slow wave bands in the symptomatic hemisphere as "high voltage slow focus: HVSF" (Yamakami et al., 1981), and special emphasis was placed upon HVSF in this study on the assessment of the effectiveness of bypass surgery.

No TIA patient had the preoperative HVSF and all patients who had the preoperative HVSF suffered from a completed stroke. Etiologically, the rCBF study has suggested that TIAs are generally based on two interrelating factors; one is a background decrease in CBF and the other is a superimposed transient drop of CBF below the critical threshold level to produce neurological deficits (Heilbrun et al., 1975; Austin et al., 1978). In the interval between the attacks, the rCBF of the ischemic area might return to normal, or at least return to the level above the critical flow, although an ischemia should have been present at the time of attack and a few hours thereafter (Kletter, 1979). In TIA patients, the neurological deficit and cerebral ischemic damage are transient, and the transient cerebral damage may not give rise to HVSF in the interval. In completed stroke patients, the ischemia is more severe than in TIAs and/or it is permanent, and therefore the cerebral ischemic damage and neurological deficit are irreversible and permanent. In this study, HVSF was seen exclusively in those patients who had permanent ischemic cerebral damage. With regard to the EEG findings in completed stroke patients, the importance of focal or unilateral slow waves has been emphasized and the CT–EEG clearly visualizes, semiquantitatively and topographically, the focal slow wave in the symptomatic hemisphere as HVSF.

A cerebral lesion near the cortical surface is apt to bring about the conspicuous focal slow wave, but a deep-seated cerebral lesion hardly produces it (Cohn et al., 1948; Roseman et al., 1952). For this reason, patients with a low density area restricted to the basal ganglia were excluded from this study. But completed stroke patients did not always show HVSF and the number of the patients who showed preoperative HVSF was fewer than half of the total. What determines whether a completed stroke patient shows HVSF or not? The rCBF studies in this series showed that the CBF of patients who had HVSF was significantly decreased compared to that of patients who did not have it. This result implies that severe ischemia produces HVSF and mild does not. The presence of HVSF in CT–EEG means severe cerebral damage by the ischemic process.

The serial CT–EEG examinations revealed that all patients who had a preoperative HVSF maintained it throughout 3 months after surgery. STA–MCA anastomosis did not correct the HVSF abnormality. The presence of preoperative HVSF means irreversible functional cerebral damage that could not be cured even by STA–MCA anastomosis. Roseman et al. (1952) stated that the focal slow waves would usually increase in frequency and decrease in amplitude as the natural course of EEG findings in cerebral infarction. In this study, the interval between STA–MCA anastomosis and the last CT–EEG study was about 3 months. If the interval had been much longer than 3 months, the HVSF would have disappeared in some cases. Disappearance of HVSF may not, however, be the result of STA–MCA anastomosis but rather the natural course of cerebral infarction.

In the rCBF study, the significant difference in CBF between patients with the preoperative HVSF and those without it did not disappear 3 months after STA–MCA anastomosis. The STA–MCA anastomosis theoretically causes an increase in CBF, but actually, as demonstrated in this rCBF study and in many other previous studies (Schmiedek et al., 1976, de Weerd et al., 1982; Laurent et al., 1982), the surgical technique is not always successful in increasing the CBF. In patients with preoperative HVSF, STA–MCA anastomosis was not successful in resolving HVSF nor in increasing CBF; moreover, in these patients the bypass surgery could not produce a noticeable neurological improvement. It is supposed that the presence of HVSF represents irreversible ischemic damage in which the CBF cannot be increased and an improvement of EEG abnormalities (i.e. resolution of HVSF) cannot be brought about, even by STA–MCA anastomosis. If this hypothesis is true, there would be no indication for STA–MCA anastomosis in completed stroke patients who have HVSF in CT–EEG.

Some of the completed stroke patients without the preoperative HVSF showed "transient" HVSF during the first postoperative week. During the first postoperative week, surgical stress may still remain, causing the slow waves near the surgical area. Pfurtscheller and Auer (1981) suggested that the transient cerebral dysfunction might cause such EEG patterns as slowing of the mu rhythm, reduced movement-related desynchronization, etc. In this CT–EEG study, the "transient" HVSF during the first postoperative week is not such a permanent finding as HVSF during the preoperative period or the third postoperative month.

The clinical "GOOD" result of STA–MCA anastomosis was achieved only in those patients who had neither preoperative HVSF nor HVSF in the third postoperative month. Mild ischemia that does not cause the appearance of HVSF might be reversible and so the neurological dysfunction might be improved if the extra-intracranial anastomotic channel is established.

The preoperative rCBF study showed that, in the asymptomatic hemisphere, the mCBF of patients with HVSF was significantly decreased compared to the mCBF of the patients without it. From this result, we may conclude that a severe unilateral cerebral ischemia gives rise to an important diaschisis, if the presence of HVSF means a severe unilateral ischemia and the absence of it means mild ischemia. The degree of diaschisis is dependent upon the severity of unilateral cerebral ischemia. Although Slater et al. (1977) could not establish a correlation between the severity of the stroke and the degree of diaschisis, the details of the severity of stroke were not clear in their study. In the study by Lavy et al. (1975), the mCBF (20 ml/100 g/min) of the asymptomatic hemisphere in patients with a disturbance of consciousness was lower than that in those without (26 ml/100 g/min). In their recent investigation with positron emission tomography, Lenzi et al. (1982) also reported that patients with impaired consciousness showed a significantly lower rCBF in the asymptomatic hemisphere than patients who were alert. If we accept the neurogenic theory of diaschisis suggested by Hoedt-Rasmussen and Skinhøj (1964), it is possible that a more severe unilateral cerebral dysfunction causes a more severe cerebral dysfunction in the contralateral hemisphere as well. Three months postoperatively, the mCBF in the asymptomatic hemisphere of patients with HVSF was significantly decreased compared to patients without it. The severe reduction of CBF in the asymptomatic hemisphere of patients with severe unilateral ischemia could not be corrected, even after bypass surgery. In recent years, several authors have advocated the importance of the reversal of intracerebral steal or redistribution of cerebral circulation by the STA–MCA anastomosis (Holbach and Wassmann, 1979; Laurent et al., 1982). However, the results of this study suggest that the reversal of intracerebral steal could not be accomplished in patients with severe preoperative cerebral damage, that is, in patients with the preoperative HVSF. Laurent et al. (1982) also stated that the improvement of decreased CBF in the asymptomatic hemisphere was related to the improved CBF in the symptomatic hemisphere. The postoperative improvement of CBF in the asymptomatic hemisphere is dependent upon the degree of preoperative ischemic damage in the symptomatic hemisphere.

Although the principle of diaschisis is applicable in patients with unilateral ischemia, the mCBF in the symptomatic hemisphere is more reduced than that in the asymptomatic one, giving rise to an asymmetry of mCBF between the symptomatic and asymptomatic hemispheres. The asymmetry of mCBF is more severe in a severe unilateral ischemia than in a mild one. In the preoperative rCBF study, the "Fl symmetry index" of patients with the preoperative HVSF (87 ± 6) was significantly smaller than in patients without it (99 ± 5) ($p < 0.005$). The presence of preoperative HVSF means a severe unilateral ischemic dysfunction and a severe asymmetry of mCBF.

According to the results of the rCBF study in the third postoperative month, the asymmetry of mCBF in patients with the preoperative HVSF is remarkably reduced, although all those patients maintained HVSF even after bypass surgery. The disappearance of asymmetry of mCBF is one thing and the resolution of HVSF is another. This result means a discrepancy between EEG and CBF, and therefore the principle of so-called "coupling of EEG and CBF" cannot be applicable in these cases.

In the pathophysiology of cerebral ischemia, the principle of so-called "coupling of EEG and CBF" can be partly applicable and partly not (Paulson and Sharbrough, 1974; Herrschaft et al., 1977). For this reason, in the serial examination of cerebral ischemic patients who underwent the STA–MCA anastomosis, the combination of EEG and rCBF studies plays a very important role. The CT–EEG, which represents the EEG activities semiquantitatively and topographically, is very helpful in the objective interpretation of EEG activities.

SUMMARY

Computerized topography of the EEG (CT–EEG) is a newly developed computer method for displaying EEG activities measured on the scalp on a two-dimensional map. In these plots the square roots of the average power for each frequency band are defined as the equivalent potential. We investigated serial CT–EEGs from 32 patients (3 TIA patients and 29 completed stroke patients) who underwent the STA–MCA anastomosis for their cerebral ischemic processes, for the purpose of objective evaluation of the effectiveness of surgery. The results of these CT–EEG studies were compared with the results of clinical evaluation and of the serial rCBF studies with the

118

133-xenon inhalation method. In preoperative CT–EEGs, 11 out of 32 patients had clearly visualized high voltage foci in slow wave bands (delta and/or theta) in the symptomatic hemisphere (which the authors defined as "high voltage slow focus: HVSF"). No TIA patient had the preoperative HVSF that was seen exclusively in completed stroke patients. The serial CT–EEG studies revealed that all of the preoperative HVSFs remained unchanged even after bypass surgery. The clinical results of bypass surgery were as follows; "GOOD" with 8 patients, "FAIR" with 24 patients and no "POOR" patient. The surgery could not offer the "GOOD" result in any one of 11 patients who had the preoperative HVSF. The CBF of patients with the preoperative HVSF was significantly decreased in both hemispheres compared to that of patients without the preoperative HVSF. This significant discrepancy of CBF remained after surgery in these two groups, although the degree of discrepancy was slightly minimized. It is supposed that the preoperative HVSF indicates the presence of severe ischemic damage irreversible even by bypass surgery, and there might be no indication for surgery in completed stroke patients who have the preoperative HVSF.

REFERENCES

Austin, G., Haugen, G. and Schuler, W. (1978) Transient ischemic attacks and metabolic aspects of their relief by microneurosurgical anastomosis. In J.M. Fein and O.H. Reichman (Eds.), *Microvascular Anastomoses for Cerebral Ischemia*, Springer-Verlag, New York, pp.94–102.

Cohn, R., Raines, G.N., Mulder, D.W. and Neumann, M.A. (1948) Cerebral vascular lesions. Electroencephalographic and neuropathologic correlations. *Arch. Neurol. Psychiat.* 60: 165–181.

De Weerd, A.W., Veering, M.M., Mosmans, P.C.M., van Huffelen, A.C., Tulleken, C.A.F. and Jonkman, E.J. (1982) Effects of the extra-intracranial (STA–MCA) arterial anastomosis on EEG and cerebral blood flow. A controlled study of patients with unilateral cerebral ischemia. *Stroke*, 13: 674–679.

Galibert, P. and Grunewald, P. (1979) Extra-intracranial anastomosis in patients with completed strokes. *Acta Neurochir.*, Suppl. 28: 306–307.

Heilbrun, M.P., Reichman, O.H., Anderson, R.E. and Roberts, T.S. (1975) Regional cerebral blood flow studies following superficial temporal-middle cerebral artery anastomosis. *J. Neurosurg.*, 43: 706–716.

Herrschaft, H., Hossmann, K.-A., Mies, G. and Zulch, K.J. (1977) Relationship between cerebral blood flow and EEG frequency content in patients with acute brain ischemia. *Acta Neurol. Scand.*, Suppl. 56: 414–415.

Hoedt-Rasmussen, K. and Skinhøj, E. (1964) Transneural depression of the cerebral hemispheric metabolism in man. *Acta Neurol. Scand.*, 40: 41–46.

Holbach, K.H. and Wassmann, H. (1979) Effect of extra-intracranial arterial bypass (EIAB) on cerebral circulation and EEG. *Acta Neurochir.*, Suppl. 28: 308.

Kletter, G. (1979) *The Extra-Intracranial Bypass Operation for the Prevention and Treatment of Stroke*, Springer–Verlag, Wien.

Laurent, J.P., Lawner, P.M. and O'Conner, M. (1982) Reversal of intracerebral steal by STA–MCA anastomosis. *J. Neurosurg.*, 57: 629–632.

Lavy, S., Melamed, E. and Portnoy, Z. (1975) The effect of cerebral infarction on the regional cerebral blood flow of the contralateral hemisphere. *Stroke*, 6: 160–163.

Lenzi, G.L., Frackowiak, R.S.J. and Jones, T. (1982) Cerebral oxygen metabolism and blood flow in human cerebral ischemic infarction. *J. Cereb. Blood Flow Metab.*, 2: 321–335.

Matsuoka, S., Arakaki, Y., Numaguchi, K. and Ueno, S. (1978) The effect of dexamethasone on electroencephalograms in patients with brain tumors. *J. Neurosurg*, 48: 601–608.

Nagata, K., Mizukami, M., Araki, G., Kawase, T. and Hirano, M. (1982) Topographic electroencephalographic study of cerebral infarction using computed mapping of the EEG. *J. Cereb. Blood Flow Metab.*, 2: 79–88.

Obrist, W.D., Thompson, H.K., Wang, H.S. and Wilkinson, W.E. (1975) Regional cerebral blood flow estimated by 133 xenon inhalation. *Stroke*, 6: 245–256.

Paulson, O.B. and Sharbrough, F.W. (1974) Physiologic and pathophysiologic relationship between the electroencephalogram and the regional cerebral blood flow. *Acta Neurol. Scand.*, 50: 194–220.

Pfurtscheller, G. and Auer, L. (1981) Computer EEG evaluation before and after extracranial to intracranial arterial bypass surgery (EIAB) in patients with completed stroke. *Electroenceph. clin. Neurophysiol.*, 52: S105.

Pfurtscheller, G. and Wege, W. (1981) Follow-up computer EEG evaluation and prognosis in patients with cerebral ischemia. *Electroenceph. clin. Neurophysiol.*, 52: S7.

Roseman, E., Schmidt, R.P. and Foltz, E.L. (1952) Serial electroencephalography in vascular lesions of the brain. *Neurology*, 2: 311–331.

Schmiedek, P., Gratzl, O., Spetzler, R., Steinhoff, H., Enzenbach, R., Brendel, W. and Marguth, F. (1976) Selection of patients for extra-intracranial arterial bypass surgery based on rCBF measurements. *J. Neurosurg.*, 44: 303–312.

Slater, R., Reirich, M., Goldberg, H., Banka, R. and Greenberg, J. (1977) Diaschisis with cerebral infarction. *Stroke*, 8: 684–690.

Tolonen, U., Ahonen, A., Sulg, I.A., Kuikka, J., Kallaranta, T., Koskinen, M. and Hokkanen, E. (1981) Serial measurements of quantitative EEG and cerebral blood flow and circulation time after brain infarction. *Acta Neurol. Scand.*, 63: 145–155.

Yamakami, I., Yamaura, A., Isobe, K., Nakamura, T., Ise, H., Date, H. and Makino, H. (1981) Computerized topography of EEG in patients with extra-intracranial bypass for cerebral ischemic vascular disease. *Electroenceph. clin. Neurophysiol.*, 52: S45.

Yasargil, M.G. (1967) Experimental small vessel surgery in the dog including patching and grafting of cerebral vessels and the formation of functional extra-intracranial shunts. In R.M.P. Donaghy and M.G. Yasargil (Eds.), *Microvascular Surgery*, C.V. Mosby, Co., St. Louis, pp.87–126.

Brain Ischemia: Quantitative EEG and Imaging Techniques, Progress in Brain Research, Vol. 62, edited by
G. Pfurtscheller, E.J. Jonkman and F.H. Lopes da Silva
©*1984 Elsevier Science Publishers B.V.*

Quantitative EEG Follow-up Study after Extracranial–Intracranial Bypass Operation for Cerebral Ischemia

G. PFURTSCHELLER[1], L.M. AUER[2] and V. KÖPRUNER[1]

[1]*Department of Computing, Institute of Biomedical Engineering, Technical University of Graz, A-8010*
Graz and [2] *Department of Neurosurgery, University of Graz, A-8036 Graz (Austria)*

INTRODUCTION

The extracranial–intracranial arterial bypass operation (EIAB) was introduced (Yasargil, 1969) to circumvent cerebrovascular occlusive lesions such as carotid occlusion and thereby improve blood flow to reversibly dysfunctional ischemic areas of the brain. Since that time, many reports have described a beneficial effect of EIAB, especially in patients with transitory ischemic attacks (TIA) and in patients with prolonged though reversible ischemic neurological deficits (PRIND) (Austin et al., 1974; Schmiedek et al, 1976; Zumstein and Yasargil, 1980). There is, however, much discussion about the indication for such surgical treatment in patients with completed stroke, i.e. cerebral infarction accompanied by irreversible neurological deficits, since reperfusion of such an infarcted area cannot induce improvement of function. The only consequence would have to be luxury perfusion, i.e. creation of a blood flow level above metabolic demands. Several blood flow follow-up studies have shown that the effect of EIAB in increasing the cerebral blood flow (CBF) in such patients is only transitory and followed by recoupling of flow to function at a lower level (Meyer et al., 1982). Nevertheless, two arguments have been considered for an indication for EIAB in this group of patients: one is the hypothesis of a peri-infarct penumbra, i.e. a zone of low perfusion in the viable brain tissue surrounding the infarct as well as in areas remote from the infarct (Lassen, 1982). The second argument is that the cerebrovascular occlusive disease that induced cerebral infarction by critically low perfusion in a circumscribed area may be the origin of further ischemic events in other brain areas, i.e. may cause reinfarction. Here, EIAB has been considered as a preventive measure for reinfarction. Presently, an international cooperative study is underway to show unequivocally which group of patients might benefit from EIAB and have a better long-term outcome compared to patients treated medically.

Another way to study the neuronal function and dysfunction and to compare possible effects of EIAB is the application of quantitative EEG (qEEG) techniques using bipolar EEG recording over the affected region during rest and under physical load. The generation of the EEG is closely linked to neuronal activity in the superficial cortical layers controlled by subcortical structures. An occlusion of the internal or middle cerebral artery therefore can result in a changed EEG pattern over the sensorimotor region. The visually evaluated EEG is scored as "normal" in a high percentage of patients with cerebrovascular insufficiency and with minor neurological deficits (Birchfield et al., 1959; Enge et al., 1980). The visually evaluated EEGs therefore are unsuitable for monitoring the effects of bypass surgery. A prerequisite for studying minor and localized changes in brain activity is the availability of a sensitive method allowing (1) the discrimination between normal and abnormal regional brain function and (2) measurement and quantification of changes in local brain dysfunction at different time intervals after revascularization surgery. Such methods are now available in the evaluation technique for sensorimotor rhythm (Pfurtscheller et al., 1982; Pfurtscheller and Auer, 1983) and in the calculation of a multiparametric asymmetry score as described by Köpruner et al. (this volume), both based on computerized EEG analysis.

We wanted to see whether qEEG methods are sensitive enough (1) to measure changes in electrical brain activity after EIAB; (2) to differentiate between such changes obtained in patients with different types of cerebral infarction; (3) to test which EEG parameters are most suitable for monitoring purposes, and (4) to describe the improvement or deterioration of brain function 12–24 months after surgery in comparison with postoperative changes in the neurological deficit, and possibly to predict reinfarction.

METHODS AND MATERIAL

In a group of 27 EIAB patients, EEGs were recorded shortly before surgery, 7 days thereafter and then approximately 1, 2, 4, 6, 9, 12 and 24 months later. EEG measurements after 7 days were available from all patients, data after 9 and 12 months from 19 and data after 24 months from 9 patients. The neurological follow-up examinations were performed at the same intervals after surgery. The age of the patients ranged from 29 to 71 years and averaged 51 years; 20 patients were male and 7 were female.

Method

EEG recording

For the EEG recording, six bipolar derivations were used in an equidistant transverse montage along the tempero-central areas and across the vertex. Six mm diameter disc electrodes (Ag/AgCl) were fixed with collodion in the following scalp positions: C_z–C_4', C_4'–C_4, C_4–T_4', C_z–C_3', C_3'–C_3 and C_3–T_3'; the primed notations indicate intermediate positions between neighboring electrodes in the 10–20 system. Because of the operation scar in the temporal region, all electrodes were moved forward by approximately 2 cm from the standard position. Recordings were made with a time constant of 0.3 sec and an upper cutoff frequency (-3 dB) of 30 Hz. Throughout the recording session the patients were sitting comfortably in a chair. The analog data, including trigger and pressure curve from a pressure transducer, were stored on a HP 3968A analog tape.

Experimental sequence

The following sequence was used:
(i)   Control situation: EEG recording with subject's eyes closed, without intentional hand movements, for a period of about 12 min.

(ii)   Right-hand movement consisting of voluntary, repeated, self-paced squeezing of a rubber ball with a diameter of 7 cm with eyes closed. Intervals between movements were at least 10 sec.

(iii)   Left-hand movement as above.

Twenty patients applied pressure on the ball with the right and 26 with the left hand. In the 19 patients able to perform movements with both hands, the right-hand movement was always done before the left-hand experiment.

The overall time for the whole recording was between half an hour and 2 hours, depending on the patients' co-operation and severity of the neurological deficit.

The rubber ball was connected to a pressure transducer (Duym and Pfurtscheller, 1984), the pressure curves were sampled, averaged and the maximal peak of the mean pressure curve was taken as a measurement for the maximal hand pressure (Pfurtscheller and Auer, 1983).

EEG data processing

The EEG signals were processed according to methods developed in our laboratory and described elsewhere (Pfurtscheller and Aranibar, 1977, 1979, 1980; Pfurtscheller and Auer, 1983). The sampling epochs had a duration of 6 sec, each including 4 sec preceding and 2 sec following the trigger generated by the onset of movement. In the control experiment, the intertrial intervals were 8 sec. In each sequence, 60 epochs were digitized at 64 samples per sec.

A very important procedure was the automatic rejection of EEG trials with artifacts after EEG data sampling (see Köpruner et al., this volume). From the remaining artifact-free trials (≤ 60), average band power versus time curves for the alpha (6–14 Hz) and beta band (14–24 Hz), and power spectra were calculated for each channel using an FFT algorithm. Delta, theta, alpha and beta power and alpha peak frequency were calculated from the power spectra, and alpha and beta ERD (ERD = Event-Related Desynchronization) from power versus time curves. A detailed description of these parameter calculations is given in Köpruner et al. (this volume). Data processing and parameter calculation were performed with a PDP 11/23 computer.

Patient material

Neurological deficits

Part of the patient material was already involved in a study reported elsewhere (Pfurtscheller and Auer, 1983). Only patients with EIAB on one side were included in this study.

In the group of 27 patients, 5 had transitory ischemic attacks (TIA) and 22 a completed stroke. From the last group, 6 had severe, 7 moderate and 9 minor neurological deficits. The average time interval between the stroke and the operation was 2.8 months (range 6 weeks to 5 months) with the exception of 3 patients who were operated more than one year after the stroke.

Angiography

A single occlusive lesion was found in 16 patients; 13 had an internal carotid artery occlusion, one a high internal carotid stenosis and 2 a middle cerebral artery occlusion. Nine patients had a combination of two occlusive lesions: in 5 cases a carotid occlusion was combined with contralateral carotid stenosis, one patient had a middle cerebral artery occlusion and an internal carotid artery stenosis, in 3 patients internal carotid artery occlusion was combined with a vertebral artery stenosis. Multiple lesions were found in 2 patients.

Computerized tomography

Cortical infarction alone was reported in 7 patients, combined cortical and subcortical infarction in 8, and infarction of basal ganglia and/or internal capsule in 5 patients. In the last group there was also one patient with a small lesion in the medial thalamus. A normal CT scan with or without mild atrophy was found in 6 patients; severe one-sided atrophy in one.

Clinical EEG

In 17 patients, abnormal EEGs were reported, in one, no clinical EEG was available. The clinical EEG was always made before the qEEG study, usually after admission to the hospital.

Neurological outcome

The deficit of two patients improved within 24 h after operation. In two patients, the preoperative neurological deficit deteriorated reversibly, normalizing within several days. The remaining 23 patients remained unchanged during their stay in hospital. On follow-up examination 4–24 months after operation, 12 patients were fully recovered, able to lead a full and independent life with no or minimal deficit. Seven patients were minimally disabled, able to lead a full independent life with minor neurological deficit. Eight patients were moderately disabled with moderate neurological deficit or intellectual impairment but were independent. None of the patients was severely disabled and none was dependent on others to perform daily activities. Recurrent stroke occurred in one patient, ipsilateral to the first stroke.

AGE-SPECIFIC FREQUENCY

The mean EEG frequency (Sulg, 1969) correlates with the cerebral oxygen uptake and with the rCBF (Obrist et al., 1963; Ingvar et al., 1976). In old age, the cerebral blood flow (Yonekura et al., 1981), the glucose metabolism (Le Poncin-Lafitte and Rapin, 1980) and the alpha frequency (Matejcek, 1980) are diminished in parallel. Not only the frequency of the alpha rhythm, but also the sensorimotor or mu rhythm, is decreased with age (Fig. 1). This can be interpreted as the result of a slow decrease in cerebral activity in the occipital and rolandic regions with age. Based on this age dependency of the occipital alpha and central mu rhythm – both with a similar negative slope – an "age-specific frequency" (ASF) can be defined for each subject: ASF = $11.95 - 0.053 \cdot$ age (Köpruner et al., this volume).

It is of interest to compare the actual measured peak frequency in the patient group with the ASF. The average peak frequencies of our patient group measured over the affected side during rest are displayed in Fig. 1. This figure shows that on the average, the actual frequency was slightly lower than the ASF; in 4 patients the actual frequency was significantly lower ($<$ASF $-2\cdot$S.D.). Of those 4 patients, 3 were suffering from completed stroke with large cortical infarctions, but one, however, had had a TIA instead of a CS. This was unexpected, because there are grounds for the assump-

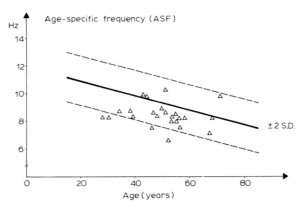

Fig. 1. The relationship between peak frequency within the alpha band and age in normals (regression line with two standard deviations is plotted), and patients with cerebrovascular insufficiency is marked by triangles. Data from 50 neurologically normal subjects; in the patient group, the frequency was measured over the affected side. All EEG recordings were done during rest.

tion that marked slowing of the EEG is due to severe impairment of perfusion combined with neurological deficits (Sulg, 1969).

Up to now no clear correlation between the deviation of the actual frequency from the ASF and clinical data, CT scan or angiographic findings has been established. However, in cases in which the frequency parameter is used for monitoring purposes, it is helpful to know the physiological range of the actual frequency.

SEVEN DAY FOLLOW-UP AFTER EIAB

Peak frequency

Characteristic for a normally functioning brain is a high degree of interhemispheric symmetry for all types of qEEG parameters (Pfurtscheller and Aranibar, 1980; Pfurtscheller et al., 1980; Van Huffelen et al., 1980). Each asymmetry above a certain level can thus be interpreted as dysfunction of neuronal tissue, for example, due to unilateral cerebral ischemia. A typical example for the strong hemispheric symmetry is displayed in Fig. 2. The bivariate distribution displays the peak frequency within the alpha band (called "peak frequency" in the following) averaged over each hemisphere in the left and right movement experiments measured in 47 neurologically normal subjects. The 80% confidence ellipse and the regression line are plotted.

The interhemispheric frequency difference and also the frequency asymmetry are enhanced in patients with unilateral cerebral ischemia, especially when the cortex is affected (Table I) and can reach 0.47 Hz on the average. This frequency asymmetry is caused mainly by a decreased frequency over the side with the cerebrovascular lesion, probably due to the lowered perfusion. Average interhemispheric frequency differences on the order of 0.20 Hz and 0.17 Hz were reported by Tolonen and Sulg (1981) and by Pfurtscheller and Auer (1983), respectively, both groups did measurements about 2 months after the cerebrovascular accident.

Bivariate frequency distributions for our patient group before and 7 days after revascularization surgery, divided into subgroups with and without cortical infarction – the latter group included the patients with infarction in the basal ganglia and/or

126

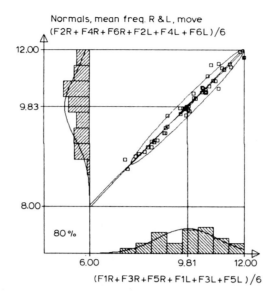

Normals, mean freq. R & L, move
(F2R + F4R + F6R + F2L + F4L + F6L)/6

(F1R + F3R + F5R + F1L + F3L + F5L)/6

Fig. 2. Bivariate distribution of the peak frequency of both centro-temporal regions in the group of 47 neurologically normal subjects. Frequency data were measured in both movement tasks and averaged for each hemisphere. The regression line and the 80% confidence ellipse are plotted.

TABLE I

MEAN INTERHEMISPHERIC PEAK FREQUENCY DIFFERENCE MEASURED IMMEDIATELY BEFORE EIAB IN A GROUP OF 26 PATIENTS. THE REFERENCE IS THE NON-OPERATED SIDE

Adapted from Pfurtscheller and Auer, 1983

	Cortical infarction (N = 15)	Non-cortical infarction (N = 11)
F ± S.D. (Hz)	−0.47 ± 0.42 $P<0.02$	+0.14 ± 0.18 N.S.

internal capsule and negative CT scan as well – are displayed in Figs. 3 and 4. The group with cortical infarction demonstrated a high interhemispheric asymmetry as compared with the frequency distribution obtained in normal subjects, displayed in Fig. 2. The frequency asymmetry of the non-cortical infarction group had values approximately between the normals and those with cortical infarction.

The comparison between pre- and postoperative frequency measurements in both groups demonstrated no difference in the subgroup without cortical infarction, but a trend to lower frequencies in the group with cortical infarction. The mean frequency difference over each hemisphere (patients with left- and right-sided ischemia mixed) was about 0.4 Hz but did not reach significance.

Measurements of the frequency change after operation separated for the affected and non-affected side in a group of 24 patients gave a significant postoperative frequency decrease over the affected (operated) side but only for the patient group with cortical infarction (Table II).

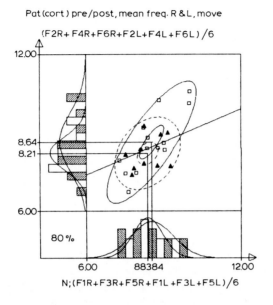

Fig. 3. Bivariate distribution of peak frequency obtained in the "cortical infarction" group before and 7 days after EIAB. Frequency parameters were averaged for each hemisphere. The 80% confidence ellipses are plotted. Data measured after revascularization are marked by black triangles.

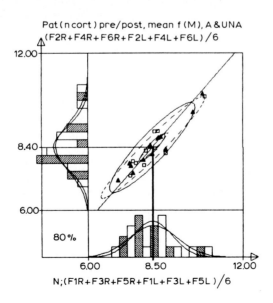

Fig. 4. As in Fig. 3, but distribution for the "non-cortical infarction" group.

TABLE II

MEAN INTERHEMISPHERIC PEAK FREQUENCY CHANGE (±S.D.) IN HZ, 7 DAYS AFTER BYPASS SURGERY COMPARED WITH THE PREOPERATIVE MEASUREMENT, FOR GROUPS OF PATIENTS WITH AND WITHOUT CORTIC-AL INFARCTION

Adapted from Pfurtscheller and Auer, 1983

	Cortical infarction (N = 14)	Non-cortical infarction (N = 10)
Operated side	-0.35 ± 0.56 $P < 0.05$	-0.09 ± 0.70 N.S.
Non-operated side	-0.18 ± 0.52 N.S.	-0.19 ± 0.76 N.S.

Frequency asymmetry index

The different degree of hemispheric asymmetry in normals, patients with cortical infarction and patients without cortical infarction, suggests the use of a suitable frequency asymmetry index to discriminate between normals and patients with mild cerebral ischemia, and to study postoperative changes in qEEG. Such an index has also the advantage of being normalized and therefore independent of the patient's age. The frequency asymmetry index (FAI) is defined in principle as the sum of the absolute values of the normalized differences of homologous derivations:

$$FAI = \sum_{i=1}^{3} \left| \frac{L_i - R_i}{L_i + R_i} \right|$$

The frequency asymmetry index measured before and 7 days after surgery, was calculated for 17 patients – spectral frequency peaks in all derivations were only detected in 17 patients – and compared with the cortical and non-cortical infarction subgroups (Table III). Seven patients demonstrated postoperatively a decreased fre-

TABLE III

CHANGES IN THE FREQUENCY ASYMMETRY INDEX (FAI), 7 DAYS AFTER BYPASS SURGERY IN THE CORTICAL AND NON-CORTICAL INFARCTION GROUP

qEEG ——————— CT	FAI decreased	FAI increased	unchanged	Σ
Cortical infarction	4	4	2	10
Non-cortical infarction	3	4	0	7
Σ	7	8	2	17

TABLE IV

FREQUENCY OF OCCURRENCE OF IMPROVEMENT (DECREASED ASYMMETRY) OR DETERIORATION (INCREASED ASYMMETRY), 7 DAYS AFTER BYPASS SURGERY IN PATIENTS SUFFERING FROM DIFFERENT CEREBRAL LESIONS. THE REFERENCE IS THE PREOPERATIVE MEASUREMENT. THE CLASSIFICATION IS BASED ON THE BIVARIATE FREQUENCY-THETA/BETA ASYMMETRY INDEX

qEEG _____ CT	Improvement	Deterioration	Equal	Σ
Cortical infarction	4	3	3	10
Non-cortical infarction	4	3	0	7
Σ	8	6	3	17

quency asymmetry; in 8 it was increased. No preference for increased or decreased asymmetry in either the cortical or non-cortical infarction group was found. This obvious contradiction – on the one hand a clear preference for a frequency decrease in patients with cortical infarction, on the other hand the same frequency of occurrence in decrease or increase of the frequency asymmetry in the cortical infarction group – can be explained by the fact that in some patients the peak frequency decreased after surgery over both hemispheres so that the frequency asymmetry was unchanged or even reduced. A frequency decrease and a reduced frequency asymmetry index can therefore be common findings after revascularization surgery; the frequency asymmetry index alone is thus an unsuitable parameter for verifying changes in neuronal dysfunction after bypass surgery.

Bivariate frequency and theta/beta asymmetry

Using the frequency asymmetry index as one parameter, another can be added for bivariate statistics. From a large group of parameters tested (Köpruner et al., this volume) the theta/beta power asymmetry index is the most suitable for discrimination between normals and patients with unilateral ischemia (Fig. 5). For this combination of parameters, specificity reached was 76% and sensitivity 82%. But the major disadvantage of this parameter combination is still that the frequency asymmetry index can only be calculated in a limited group of subjects, that is, in those showing clear peaks in the spectrum.

Using the bivariate distribution and a linear discriminant analysis, a distance function can be calculated for every pair of parameters. If this distance function is positive, the measurement is classified as "normal", if it is negative, as "abnormal". Comparison between pre- and postoperative measurements can be done by direct comparison of both distance functions. A shift of the distance function to more negative values is interpreted as deterioration, and a shift to less negative or even positive scores as normalization of brain dysfunction. The classification of the pre- and postoperative data in the cortical and non-cortical subgroups is summarized in Table IV.

130

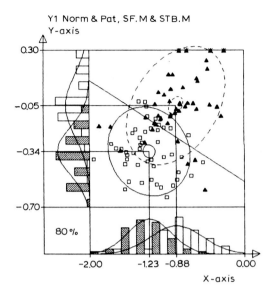

Fig. 5. Bivariate distribution of the frequency asymmetry index (*X*-axis) and the theta/beta asymmetry index (*Y*-axis) for the group of neurologically normal subjects (marked by squares) and patients with cerebrovascular insufficiency (marked by black triangles). EEG data from both movement experiments. The linear discriminant function and the 80% confidence ellipses are plotted.

TABLE V

ANALOGOUS TO TABLE IV, BUT CLASSIFICATION BY THE ERD-THETA/BETA ASYMMETRY INDEX

qEEG CT	Improvement	Deterioration	Equal	Σ
Cortical lesion alone	1	5	1	7
Subcortical lesion alone	4	1	0	5
Cortical + subcortical lesion	2	3	3	8
Atrophy	1	0	0	1
Neg. CT scan	2	3	1	6
Σ	10	12	5	27

Bivariate ERD and theta/beta asymmetry

To overcome the problem that peak frequency measurements were not possible in all patients, an ERD asymmetry index was introduced, which was measurable in all

131

subjects. The ERD data of both movement experiments, if available, are averaged, otherwise the data of the single hand movement experiment were used. The calculation of this asymmetry index (ETB) is done according to the following formula:

$$\text{ETB} = \sum_{i=1}^{3} \left(1 - \left|\frac{R_i - L_i}{R_i + L_i}\right|\right)(R_i + L_i),$$

where R and L stand for the ERD of homologous derivations. A large bilateral symmetrical ERD results in a high ETB value, whereas a small bilateral symmetrical ERD or an abolished ERD or an asymmetrical ERD – all characteristic of some abnormal brain function – results in a low ETB value. The ETB index is only valid for positive ERD values. Using this bivariate ERD theta/beta asymmetry distribution and a linear discrimination function, the specificity was 85% and sensitivity 84% (Fig. 6). As can be seen in the bivariate distribution, the theta/beta asymmetry index displayed on the x-axis is much stronger for the discrimination between normals and patients than the ERD asymmetry index as displayed on the y-axis.

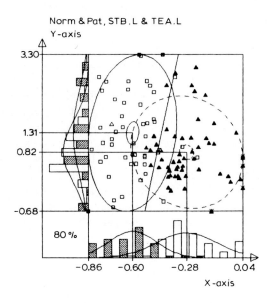

Fig. 6. See Fig. 5, but ERD asymmetry index (Y-axis) versus theta/beta asymmetry (X-axis).

To assess in detail the influence of cortical or subcortical ischemia on normalization or deterioration of brain function after EIAB, the 27 patients were divided into five groups according to the results of the CT scan: (a) patients with cortical infarction alone; (b) patients with subcortical infarction alone (infarction in basal ganglia and/or internal capsule); (c) patients with both cortical and subcortical infarction; (d) extensive atrophy only; (e) normal CT scan. The interrelationships between the morphological and functional data are summarized in Table V. Ten patients displayed a trend toward normalization and 12 a deterioration 7 days after revascularization surgery.

The only findings of interest in Table V are the relatively close correlations between pure cortical ischemia and increased hemispheric asymmetry and between pure

TABLE VI

ANALOGOUS TO TABLE IV, BUT DATA CLASSIFICATION BY THE MULTI-PARAMETRIC ASYMMETRY SCORE (MAS)

qEEG / CT	Improvement	Deterioration	Equal	Σ
Cortical lesion alone	0	6	1	7
Subcortical lesion alone	3	2	0	5
Cortical + sub-cortical lesion	3	3	2	8
Atrophy	1	0	0	1
Neg. CT scan	1	3	2	6
Σ	8	14	5	27

subcortical lesions and decreased asymmetry, respectively. This points to a trend toward normalization of brain dysfunction after revascularization surgery in patients with localized ischemia in the basal ganglia and/or internal capsule, and to a deterioration in patients with cortical ischemia without involvement of subcortical structures.

Infarction in the watershed area between the territory of the middle and anterior carotid artery was reported in the CT scan in 9 patients. Six of them displayed deterioration after surgery and only one displayed a trend toward normalization in brain dysfunction. Patients with a cortical watershed infarction thus have a risk of a postoperative deterioration of brain function.

It is of interest that the classification of the pre- and postoperative data with the frequency-free bivariate ERD-theta/beta asymmetry index produces about the same result as achieved by measuring the peak frequency alone over the operated side (Pfurtscheller and Auer, 1983). To summarize EIAB in patients with cortical ischemia usually results in a deterioration of brain function 7 days after surgery.

Multiparametric asymmetry score (MAS)

The multiparametric asymmetry score (MAS) is based on multiple asymmetry measurements using the following qEEG parameters: theta/beta power, peak frequency within the alpha band, absolute delta and theta power and the movement related blocking response (ERD). The MAS can be calculated with and without frequency measurements, from the control experiment alone or from control and movement tests together (an exact description is given in Köpruner et al., this volume). A positive MAS indicates hemispheric symmetry and a negative MAS hemispheric asymmetry. A positive score can also be interpreted as characteristic of a "normal" EEG and a negative score for an "abnormal" EEG. A shift from a positive to a negative score or from a negative to an even more negative score indicates an increased hemispheric asymmetry and a deterioration of brain function. In contrast, a less negative score or even a positive score in the postoperative measurement indicates reduced hemispheric asymmetry and a trend toward normalization of brain function. Improvement or deterioration was given only when the change of the distance function (score) was larger than 1. With the application of linear discriminant analysis and the MAS in our normal and patient data, the specificity reached 89% and the sensitivity 94%. The results of classifying patients with different types of ischemia using the MAS are summarized in Table VI.

TABLE VII

PERCENTAGES OF NEGATIVE MAS, INCREASED INTERHEMISPHERIC FREQUENCY DIFFERENCE ($\Delta f > 0.4$ Hz) AND SLOWED PEAK FREQUENCY (f < ASF$-2\cdot$S.D.) DURING THE FOLLOW-UP STUDY

		Abnormal qEEG			
	N	MAS<0	MAS<−5	Δf>0.4 Hz	f<<ASF
Pre	27	89	44	42	15
7 days	27	93	52	46	15
12 months	19	95	63	39	17
24 months	9	89%	67%	44%	11%

The data in Table VI demonstrate that 6 of the 7 patients with cortical infarction displayed postoperative deterioration and none EEG improvement. Three cases with a trend to EEG normalization were found in the subgroup with subcortical ischemia. These results are similar to those obtained by the bivariate ERD-theta/beta asymmetry index.

The classification of the 9 patients with watershed infarction demonstrated deterioration in 5 and trend towards normalization in 2 cases.

This multiparametric classification of qEEG data before and after bypass surgery demonstrates a clear preference for a postoperative deterioration in patients with cortical ischemia. This confirms the results obtained by measuring a single simple EEG parameter, namely the peak frequency within the alpha band, over the affected side (Pfurtscheller and Auer, 1983). Postoperative deterioration of brain function can therefore be detected not only by bivariate or multivariate discriminant analysis, but also by simple peak frequency measurement of the central mu rhythm.

LONG-TERM FOLLOW-UP AFTER EIAB

Peak frequency

Follow-up data up to 24 months were available in 9 patients. Serial frequency measurements from the centro-temporal derivation over the operated side obtained in 5 subjects are displayed in Fig. 7. Three patients, all with cortical ischemia (KER, GUT, KOE) demonstrated a frequency decrease 7 days after surgery. A slight frequency increase was seen in one patient with subcortical infarction (LAN). Twenty-

134

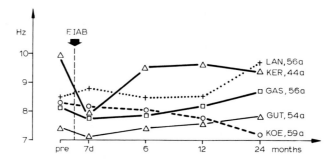

Fig. 7. Follow-up measurements of the peak frequency recorded over the affected centro-temporal region. Data from five patients after the EIAB, frequency measured during the hand movement task. Patient KOE suffered a second stroke 6 months after bypass operation.

four months after surgery, 3 patients displayed a higher and 2 a lower frequency compared with the preoperative control. One patient with a continuously decreasing frequency (KOE) suffered a second stroke 6 months and a third stroke 25 months after the anastomosis.

Fig. 8 shows frequency measurements in the mid-central channels over the operated and non-operated side in a patient with widespread cortical ischemia (KER). The early postoperative frequency decrease occurred not only over the affected but also over the unaffected side. This kind of EEG diaschisis is also found after experimental unilateral ischemia in monkeys (Jonkman et al., this volume).

The electronic measurement of the hand pressure during both voluntary hand movement experiments (Pfurtscheller and Auer, 1983) also demonstrated some decrease in left- and right-hand pressure immediately after the operation.

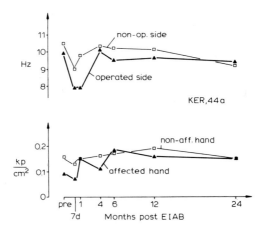

Fig. 8. Peak frequency (upper panel) and hand pressure (lower panel) follow-up measurements in one patient (KER) with extensive cortical infarction. Peak frequency measurements obtained during left hand movements in mid-central derivation, hand pressure measurements from both hands.

Bivariate frequency and theta/beta asymmetry

The bivariate data from patient KER as displayed in Fig. 9 are directly comparable with the peak frequency curves in Figs. 7 and 8. In both cases the deterioration 7 days after the revascularization and the following recovery is clearly visible. In the bivariate distribution based on data from the control experiment, the preoperative measurement had a slightly negative distance function and was therefore classified as "abnormal"; the data 24 months later had a positive distance function and were classified as "normal'.

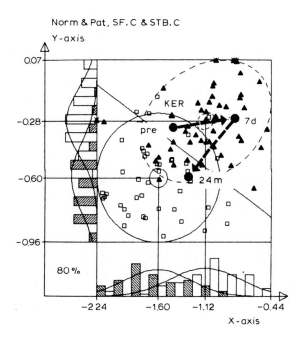

Fig. 9. Variation of the distance function (peak frequency-theta/beta asymmetry index) after EIAB in the patient KER. For further explanation see Fig. 5.

Multiparametric asymmetric score (MAS)

Follow-up EEG measurements and serial calculation of the MAS give an impression of the behavior of brain function after revascularization surgery (Figs. 10, 11 and 12).

The MAS was calculated from EEG data recorded during rest alone (stippled line) and during right- and left-handed squeezing (continuous line). The latter condition was called "physical load". In all three examples the MAS was more pronounced during load than during rest; this underlines the importance of recording the EEG not only during rest alone but also during a controlled condition, such as voluntary movement.

136

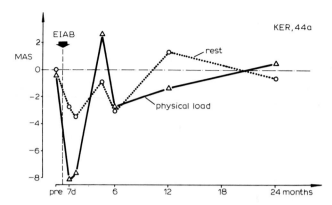

Fig. 10. Multivariate asymmetry score (MAS) measured after EIAB in one patient (KER). In one case (stippled line), the MAS was calculated from the control experiment alone (rest) *without* using the frequency parameter, in the other case (continuous line), from the control and both movement experiments (physical load) *with* the use of the peak frequency parameter. Positive MAS indicates normal, negative MAS abnormal hemispheric asymmetry.

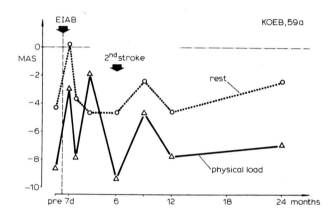

Fig. 11. MAS follow-up measurements from a patient (KOE) with cortical and subcortical infarction, who suffered further episodes. For further explanation see Fig. 10.

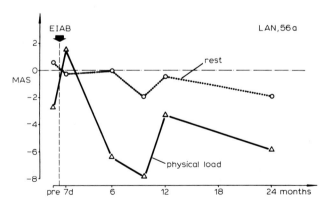

Fig. 12. MAS follow-up measurements from a patient (LAN) with a small subcortical lesion. For further explanation see Fig. 10.

The temporary deterioration after the bypass surgery in a patient with widespread cortical infarction (KER) is clearly visible in Fig. 10. In another patient (KOE) with recurrent strokes 6 and 25 months after revascularization surgery the MAS increased 7 days after surgery, but reached its lowest value 6 months later at the time of the second stroke (MAS = −9.5) and was still very low at the 24-month follow-up (MAS = −7). These low MASs 1, 6, 12 and 24 months after surgery indicate severe brain dysfunction essentially unchanged by revascularization surgery.

Normalization of brain function 7 days after bypass surgery followed by a trend to impaired brain function was found in a patient with a subcortical infarction (LAN, Fig. 12). In this patient no change in the neurological status was reported during the follow-up. Whether this more negatively directed trend of the MAS serves as risk factor for a further stroke or is the result of multi-infarct dementia, cannot be determined at this time.

The percentages of patients with a negative MAS during the follow-up study are summarized in Table VII. The number of patients with abnormal brain function (negative MAS) was about 90% in all follow-ups before and after bypass surgery. Considering only patients with a MAS < −5 (interpreted as moderate to severe brain dysfunction, cf. Köpruner et al., this volume), the percentages increase slightly from 44% to 67%, indicating a trend to more impaired brain function 24 months after the bypass operation.

In comparison to this relatively high percentage of abnormal EEGs using the multiparametric asymmetry score, an interhemispheric peak frequency difference of more than 0.4 Hz (this threshold was chosen according to the proposal of Van Huffelen et al., 1980) was found in about 40% of the patients. Comparison with the age-specific frequency (ASF) revealed a slowed central mu rhythm (f < ASF−2·S.D.) in about 15% of the patients. These three different ways of classifying an abnormal qEEG – peak frequency, interhemispheric frequency difference and multiparametric asymmetry score – demonstrate (1) the classification power of the MAS and (2) the same numbers of abnormal qEEGs before and after bypass surgery using different classification criteria.

Comparison of EEG measurements before and 12 months after surgery revealed an improvement in 6 patients (32%) and a deterioration in 10 (Table VIII). No correlation with the localization of the ischemic lesion, reported in the CT scan, could be established.

TABLE VIII

ANALOGOUS TO TABLE IV, BUT DATA CLASSIFICATION BY THE MULTI-PARAMETRIC ASYMMETRY SCORE 12 MONTHS AFTER EIAB

qEEG CT	12 months after EIAB			
	Improvement	Deterioration	Equal	Sum
Cortical lesion	4	4	1	9
Non-cortical lesion	2	6	2	10
Sum	6	10	3	19

Twenty-four-month measurements were available from only 9 subjects; here 4 patients demonstrated a trend toward normalization and 4 a deterioration compared with the preoperative control measurements. In this small group, only one patient displayed hemispheric symmetry within the range of normals (positive MAS); all others showed abnormal hemispheric asymmetry as demonstrated in Table VII.

These long-term follow-up measurements, based on the multiparametric asymmetry score, give evidence that in the majority of the patients the neuronal function in the ischemic tissue in the supply territory of the MCA has not improved, as long as it is assumed that a certain degree of hemispheric symmetry is characteristic of normal brain function, and a decreasing asymmetry characterizes normalization of neuronal function.

COMMENTS

In some patients, a contradiction exists between simple frequency measurements and the multiparametric asymmetry score (MAS) in the determination of normalization or deterioration of cerebral functioning. The frequency over the operated side was sometimes clearly increased 24 months after the ictus (an example for this is patient LAN in Fig. 7), whereas the frequency over the non-affected side remained nearly unchanged; the MAS in the same patients was more negative (example in Fig. 12) because of the increased hemispheric frequency asymmetry. The latter result is interpreted as deterioration of neuronal function whereas in the former, the frequency increase represents a trend toward normalization. This unilateral frequency increase probably indicates reperfusion of ischemic tissue in one side and thus a partial recovery of neuronal activity, whereas the increased asymmetry score still indicates a considerable degree of global or diffuse interhemispheric dysfunction. Other examples of contradiction are given by the patients KER and KOE. In both of them, the frequencies were decreased in 24 months' follow-up (Fig. 7), but the MASs during physical load were slightly less negative (Figs. 10 and 11) compared with the preoperative scores.

Frequency measurements are based on the detection of spectral peaks within the alpha band and this introduces problems. These peaks can be small or unclear (double peaks) and not always consistent in all three derivations over one side or they can even be significantly different in vertex and centro-temporal recordings. Furthermore, the frequency also changes with the state of consciousness and decreases when vigilance or attention is reduced; this means the frequency can be considerably different between the control and the left hand movement experiment when the whole recording session lasts more than one hour. All these different types of variability in frequency measurements can influence the follow-up studies and should be taken into consideration when absolute frequency measurements are interpreted and compared with the MAS. A bilateral slowing of the central alpha band activity, as is typical for a state of decreased alertness, has no influence on the MAS.

Comparisons between follow-ups of single frequency measurements and hemispheric frequency averages have shown that the former are more consistent in trend studies (compare Figs. 7 and 8) than the latter. This is somewhat surprising, but probably demonstrates the close linkage between frequency measurements using closely spaced electrodes and neuronal function in a limited region below both electrodes.

Concerning the question as to which parameter – the peak frequency or the MAS – is more suitable for monitoring cerebral functioning in follow-up studies, the preference should be given in general to the frequency, because this parameter is an absolute measurement and directly related to the physiological properties of neuronal tissue and metabolism. In this context the close correlation should again be emphasized between EEG frequency, metabolism and rCBF in normal healthy brain tissue (Obrist et al., 1963; Ingvar et al., 1979; Sulg et al., 1981). The peak frequency measurement, however, has a lot of disadvantages, as discussed above: it is only possible in a limited number of patients and it is nearly impossible in severe cerebrovascular insufficiency with dominant theta and delta activity. In these cases, the frequency-free MAS must be used.

Interhemispheric asymmetry measurements are influenced by the unilateral slowing of the sensorimotor, or mu rhythm primarily observed in the cortical-infarction group, with a maximal magnitude 7 days after surgery, followed by slow recovery. In this group of patients unilaterally enhanced sensorimotor activity was very often found in parallel with the frequency decrease, which reached a maximum not 7 days after the bypass operation, but 1 month thereafter (as can be seen in Fig. 13). This enhanced sensorimotor rhythm is in agreement with the observations of Fischgold et al. (1952), and probably identical with the "breach rhythm" reported by Cobb et al. (1979).

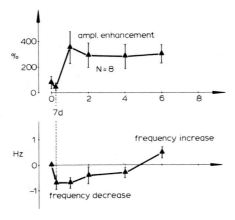

Fig. 13. Follow-up measurements of peak frequency (lower curve) and unilateral amplitude enhancement (upper curve) in eight patients with preoperative cortical infarction; means ± standard errors are displayed. (Adapted from Pfurtscheller et al., 1982.)

In contrast to the declining frequency asymmetry, the unilateral amplitude enhancement can persist much longer. These characteristic asymmetries, as reported by Pfurtscheller et al. (1982), affect essentially the multiparametric asymmetry score and probably contribute to the dissociation observed in some cases between frequency measurement and the MAS, especially in the 12- and 24-month follow-up measurements.

The meaning of a strongly negative MAS 24 months after the ictus as found in two patients with a negative CT scan and without neurological deficits and in one patient with a minor deficit (LAN, Fig. 12) is unclear and requires further observation. Whether such an increased interhemispheric asymmetry serves as a risk factor for a further stroke or is the result of multi-infarct dementia can only be answered after further qEEG and neurological follow-up studies in these patients.

The large number of patients with abnormal qEEG 12 and 24 months after the bypass operation is evidence that a functional recovery did not take place. This is confirmed by measurements of the regional cerebral blood flow 24 months after the bypass operation (Meyer et al., 1982) showing that the flow remained still lower as compared with the preoperative or initial measurement.

The MAS does not work when the perfusion is bilaterally diminished and the ischemic zones in both hemispheres are equal. This case is very unlikely because in nearly all patients occlusion and/or stenosis of cerebral vessels are never exactly symmetrical.

The ability of the MAS to detect cerebrovascular insufficiency is demonstrated by the low numbers of false negatives (3 out of 27) in our patient group and false positives (3 out of 50) in our normal reference group, although we had 5 patients with TIAs in our group. From the 9 patients with negative clinical EEG only one had a normal asymmetry score.

Besides the advantage of the MAS in discriminating between normals and patients, the MAS is also very sensitive for the detection of minor functional changes in neuronal tissue. This is demonstrated by the finding of a subgroup of patients with impairment of neuronal tissue after reperfusion of an ischemic zone, all of them with cortical infarction in the CT scan. This correlation between morphological and functional findings is not just chance, but for the first time gives evidence for the disturbance of neuronal tissue in the region of reperfused cortical ischemic zones.

We believe that around a cortical infarct a zone of hypoperfused brain tissue may exist that is more vulnerable to a further reduction of perfusion during clamping of an MCA branch and performance of the anastomosis, as compared to normal brain tissue. After the unclamping of the anastomosed MCA branch, the ischemic brain tissue is reperfused and the perfusion pressure suddenly increases. This could result in edema and thus affect neuronal activity. This phenomenon has been called "normal perfusion-pressure breakthrough" under the similar pathophysiological circumstances of arteriovenous malformations (Spetzler et al., 1978).

The impairment of neuronal tissue as a result of an EIAB can be either of short duration (weeks) or long lasting (up to 12 months), as found in one patient (Pfurtscheller and Auer, 1983). The latter case, however, most likely represents a combination of the above-mentioned hypothesized pathophysiological events with other unknown processes. We do not know which factors – such as age, duration of the clamping, size of the cortical infarction, etc. – are responsible for a fast, slow or even an absence of recovery after local neuronal impairment due to an EIAB. It must be stressed, however, that this deterioration in EEG and brain function was never accompanied by clinical deterioration, thus suggesting the assumption of very faint edema formation, resolved in the course of 1–2 weeks.

Measurements of regional cerebral blood flow (rCBF) following EIAB have shown a statistically significant increase of 12.8% on the bypassed side and 8% on the contralateral side 3 months after surgery (Meyer et al., 1982). A similar flow increase several months after surgery was also reported by Halsey et al. (1982) and Hungerbuhler et al. (1981). But there are also reports showing no significant increase of rCBF either 10 days or 3 months after the operation (Veering et al., 1983). These blood flow measurements, all performed with the 133-xenon technique, give no clear evidence for a redistribution of blood flow after EIAB with increases in both hemispheres.

rCBF measurements may indirectly represent the level of neuronal activity, but they are only valid in non-ischemic, non-hypoxic brain tissue. In ischemic tissue, however, this coupling between flow and function of nervous tissue can be disturbed (Baron et al., 1981; Ingvar, 1981), a phenomenon also known as "luxury perfusion syndrome" (Lassen, 1966). Under certain circumstances a discrepancy can exist between the EEG, directly reflecting neuronal activity and metabolism and the rCBF, as an indirect measurement of neuronal activity. This discrepancy may well be possible within the first week after EIAB, that is, an assumed increased rCBF and deterioration of brain function as indicated by our qEEG measurements. This decoupling between flow and function of nervous tissue seems to occur more frequently in patients with cortical ischemia than in all other types of patients. This will confirm the hypothesis that in the patients with cortical infarction, nervous tissue is disturbed temporarily by tissue hypoxia caused by clamping and/or reperfusion during EIAB operations.

SUMMARY

In a group of 27 patients, most of them with minor unilateral cerebral ischemia, and all undergoing extracranial–intracranial arterial bypass operation (EIAB), qEEG follow-up studies were made before and after revascularization. Peak frequencies within the alpha band and different hemispheric asymmetry parameters were calculated from centro-temporal EEG recordings and used for the assessment of postoperative changes in bioelectrical brain activity. Increased peak frequency or decreased hemispheric asymmetry was defined as an improvement, and decreased peak frequency or increased asymmetry as deterioration of brain function. Peak frequency asymmetry, bivariate frequency-theta/beta asymmetry, ERD (blocking response due to movement)-theta/beta asymmetry and the multiparametric asymmetry score (MAS) based on the parameters theta/beta, peak frequency, absolute delta and theta power and ERD, were used and compared before and after surgery. The most effective parameter for the differentiation between normal and ischemic brain was the MAS, reaching a specificity of 89% and a sensitivity of 94%. Seven days after EIAB, a clear deterioration was found in the subgroup of patients with cortical infarction, probably due to clamping of a branch of the MCA and/or reperfusion of an ischemic area. Twelve months after surgery only 6 patients out of 19 (32%) demonstrated improved brain function, and 24 months after surgery only 4 patients out of 9; only one patient displayed hemispheric symmetry within the range of the normal subjects 24 months after surgery.

Both the multiparametric asymmetry score and the simple peak frequency measurement of the sensimotor (mu) rhythm are sensitive qEEG parameters, and are therefore suitable for follow-up studies after EIAB and perhaps also for detecting minor changes in localized brain function due to revascularization surgery.

ACKNOWLEDGEMENT

The authors wish to thank G. Lindinger, W. Reczek and Mrs. E. Mandl for the

142

EEG recordings, Dr. H. Schneider for doing the CT reports, Dr. R. Oberbauer for clinical examinations and some of the operations and M. Wlasich for preparation of the figures. The investigation was supported by the "Fonds zur Förderung der wissenschaftlichen Forschung", Projekt Nr. 4593.

REFERENCES

Austin, G., Laffin, D. and Hayward, W. (1974) Physiological factors in the selection of patients for superficial temporal artery to middle cerebral artery anastomosis. *Surgery*, 75: 861–868.

Baron, J.C., Bousser, M.G., Comar, D., Soussaline, F. and Castaigne, P. (1981) Noninvasive tomographic study of cerebral blood flow and oxygen metabolism in vivo. Potentials, limitations and clinical applications in cerebral ischemic disorders. *Europ. Neurol.*, 20: 273–284..

Birchfield, R.I., Wilson, W.P. and Heyman, A. (1959) An evaluation of electroencephalography in cerebral infarction and ischemia due to arteriosclerosis. *Neurology*, 9: 859–870.

Cobb, W.A., Guiloff, R.J. and Cast, J. (1979) Breach rhythm: The EEG related to skull defects. *Electroenceph. clin. Neurophysiol.*, 47: 251–271.

Duym, B.W. and Pfurtscheller, G. (1984) Measurement of the quality of hand contractions. *Med. Biol. Eng. Comp.*, in press.

Enge, S., Lechner, H., Logar, Ch. and Ladurner, G. (1980) Clinical value of EEG in transient ischemic attacks. In H. Lechner and A. Aranibar (Eds.), *EEG and Clinical Neurophysiology*, Excerpta Medica, Amsterdam–Oxford–Princeton, pp. 173–180.

Fischgold, H., Pertuiset, B. and Arfel-Capdeveille, G. (1952) Quelques particularités électroencéphalographiques au niveau des brèches et des volets neurochirurgicaux. *Rev. neurol.*, 86: 126–132.

Halsey, Jr., J.H., Morawetz, R.B. and Blauenstein, U.W. (1982) The hemodynamic effect of STA–MCA bypass. *Stroke*, 13: 163–167.

Hungerbuhler, J.P., Younkin, D., Reivich, M., Obrist, W.D., O'Conner, M., Goldberg, H., Gordon, J., Gur, R., Hurtig, H. and Amarneck, W. (1981) The effect of STA–MCA anastomosis on rCBF, neurologic and neurophysiologic function in patients with completed strokes. In J.S. Meyer, H. Lechner, M. Reivich, E.O. Ott and A. Aranibar (Eds.), *Cerebral Vascular Disease, Vol. 3*, 10th Salzburg Conference, Excerpta Medica, Amsterdam, pp. 73–75.

Ingvar, D.H. (1981) Measurements of regional cerebral blood flow and metabolism in psychopathological states. *Europ. Neurol.*, 20: 294–296.

Ingvar, D.H., Sjölund, B. and Ardö, A. (1976) Correlation between dominant EEG frequency, cerebral oxygen uptake and blood flow. *Electroenceph. clin. Neurophysiol.*, 41: 268–276.

Ingvar, D.H., Rosen, J. and Johannesson, G. (1979) EEG related to cerebral metabolism and blood flow. *Pharmakopsychiat.*, 12: 200–209.

Lassen, N.A. (1966) The luxury-perfusion syndrome and its possible relation to acute metabolic acidosis localized within the brain. *Lancet*, ii: 1113–1115.

Lassen, N.A. (1982) Incomplete cerebral infarction – focal incomplete ischemic tissue necrosis not leading to emollision. *Stroke*, 13: 522–523.

Le Poncin-Lafitte, M. and Rapin, J.R. (1980) Age-associated changes in deoxyglucose uptake in whole brain. *Gerontology*, 26: 265–269.

Matejcek, M. (1980) Cortical correlates of the aging process as revealed by quantitative EEG, the value of quantitative EEG in evaluating the effects of treatment. *Proc. Int. Cerebrovasc.* Diseases SIR, Pergamon, Oxford, 55–66.

Meyer, J.S., Nakajima, S., Okabe, T., Amano, T., Centeno, R., Lee, Y.Y., Levine, J., Levinthal, R. and Rose, J. (1982) Redistribution of cerebral blood flow following STA–MCA by-pass in patients with hemispheric ischemia. *Stroke*, 13: 744–784.

Obrist, W.D., Sokoloff, L., Lassen, N.A., Lane, M.H., Butler, R.N. and Feinberg, I. (1963) Relation of EEG to cerebral blood flow and metabolism in old age. *Electroenceph. clin. Neurophysiol.*, 15: 610–619.

Pfurtscheller, G and Aranibar, A. (1977) Event-related cortical desynchronization deteced by power measurements of scalp EEG. *Electroenceph. clin. Neurophysiol.*, 42: 817–826.

Pfurtscheller, G. and Aranibar, A. (1979) Evaluation of event-related desynchronization (ERD) preceding and following self-paced movement. *Electroenceph. clin. Neurophysiol.*, 46: 138–147.

Pfurtscheller, G. and Aranibar, A. (1980) Voluntary movement ERD: normative studies. In G. Pfurtscheller, B. Buser, F.H. Lopes da Silva and H. Petsche (Eds.), *Rhythmic EEG Activities and Cortical Functioning*, Elsevier, Amsterdam, pp. 151–177.

Pfurtscheller, G. and Auer, L. (1983) Frequency changes of sensorimotor EEG rhythm after revascularization surgery. *Electroenceph. clin. Neurophysiol.*, 55: 381–387.

Pfurtscheller, G., Wege, W. and Sager, W. (1980) Asymmetrien in der zentralen Alpha-Aktivität (My-Rhythmus) unter Ruhe- und Aktivitätsbedingungen bei zerebrovaskulären Erkrankungen, *Z. EEG-EMG*, 11: 63–71.

Pfurtscheller, G., Auer, L. and Oberbauer, R. (1982) The influence of skull defects and reperfusion after extra-intracranial arterial bypass surgery on the sensorimotor EEG rhythm. *Neurology*, 45: 1106–1112.

Schmiedek, P., Gratzl, O., Spetzler, R., Steinhoff, H., Enzenbach, R., Brendel, W. and Marguth, F. (1976) Selection of patients for extra-intracranial arterial by-pass surgery based on rCBF measurements. *J. Neurosurg.*, 44: 303–312.

Spetzler, R.F., Wilson, C.B., Weinstein, P., Mehdorn, M., Townsend, J. and Telles, D. (1978) Normal perfusion pressure breakthrough theory. *Clin. Neurosurg.*, 25: 651–672.

Sulg, I.A. (1969) The quantitated EEG as a measure of brain dysfunction. Thesis. *Scand. J. clin. Lab. Invest.*, 23, Suppl: 1–110.

Sulg. I.A., Sotaniemi, K.A., Tolonen, U. and Hokkanen, E. (1981) Dependence between cerebral metabolism and blood flow as reflected in the quantitative EEG. *Advanc. biol. Psychiat.*, 6: 102–108.

Tolonen, U. and Sulg, I.A. (1981) Comparison of quantitative EEG parameters from four different analysis techniques in evaluation of relationships between EEG and CBF in brain infarction. *Electroenceph. clin. Neurophysiol.*, 51: 177–185.

Van Huffelen, A.C., Poortvliet, D., Van der Wulp, C. and Magnus, O. (1980) Quantitative EEG in cerebral ischemia. A. Parameters for the detection of abnormalities in "normal" EEGs in patients with acute unilateral cerebral ischemia. In H. Lechner and A. Aranibar (Eds.), *EEG and Clinical Neurophysiology*, Excerpta Medica, Amsterdam, pp. 125–130.

Veering, M.M., Mosmans, P.C.M., de Weerd, A.W. and Jonkman, E.J. (1983) Effect of STA–MCA anastomosis (EC-IC bypass) and carotid endarterectomy on rCBF. *J. Cereb. Blood Flow Metab.*, 3, Suppl. 1: 604–605.

Yasargil, M.G. (1969) Diagnosis and indications for operations in cerebrovascular disease. In M.G. Yasargil (Ed.), *Microsurgery Applied to Neurosurgery*, Thieme, Stuttgart, pp. 95–119.

Yonekura, M., Austin, G., Poll, N. and Hayward, W. (1981) Evaluation of cerebral blood flow in patients with transient ischemic attacks and minor stroke. *Surg. Neurol.*, 15: 58–65.

Zumstein, B. and Yasargil, M.G. (1980) Verbesserung der Hindurchblutung durch mikrochirurgische Bypass-Anastomosen. *Bull. Schweiz. Akad. Med. Wiss.*, 36: 209–222.

Brain Ischemia: Quantitative EEG and Imaging Techniques, Progress in Brain Research, Vol. 62, edited by
G. Pfurtscheller, E.J. Jonkman and F.H. Lopes da Silva
©1984 Elsevier Science Publishers B.V.

EEG and CBF in Cerebral Ischemia. Follow-up Studies in Humans and Monkeys

E.J. JONKMAN[1], A. VAN DIEREN[2], M.M. VEERING[1], L. PONSEN[1], F.H. LOPES DA SILVA[3] and C.A.F. TULLEKEN[4]

[1]*Research Group for Clinical Neurophysiology, TNO, Westeinde Ziekenhuis, Lijnbaan 32, 2512 VA, The Hague,* [2]*Institute of Medical Physics, TNO, Utrecht,* [3]*Neurophysiology Group, Department of Zoology, University of Amsterdam, Kruislaan 320, Amsterdam, and* [4]*Department of Neurosurgery, University Hospital, Utrecht (The Netherlands)*

INTRODUCTION

The necessity of follow-up studies in humans and animals

It would be useful when the changes in cerebral function occurring during cerebral ischemia and/or during the recovery period after cerebral ischemia could be monitored in an objective way. Such monitoring profiles could be important in evaluating the effect of proposed therapeutic measures such as induced metabolic changes, administration of drugs and surgical procedures, e.g. superficial temporal artery (STA) – middle cerebral artery (MCA) anastomoses.

In monitoring aspects of cerebral function during ischemia we should consider not only the group of stroke patients but also those patients in whom a cerebral ischemia either is induced over a short period of time (e.g. during carotid surgery or open-heart surgery), or occurs over a very long period of time (e.g. patients with multi-infarct dementia).

The techniques for short- or long-term monitoring should be non-invasive, atraumatic and not too expensive. The EEG and evoked potential (EP) measurements as well as some methods of CBF measurement fulfill these requirements.

For the individual patient, only the clinical outcome is of importance. Clinical scales, such as the one proposed by Valdimarsson (1982) are important instruments for follow-up studies. However, such scales have two major drawbacks. An observer-bound subjective element is always present, while the inter-observer reliability of such scales is often not consistent. Moreover, these clinical scales are not applicable to animals.

"Certain physiological and chemical studies cannot be done in humans. Thus it is important to known in what way experimental models of ischemia are similar to or differ from strokes in humans" (Waltz, 1979). This applies also to the technical aspects of follow-up studies: we have to ascertain whether the follow-up parameters we want to use in animals are applicable to humans.

Apart from a short literature review, this preliminary study will deal with the follow-up study of EEG and CBF in patients with strokes in the territory of the MCA compared with monkeys studied before and after occlusion of the middle cerebral artery. One of the aims of these experiments was to establish whether the induced ischemia in monkeys could be considered an appropriate model for the spontaneous ischemia occurring in man.

EEG follow-up studies, a short literature review

The value of EEG follow-up studies (monitoring) during carotid endarterectomy is well established. Sundt et al. (1974) studied 93 patients during carotid clamping. Twenty-five patients developed major ipsilateral EEG changes during the procedure. These changes were reversible after shunting and the patients awoke without new neurological deficits. In all these cases the CBF appeared to be $\leq$ 18 ml/100 g/min. In this situation the EEG was a reliable predictor for an important decrease in CBF (see also Trojaborg and Boysen, 1973). In a larger series, Chiappa et al. (1979) confirmed that EEG abnormalities during clamping were reversible after shunting except in one patient (out of 32), who had indeed a poor outcome. These authors considered the use of EEG spectral analysis as an important improvement, notwithstanding the fact that the spectra were only interpreted visually.

An extensive survey of the possibilities of EEG monitoring during open-heart surgery was recently published by Pronk (1982). The different approaches for detecting EEG abnormalities were carefully analyzed but the value for the individual patient has not yet been determined.

The literature concerning serial EEG recordings in stroke patients is surprisingly limited. Original studies (visual inspection only) were done by Roseman et al. (1951) and Silverman (1960) among others. Cohen et al. (1976) studied 26 CVA patients and 26 controls. Serial EEGs for all patients were recorded at 72-h intervals. Frequency bands were determined by the zero-crossing technique. The greatest deviation from controls was found in the delta band (occipital and temporal derivations). In all CVA patients, the delta activity decreased with recovery, increased in those patients who became worse or died, and remained relatively unchanged in patients with a stable clinical condition. It appeared that the changes in delta activity preceded the changes in clinical course. Kayser-Gatchalian and Neundorfer (1980) did a prospective study of 79 stroke patients. All patients were examined within 2 days after the CVA, on the 10th day and on the 22nd day. It became evident that background changes in the initial EEG (visual inspection) gave reliable information about the clinical course of the ischemic accident. The EEG course correlated significantly with the clinical course. Focal EEG changes had no prognostic value.

Analyzing the spectra of 20 stroke patients, van Huffelen et al. (1980) came to the conclusion that parameters valuable for follow-up studies appeared to be the relative delta 2 power asymmetry (2–3.4 Hz) and the peak frequency of the alpha rhythm.

The effect on the EEG of STA–MCA anastomosis was studied by de Weerd et al. (1982) and compared with the EEG changes occurring in a group of non-surgical stroke patients. The only EEG parameter showing more improvement in the operated group was the relative alpha 2 power: alpha 2/(alpha 1 + alpha 2).

To our knowledge there is no literature available on EEG follow-up studies over longer time intervals, e.g. in normal aging vs. Alzheimer or multi-infarct dementia.

Some literature on CBF follow-up studies

The reproducibility of CBF measurements with the inhalation method can be described as satisfactory, although the error of measurement is higher than in studies with the intra-arterial method (Ingvar, 1975). However, nowadays repeated studies on separate days with the intra-arterial method are considered impermissible on ethical grounds. On the other hand, the inhalation method can be used in serial measurements bilaterally without any danger to the patient. Therefore we shall restrict ourselves here to describing a few follow-up studies done with the inhalation method.

Follow-up studies in stroke patients were done by several authors including Slater et al. (1977), who were especially interested in flow changes occurring in the non-ischemic hemisphere. They could prove that a decrease in CBF in the contralateral hemisphere occurred in 12 out of 15 patients. This CBF diaschisis did not reach its peak at the onset of the stroke but appeared to increase during the first week. A similar time course was found in the decrease in flow in the ischemic hemisphere and the flow changes appeared to take place in parallel in both hemispheres ($r = 0.846$; $p<0.001$).

Tolonen et al. (1981) studied the changes in rCBF in non-surgical patients with unilateral ischemia. They found no changes in the rCBF in the 3 months following the ischemia. This finding was confirmed by Demeurisse et al. (1983), who studied 30 stroke patients until 90 days after the stroke. The clinical improvement was not accompanied by a progressive normalization of the CBF at rest. No relation was found between the clinical data and the CBF values.

Many authors have used CBF follow-up studies to determine the effect of STA–MCA anastomoses. After bypass operations, Halsey et al. (1982) found a gradual progressive increase in flow in both hemispheres, but more pronounced on the operated side. These authors concluded however, that bypass surgery does not substantially affect the flow changes. They considered the flow increase to depend more on progressive recovery from the original disability than on the surgical intervention. Meyer et al. (1982) found a significant flow increase 1–2 weeks after bypass operations. Three months after the operation the trend toward increased flow was still present, but not thereafter. In a control group (medically treated stroke patients), serial flow values showed no significant increase but a trend toward decrease at 30 months was evident in both operated and non-operated groups.

In our laboratory, de Weerd et al. (1982) also did a controlled study on the effect of STA–MCA anastomoses. They found no difference in the rCBF parameters (Initial Slope Index, Initial Slope Index Asymmetry) between the operated and non-operated groups after 3 months. Veering et al. (1983) did a prospective study to measure changes in rCBF after surgical intervention (STA–MCA anastomoses and carotid endarterectomies). The patency of the anastomoses and the reconstructed carotid arteries could be proven by ultrasound at the time of the last CBF measurements (3 months after operation). A consistent beneficial effect of the surgery on the rCBF parameters could not be proven for either of the two operated groups.

The publications mentioned above are only to be considered as examples (for a complete list of relevant literature see Veering et al., 1983). We just want to stress the fact that follow-up rCBF studies are now possible but do not always lead to the results expected on clinical grounds. Moreover, especially in the STA–MCA bypass studies, the results presented by different authors are sometimes contradictory.

Electrophysiological function and cerebral blood flow

For follow-up studies on the effect of spontaneous and experimental ischemia it is important to decide whether it is necessary to monitor both the EEG and CBF. If a very close correlation between both methods does exist, then it would suffice to measure either the EEG parameters or the CBF parameters. In such a situation, especially in ischemic patients, the EEG would presumably be the method of choice, taking into consideration the ease of EEG recording.

It is well known that severe ischemia produces deterioration of the EEG pattern. In man, slowing of the EEG occurs when rCBF falls to 16–22 ml/100 g/min and flattening is seen when the rCBF decreases to 11–19 ml/100 g/min (Trojaborg and Boysen, 1973). These findings are in accordance with those of Sundt et al. (1974): to sustain a normal EEG, the CBF must be at least 18 ml/100 g/min at a PCO_2 of 40 torr. Such a threshold level does not, however, exclude a linear relationship.

In a small group of patients with occlusion of the MCA, Sulg and Ingvar (1968, see also Ingvar and Sulg, 1969) found that the rCBF correlated with the frequency index of the EEG ($r = 0.5$). Mosmans (1974) studied the rCBF and EEG simultaneously in 36 patients. In patients with diffuse EEG abnormalities, a correlation coefficient of 0.624 ($p<0.003$) between CBF values and EEG score was found. In patients with local EEG disturbances the correlation between local EEG scores and mean regional rCBF was weaker than for the cases with diffuse abnormalities ($r = 0.351$; $p<0.005$). Mosmans concluded that as could be expected, a deterioration of the brain by either diffuse or local pathological processes, tends to lead to a decrease in blood flow and an increase in EEG abnormality, but beyond this there seemed to be no direct coupling between the results of the EEG and CBF measurement methods.

Ingvar et al. (1976) established a good correlation ($r = 0.76$; $p<0.001$) between the CBF and the mean EEG frequency in chronic, mainly psychiatric, patients.

In patients with one-sided ischemic lesions, Tolonen et al. (1981) found a correlation of $r = 0.60$; $p<0.01$ between the mean rCBF and the power spectral density frequency and a negative correlation between mean rCBF and percentage of delta activity ($r = -0.75$; $p<0.001$). Over the non-infarcted hemisphere, however, no significant correlations were found between mean rCBF and diverse EEG parameters.

From these publications we gather the impression that with diffuse cerebral disturbances there is a correlation between EEG and CBF. If one studies local disturbances, this relation is less evident. Such a divergence could be due to a luxury-perfusion syndrome, but other factors may also be of importance, such as the type of lesion, the rapidity of onset and the delay between onset of the lesion and the time of the measurement (Jonkman et al., 1970; Mosmans, 1974).

In experimental ischemia in cats (Tulleken et al., 1978, 1982), it appeared that a significant decrease in rCBF was in almost all experimental situations accompanied by a significant decrease in EEG mean power. Amazingly, a significant increase in delta activity could not be demonstrated in these anesthetized cats. In anesthetized ischemic cats, Hossmann and Schuier (1980) also found a gradual decrease of EEG intensity over the whole range of flow values studied. A definite threshold for the appearance of EEG changes could not be established because of the great scatter of individual values. In contrast, the EEG frequency index was little affected, indicating that the EEG flattened but did not slow down. Date et al. (1983) found that in cats the EEG intensity began to decrease at about 30 mm Hg pial pressure (i.e. 47% of control pial pressure).

The evoked responses, especially the somatosensory evoked responses, are easier to quantify than the EEG. In 1974, Branston et al. found that the evoked potential was not affected in baboons if the flow was greater than about 16 ml/100 g/min but was abolished at flows less than about 12 ml/100 g/min. The rate of depression was highly and significantly correlated with the residual flow. As Symon (1975) pointed out, this flow level agrees reasonably with the CBF necessary for maintaining the spontaneous EEG in man. In baboons (and in man) the incomplete recovery of evoked responses after ischemia may be used as an indicator for irreversible anoxic damage (Branston et al., 1976). Strong et al. (1977) found that in baboons, lowering of the rCBF was accompanied by evoked potential failure before any massive increase in extracellular potassium occurred.

Apart from amplitude changes, latency changes in the evoked potential can occur during ischemia. Early changes seen in ischemia are conduction delays which correlate well with mild white matter ischemia; amplitude reductions in the cortical component of the evoked potential begin when significant cortical ischemia occurs (Lesnick et al., 1983). Finally, it must be noted that the thalamus and medial lemniscus are, at least as judged by evoked potential studies, less sensitive to ischemia than cortical structures (Branston et al., 1983, see also Lopes da Silva et al., this volume).

In summary, there may be a good relation between EEG and evoked potentials on the one hand, and the mean rCBF on the other, but only at very low rCBF values (< 20 ml/100 g/min). At higher rCBF values, the correlation is generally too weak to permit use of one parameter to make a reliable prediction of the other. Both types of measurement should be used simultaneously in the study of spontaneous or experimental ischemia.

The ischemic "penumbra" can be defined as the condition of the ischemic brain with a flow between the threshold of electrical failure and the threshold of energy failure and ion pump failure (Astrup et al., 1981). In primates, this CBF interval will be rather small, as we can conclude from Branston's work. However, the important clinical implications of the existence of such a "penumbra" are an extra reason for combining electrophysiological and CBF parameters in experimental ischemia.

METHODOLOGY

EEG methodology

It is beyond the scope of this article to give a complete review of the many computerized techniques for quantification of the EEG. Notwithstanding the substantial effort of many research centers in this field, it must be pointed out that there is as yet no general agreement about the relative values of some of these methods (Tolonen, 1981). It seems a well-established fact that some ways of quantifying the EEG lead to results that are in good agreement with the visual assessment of the EEG and often are more sensitive indicators for detecting cerebral lesions in the EEG, especially in patients with small vascular lesions or non-destructive space-occupying lesions (Gotman et al., 1975; Binnie et al., 1978; van Huffelen, 1980).

In most cases the search for optimal parameters is guided by the need for improvement of diagnostic possibilities of the EEG. It is by no means certain that parameters that attain a good score in such studies are also the best ones for follow-up studies. In the following paragraphs we shall limit ourselves to a few remarks concerning some methods now in general use.

Spectral parameters

A large number of parameters can be obtained from the spectral values obtained by FFT of the EEG signal. We mention among others the absolute and relative band power values, the quotients of different band power values, asymmetry values of band powers, total or mean power, peak frequencies, peak asymmetries and coherence functions. A major drawback of the absolute power per frequency band is that the interindividual variations are rather large. Taking into account the age of the patient, the relative power per frequency band shows a smaller spread and this parameter has proven to be useful for diagnostic procedures. However, a major disadvantage is that this parameter is less interesting when an (ischemic) disorder results in an increase or decrease of power in all frequency bands. Both measures can be used per electrode position or for each electrode position compared with the same position on the contralateral hemisphere. Such asymmetry indices have the advantage that they are useful for the detection of one-sided ischemia but they can produce misleading results when a one-sided lesion induces severe abnormalities on the contralateral side as well.

Quotients of band power values and asymmetry values of these quotients have proven their value in the detection of one-sided supratentorial brain lesions (Gotman et al., 1975). A difficulty in the use of spectral band power parameters is that these parameters do not show a normal distribution in a normal population. Thanks to the studies of John (1980) and Gasser et al. (1982), it seems clear that a transformation of the sample data may bring them much closer to a normal distribution. For the relative band power the $\ln X(1-X)$ transformation is suggested by both authors mentioned above (X being the relative band power). For the absolute band power (Y), was $\ln (Y)$ the best transformation found, but this transformation was not fully satisfactory for all frequency bands (Gasser et al., 1982).

The asymmetries of peak frequencies are extremely useful for the diagnosis of (ischemic) lesions (van Huffelen 1980; van Huffelen et al., this volume). For follow-up studies, peak frequencies and peak frequency asymmetries are interesting parameters in some patients, but in other patients apparently do not change over a long period after the ischemic insult (van Huffelen, 1980). Moreover, these parameters cannot be used in animal studies when the animal is awake and alert with the eyes open.

As yet, interhemispheric coherence values do not seem to have any value for diagnosis or follow-up.

Finally, we must draw attention to the importance of changes in spectral power values caused by external influences. "Event-related desynchronization" can be described as such; this is the reactivity of the central mu rhythm to sensorimotor activation and the reactivity of the alpha rhythm to visual activation. The first type of desynchronization was studied by Pfurtscheller (Pfurtscheller et al., 1981; Pfurtscheller and Auer, 1983), the second by van Huffelen et al. (this volume).

Time domain parameters

Hjorth (1970, 1973) made a major contribution to automatic EEG analysis by introducing the normalized slope descriptors "activity", "mobility" and "complexity". These parameters are derived from the signal description in the time domain but may also be calculated in the frequency domain from spectral moments of the power density spectrum or autospectrum. One of the advantages of this method is the possibility for on-line measurements in multichannel recordings using equipment that is relative simple and inexpensive.

In the work of Tolonen and Sulg (1980), the Hjorth parameters were compared with spectral density and other variables. The correlation between mean rCBF with the mean frequency of the power density estimation was higher than the correlation with the mobility (0.60 and 0.46, respectively). The correlation of activity and complexity with the mean rCBF was low (−0.11 and −0.39). This seems to devaluate the method but one has to realize that in this study the mean rCBF is taken as the "golden standard", which is disputable because of the well-known divergences between rCBF and EEG results (see section on Electrophysiological function and cerebral blood flow, p. 148).

The relative value of parameters may to a large extent depend on the clinical or experimental situation. Pronk (1982) made a very comprehensive evaluation of EEG processing in cardiac surgery. Four processing methods were used: zero-crossing analysis, spectral analysis, analysis by Hjorth's slope descriptors and autoregressive filtering (Kalman coefficients). The total percentage of correctly classified normal and abnormal EEG patterns was about the same for the Hjorth descriptors and the period/amplitude features and slightly poorer for the spectral features and the Kalman filter coefficients. In such a situation, the use of zero-crossing techniques or the use of Hjorth's parameters is preferable but as Pronk rightly points out, "the lack of specificity of the analysis methods can be explained by the fact that during open heart surgery the abnormal patterns have rather simple characteristics, namely a decrease in frequency and/or a decrease in amplitude".

Multidimensional parameter scoring

The spectral analysis of a multichannel recording leaves us with a huge amount of data (see section on spectral parameters, p. 150). John (1981) established one way to achieve a data reduction. To apply multidimensional parameter analysis, it is necessary to examine the parameters of possible interest in a normal population. For each feature (if necessary after transformation, see p. 150), mean and standard deviations are calculated for all age groups. When these data are known, each value from each individual patient can be Z-transformed relative to these norms. An "abnormality matrix" can be constructed with the resulting Z-values. From this matrix abnormality indices can be calculated taking into account the correlations between different features for different electrode positions as established in the normal population. Relative power values, coherences and asymmetry values for example, can be so combined for one or several electrode positions.

In our laboratory, Poortvliet was able to prove that the age regression coefficients for the different parameters show only minor differences when studied in the U.S.A. and The Netherlands with different populations of normals. Gasser and Mocks (1983) recently published their results with non-metric multidimensional scaling and principal component analysis in order to achieve a general means of comparing groups and

152

identifying subgroups.

Although good results have been obtained by John in identifying groups of normal children vs. groups of children with learning disorders, it is not known yet if this approach is reliable in the diagnosis of cerebral ischemia and suitable for follow-up studies.

Conclusion

It is not yet clear which method should be preferred for EEG follow-up in spontaneous and experimental ischemia. Since all the methods discussed above are interrelated (Lopes da Silva, 1982) it seems wise to use the more general one: spectral analysis. The time domain analysis techniques are certainly valuable but the resulting information is more limited. In the long run, one would expect the best results from multidimensional scoring techniques.

CBF Methodology

CBF studies in humans

Since the clinical benefit to the individual patient derived from intra-arterial CBF studies is as yet extremely small, we consider it unethical to use such methods for follow-up studies. This leaves us with those methods that are based on the inhalation technique or on the intravenous administration of xenon-133. At the moment there are four methods available which could be used for follow-up studies:

1) Flow measurements based on the contrast properties of stable xenon gas as measured by CT scanning (Drayer et al., 1978; Meyer et al., 1981). This technique has the advantage of measuring superficial as well as deep structures of the brain and like all other tomographic techniques, it is not bothered by the "look-through" phenomenon. Problems are, however, the signal to noise ratio, the cost of xenon, the anesthetic properties of xenon of high concentrations and the limited time available for research in most CT departments.

2) Positron emission tomography (PET), which can provide data on CBF as well as on metabolism. The high cost involved in PET scanning is still prohibitive for most clinical centers.

3) Single photon emission tomography based on xenon-133 clearance is a very promising technique and is relatively cheaper. The spatial resolution, however, is still limited (Lassen, 1981).

4) The inhalation/intravenous method with xenon-133 and fixed detectors as originally developed by Mallet and Veal and made suitable for practical clinical use by Obrist et al. (1975) and Risberg et al. (1975). This technique is very simple and can be used for routine examinations but has severe limitations. The most important limitation is caused by the "look-through" phenomenon. Halsey et al. (1981) proved that it was necessary to combine many parameters derived from this kind of flow measurement to make an acceptably accurate lateralization in patients with one-sided ischemia. Indeed, we agree with Halsey that asymmetries in flow measurements may be more important for diagnostic purposes than measurements of absolute values.

Notwithstanding the limitations of the inhalation technique it appears that this technique may be useful for various clinical purposes (Meyer, 1978). For our study it was especially important that Slater et al. (1977) found indications of the existence of a flow decrease over the contralateral hemisphere after a one-sided stroke. This observation was made with the use of Initial Slope Index (ISI; Risberg et al., 1975). This parameter also proved to be the most useful of all available flow parameters in our laboratory.

CBF measurements in animals

There are several acceptable methods for measuring the CBF in the acute animal experiment (e.g. the microsphere technique). For the chronic experiment, however, the hydrogen clearance as measured by platinum or platinum-iridium electrodes seems to be the only appropriate method. Especially in unanesthetized animals with a minimum of physical restraint, the hydrogen clearance measurement is the method of choice. Technically, the method has hardly changed since the original description by Aukland et al. (1964). The hydrogen clearance can be used for local intracerebral measurements, but also for measurements of total CBF or hemispheric blood flow (Shinohara et al., 1969; Martins et al, 1974). Using the hydrogen method, Doyle et al. (1975) found a very high ($r = 0.928$) correlation between the two compartmental analyses and the flow values derived from initial slope measurements. This may indicate that in most cases a very simple curve analysis is admissible.

It seems probable that with the commonly used platinum electrodes the average flow is estimated for a few cubic millimeters around the electrode tip (Halsey et al., 1977). This very small recording volume could explain the poor correlation found between the flow values measured with the hydrogen method and those measured with the microsphere technique (Heiss and Traupe, 1981).

Owing to the differences in flow in different parts of the normal cortex, regional differences can be rather large. This is revealed in the variance of the mean cortical CBF. Pasztor et al. (1973) found values of 82.2 (S.D. = 18.0) for cortical electrodes in the monkey. Morawetz et al. (1978) found values ranging from 34 to 101 ml/100 g/min in the basal ganglia and insular cortex of the baboon. The normal value for cortical electrodes is estimated by Symon et al. (1979) at 40.1 ml/100 g/min (S.D. = 11.8).

Hydrogen measurements have proven their practical utility in all situations where local measurements are essential for the interpretation of the results (Branston et al., 1974; Symon et al., 1975). After favorable results in cats (Tulleken et al., 1982), we decided to use the hydrogen method for our studies in monkeys as well.

OBSERVATIONS IN STROKE PATIENTS

Description of patients

For this study we examined 25 patients with an acute one-sided cerebrovascular lesion (10 females, 15 males, mean age 52.8 years, range 21–68 years). All patients were admitted to the hospital for observation in the initial phase of the disease. Only those patients who had suffered from an ischemia in the region of the MCA were included in the study group. Each patient was examined three times: approximately 1 week, 3 weeks and 3 months after the onset of the ischemia (see section on Methods p. 154). At the time of the neurophysiological studies, the clinical score was determined according to the method of Valdimarsson et al. (1982). The clinical scores are presented in Table I.

It appears that in most cases there was only a limited neurological deficit (six

154

TABLE I

CLINICAL SCORE OF INDIVIDUAL PATIENTS

Clinical score	1 week	3 weeks	3 months
0– 5	9	17	21
6–10	6	4	2
11–20	7	3	1
21–50	1	0	1
> 50	2	1	0
Mean score	11.9	6.7	3.0

patients could be classified as TIA patients). There are two reasons why patients with a major neurological deficit are poorly represented in this group. First of all, we limited ourselves to patients under 70 years of age; furthermore, it appeared that patients in a poor condition (with a high score) were not suitable candidates for reliable CBF studies with the inhalation method.

In the first 3 months after the accident all patients with a clinical deficit improved to a considerable degree except for one who showed a minor deterioration. At the end of the observation period no neurological signs or symptoms of cerebral ischemia could be detected in 11 out of 25 patients. During the observation period the patients were treated with anticoagulants or anti-aggregation compounds only. No surgery (carotid endarterectomy or STA–MCA bypass operations) was undertaken in any of these patients. Apart from these 25 patients, two additional patients were studied in more detail. The results from one of these patients will be presented in the Case study, p. 155).

Methods

One week, 3 weeks and 3 months after the stroke a CBF measurement and a computerized EEG were performed on all patients. The interval between CBF studies and EEG was at most 24 h. The EEG was studied at rest (eyes open and eyes closed) and during photic stimulation. A montage of all electrodes of the 10–20 system was used with C_z as a common reference. For all derivations, four power spectra were computed from periods of 100 sec of spontaneous EEG (averaging 19 epochs of 10 sec with an overlap of 50%). Two power spectra were made from the EEG at rest with eyes closed, one from the EEG with eyes opened and one from the EEG with eyes opened during tactile stimulation (see van Huffelen et al., this volume). The voltage spectra as well as their differences for the homotopical derivations were plotted. The following parameters were calculated: significant differences between the power on the left and right side, peak frequencies and amplitudes, absolute and relative powers in the delta, theta, alpha and beta bands, and asymmetries in the peak amplitudes as well as in the power per frequency band (for the width of the bands see Table II). The EEG taken during photic stimulation was also subjected to computer analysis. For this study, only the parameters derived from the spectra made from the EEG at rest with the eyes open were taken into account. This was done in order to compare these results with those of the EEGs of the experimental animals (see section on Animal experiments, p. 160).

A Novo Cerebrograph (inhalation technique) was used; this apparatus enables simultaneous measurements of the CBF in 16 homologous regions of both hemispheres. For technical reasons the values derived from the three detectors in the lower temporal region on each side were not used in the present study (see Mosmans et al., 1982). During the CBF measurement the patient was in a supine position, in a quiet environment, with the eyes closed. The end-tidal pCO_2 values were used to detect changes in pCO_2 values and evaluate the breathing pattern of the patient. The CBF values were not corrected for the slightly varying pCO_2 values. In the present study only Initial Slope Index (ISI) values as defined by Risberg et al. (1975) were used. For each hemisphere the mean ISI for the 13 detectors was calculated. A right/left ratio was used to indicate the difference in flow values between the two hemispheres. R/L ratio = |(ISI right − ISI left)/(ISE right + ISI left)| A ratio ≥ 0.025 was considered abnormal (de Weerd et al., 1982).

Case study

A 25-year-old Hindustani female patient had a mitral and tricuspidal commissurectomy in 1978. After the operation she used anticoagulants which had to be stopped after a suicide attempt using these drugs. In 1982 she was admitted to hospital after an acute cerebrovascular accident resulting in a severe right-sided hemiparesis and aphasia. Two days after the stroke the CT scan showed pronounced ischemia in the whole region of the left MCA. Selective angiography did not reveal abnormalities in the territories of the carotid artery or MCA. Clinically, the patient improved gradually and one month after the stroke there was only a slight hemiparesis and hemihypesthesia. The cause of the stroke was thought to be an embolism originating from the enlarged left atrium. The anticoagulant therapy was restarted.

The EEG and CBF data during the first month after the stroke are presented in Figs. 1–3. These figures show the following:
– Power was almost always greater on the diseased side than on the contralateral side. This difference in power was not only present (as could be expected) for the lower frequencies, but also for the alpha frequency.
– In the course of time, the power decreased but this decrease did not take place symmetrically over the two hemispheres: it occurred more rapidly over the non-ischemic hemisphere than over the ischemic hemisphere; therefore the power asymmetry was not maximal shortly after the stroke but was maximal only on the 15th day after the stroke. This is more obvious from Fig. 2, where the power ratio r = (right − left)/(right + left) for the alpha 1 and delta 2 band has been depicted.
– The CBF decreased in both hemispheres in the period after the accident (Fig. 3). This decrease is not amazing, considering the observations of Slater et al. (1977). It is striking, however, that the CBF values did not increase in the second half of the observation period, although there was a satisfactory clinical improvement (such a discrepancy was also observed by Demeurisse et al., 1983).
– The maximal asymmetry of the CBF values was not reached before the 22nd day after the stroke.

From this case study one could get the impression that in EEG follow-up studies absolute power values are indeed an important measure. However, owing to the overall increase in power over all the frequency bands, relative power values can be misleading. The asymmetry of EEG and CBF was time dependent and certainly not

156

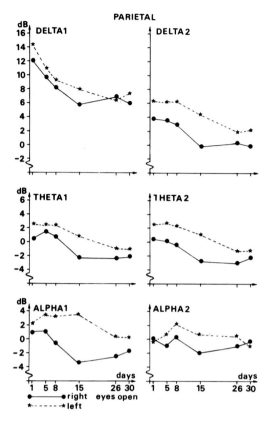

Fig. 1. Changes in mean power per frequency band in the EEGs of the patient described in the Case study, on p. 155 (left side is diseased side; parietal derivations).

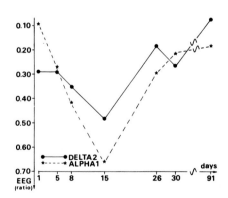

Fig. 2. Power ratio of the alpha 1 and delta 2 band (same patient as Fig. 1, parietal derivations). Ratio = (right − left)/(right + left). A perfect symmetry corresponds to a ratio = 0; the ratio increases as the asymmetry increases (max. = +/− 1).

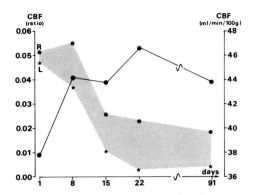

Fig. 3. CBF ratio ●—● and mean ISI values of the same patient as in Figs. 1 and 2. Right and left mean ISI indicated by upper and lower border of shaded area.

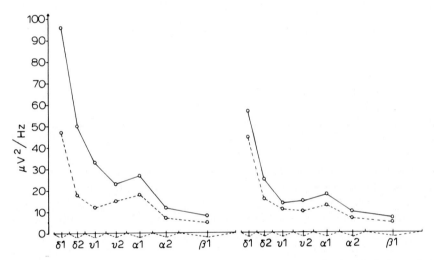

Fig. 4. Mean power for all frequency bands 1 week (solid line) and 3 months (broken line) after an ischemic accident for a group of 25 patients. (Left side: ischemic hemisphere, right side: non-ischemic hemisphere.)

maximal shortly after the stroke. The EEG as well as the CBF values pointed to a considerable neurophysiological diaschisis. The non-ischemic hemisphere showed the same changes as the ischemic hemisphere but to a lesser degree and with a more rapid recuperation.

Group results

The results of the 25 patients described in section on Description of patients, p. 153 were combined in order to evaluate whether this group as a whole showed the same tendencies for EEG and CBF changes as seen in the illustrative case described in the Case study on p. 155. The changes in time for all cases and for all frequency bands are shown in Fig. 4. On the diseased side, the mean power in all frequency bands was substantially larger one week after the cerebrovascular accident than 3 months after the stroke. On the normal side, a decrease of power in all frequency bands was also seen, but to a lesser degree than on the diseased side. Three months after the stroke

158

TABLE II

DECREASE IN POWER PER FREQUENCY BAND OVER THE FIRST 3 MONTHS AFTER THE STROKE

I.H. = ischemic hemisphere, N.I.H. = non-ischemic hemisphere. Chance of misclassification: $p<0.05 =$*; $p<0.005 =$ **; $p<0.0005 =$ ***

		2.0–3.4 Hz (%)	3.5–5.4 Hz (%)	5.5–7.4 Hz (%)	7.5–9.9 Hz (%)	10.0–12.4 Hz (%)
Temporal	I.H.	31.4 ***	27.6 ***	21.5 ***	25.0 ***	28.7 ***
Temporal	N.I.H.	24.6 ***	15.0 **	17.6 *	6.5 n.s.	16.8 **
Occipital	I.H.	22.2 **	14.0 *	16.5 *	11.8 n.s.	15.5 **
Occipital	N.I.H.	23.1 ***	14.5 *	14.7 *	3.0 n.s.	18.8 **

there was hardly any difference between both hemispheres for the mean values of the whole group. In order to ascertain the significance of this decrease in power, the percent decrease in power for each frequency band was measured for each patient in temporal and occipital derivations. The mean decrease as a percentage of the original power values was calculated. The results are presented in Table II.

Application of the Wilcoxon distribution free rank test indicated that all decreases on the ischemic side as well as on the non-ischemic side were significant ($p<0.05$ or less), except for the alpha 1 band on the non-ischemic side in the temporal derivation and the occipital derivations on both sides. In this band, the majority of patients showed a considerable decrease in power over the observation period but in some cases there was an increase in power after 3 months which was due to the development of a (pathological ?) alpha activity not suppressed by the opening of the eyes.

So we must conclude that in this group the (moderate) ischemia resulted in an increase in power in all frequency bands on the ischemic side. A lesser, but also significant, effect could be detected for most frequency bands over the non-ischemic hemisphere. From the spectral data obtained 3 weeks after the stroke (not presented here), it became apparent that over the diseased as well as over the non-diseased hemisphere most of the decrease in power took place in the first 3 weeks. The asymmetry (as measured by the right/left ratio), however, decreased only slightly in the first 3 weeks but decreased to a mean normal value in the period thereafter. The absolute temporal delta 2 power ratio, for instance, showed the following values: after 1 week: 0.33; after 3 weeks: 0.26; after 3 months: 0.06.

In several cases the original EEGs and spectra were considered to be within normal limits for both sides. A decrease in overall power nevertheless could be measured in these cases. Thus electrophysiological disturbances could only be proven retrospectively.

For the whole group there seemed to be an association between the decrease in power and the clinical score (see Table III). This correlation could not be proven for

TABLE III

MEAN TEMPORAL DELTA 2 POWER AND MEAN CLINICAL SCORE 1
WEEK, 3 WEEKS AND 3 MONTHS AFTER THE STROKE

N = 25	1 week	3 weeks	3 months
Mean temporal delta 2 power	74.9	39.8	27.3
Mean clinical score	11.8	6.0	3.0

TABLE IV

MEAN ISI VALUES AND STANDARD DEVIATIONS 1 WEEK, 3 WEEKS AND
3 MONTHS AFTER THE STROKE

N = 25	1 week	3 weeks	3 months
Ischemic hemisphere	45.4 (7.5)	42.3 (4.6)	43.6 (7.7)
Non-ischemic hemisphere	46.0 (7.5)	42.9 (4.6)	44.0 (7.5)

TABLE V

MEAN ISI VALUES AND RATIOS COMPARED WITH THE FINAL CLINICAL
SCORE

N = 25	Final clinical score > 2	Final clinical score ≤ 2
Mean ISI and/or ratio abnormal	7	2
Mean ISI and ratio normal	2	14
$p < 0.005$		

individual patients, nor was there a significant correlation between the original EEG abnormalities and the original or final clinical score.

The results of the CBF examinations for this group were not illuminating. The mean ISI values and standard deviations are presented in Table IV. As in our case study, an increase in CBF after the stroke could not be proved. There was only a slight (non-significant) decrease. Seven patients had low ISI values (<40) over the ischemic hemisphere. Only one of these patients recovered without neurological deficit. (In the entire group 10 out of 25 patients had a final clinical score of 0). Individual increases or decreases of mean CBF values did not correlate with individual clinical improvement or deterioration. Three patients showed a pathological asymmetry of the CBF ratio (ratio ≥ 0.025). The prognosis in these three patients was not optimal. Although the CBF measured in this way seems to have no value for follow-up studies, there is some indication of a prognostic value (see Table V).

The lack of asymmetry in the CBF values in most cases (22 out of 25) is not due to an excessive "contamination" of the clearance curves by the contralateral side. This could be proved by the study of a group of patients with one-sided carotid occlusion (Mosmans et al., 1983) and a group of patients with one-sided occlusion of the MCA (to be published). There was no correlation between the decrease in EEG power and the changes of the CBF values either for the group or for the individual patients.

160

ANIMAL EXPERIMENTS

Material and methods

Ten adult rhesus monkeys (*Macaca mulatta*) were used in this study. Under general anesthesia, electrode bundles consisting of 4–5 stainless steel and platinum/iridium wires (bare tip 200 μ*m*) were inserted with the aid of a stereotactic apparatus. The electrode bundles were placed in the frontal, parietal and occipital cortex of the right hemisphere and one bundle in the parietal cortex of the left hemisphere (in the Regions B and C according to Symon et al., 1974). Moreover, electrodes were inserted in the caudate nucleus and thalamus (VPL) on both sides (for details see Tulleken et al., 1978, 1982). The electrodes were attached to a connector, which was fixed to the skull with acrylic.

In the weeks after this first operation, rCBF and EEG measurements were taken without anesthesia or sedation of the animal. After this observation period, the right MCA was approached by the transorbital route. In four animals the vessel was occluded directly, resulting in the death of three animals, probably due to massive brain edema. In the remaining six animals a ligature was placed around the MCA. The vessel was occluded 1–2 weeks after the placement of the ligature.

Several combined EEG and rCBF studies were performed during a period of at least 4 weeks after the occlusion of the MCA. The CBF was calculated from the hydrogen-clearance curves according to the formula rCBD = $\lambda \cdot 69.31/T_{1/2}$ in which $\lambda = 1$ (because hydrogen was used). The power in the EEG was calculated using the same bands as determined for the measurements in humans (see Table II).

Half an hour before the termination of the experiment 2-deoxy-D-[^{14}C]glucose was given intravenously (50 μC/kg). The animal was sacrificed with an overdose of barbiturates and the brain was removed and frozen at $-55°C$. Coronal sections were cut in a cryostat and used for autoradiography (see Fig. 6) and microscopic determination of the localization of the electrodes.

Clinical results

Acute occlusion of the MCA resulted in the death of three out of four animals. All six animals in which the MCA was occluded by a previously placed ligature survived. A neurological deficit developed in six out of the seven surviving animals. The extent of the deficit varied in the individual animals (cf. Morawetz et al., 1978) but was entirely compatible with the descriptions given by Symon (1975) and Watanabe et al. (1977).

The MCA occlusion did not cause any neurological symptoms only in one animal. It is interesting to note that in this animal, a hemiplegia developed after an attempt to construct an extracranial/intracranial bypass. Probably there was only a marginal blood supply after the MCA occlusion which became insufficient during the last operation.

The autoradiographic results from four animals showed that occlusion of the MCA gave rise to a massive hemispheric infarct (see also Waltz, 1979).

A case study (monkey E)

The placement of the electrodes did not give rise to neurological symptoms. The data obtained from one electrode are presented in Fig. 5. This electrode was situated in the parietal cortex, approximately 4 mm behind the central sulcus and 8.5 mm to right of the midline.

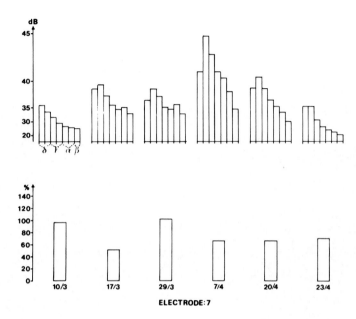

Fig. 5. Above: changes in EEG power per frequency band. Below: changes in rCBF for one electrode in monkey E.

The last of the control measurements was done on day 10/3. At that time the rCBF was 97% of the mean of all previous values. Immediately thereafter a ligature was placed around the MCA. The animal did not show any neurological deficit after this operation. However, the EEG and rCBF showed important changes: the rCBF decreased to 51% whereas the power in all frequency bands increased. These changes were probably due to spasm of the MCA. At day 29/3 the rCBF had returned to normal (102%) but the EEG had recovered only slightly.

The MCA was occluded after these measurements on day 29/3. This resulted in a further increase in power in all frequency bands and once again a decrease in rCBF (to 66%). At this time the monkey showed an almost complete left-sided hemiplegia with only a limited function of the left foot. In the weeks thereafter the neurological condition improved but recovery was incomplete. The use of the left hand remained especially restricted until the end of the experiment. In this period there was hardly any recovery of the rCBF but an important decrease in power in the EEG. So this electrode, placed in a region of moderate ischemia, showed the same EEG changes as seen in the patient group (see section on Observations in stroke patients, p. 158).The regional flow values appeared to be more informative than the mean hemispheric flow values as used in our patient studies. On the contralateral side a cortical electrode

162

revealed the same changes but to a lesser degree (for the EEG as well as for the rCBF).

The experiment was terminated on day 12/7. An autoradiogram of a brain section is shown in Fig. 6. There appeared to be a large central infarct and, as compared with the contralateral side, a diminished glucose uptake over a large part of the right hemisphere (involving superficial as well as deep structures).

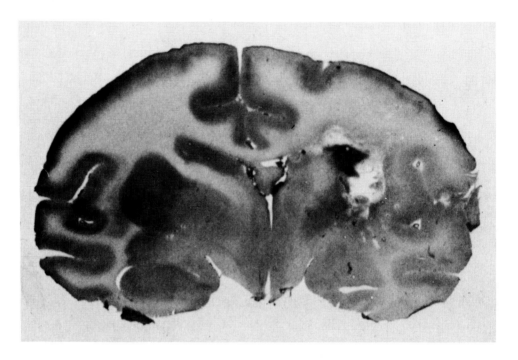

Fig. 6. One autoradiogram from monkey E. Note the central infarct in the right hemisphere and the diminished glucose uptake in the whole right hemisphere.

Group results

It seemed questionable whether the EEG measurements of the different electrodes of one bundle could be considered as independent observations because the changes in the EEG induced by the ischemia were almost the same in all the electrodes of one bundle. We therefore decided to use only one electrode per bundle (the same electrode was used for the EEG as well as for the rCBF measurements). In each of the six monkeys that survived the acute phase of the experiment four cortical electrodes were available on the ischemic side, two electrodes in the basal ganglia on the affected side and one cortical electrode on the contralateral side (the depth electrodes on the contralateral side have not yet been evaluated). Although many more measurements were done in each animal (Fig. 5 shows only a selection of the data available from electrode 7 in monkey E) we limited ourselves to three measurements per animal:
  (1) the mean values of the EEG parameters and the mean value of the rCBF of all experiments before the onset of ischemia (expt. I);

(2) one experiment in the period between 7 and 14 days after the first clinical signs became obvious (expt.II);

(3) one experiment in the period between 24 and 31 days after the onset of the neurological signs (expt.III).

In Fig. 7 the EEG results are presented for six animals (see section on Clinical results, p. 160). The data of the four cortical electrodes on the ischemic side have been averaged for each animal. It appears that in animals C, D, E and H there is an increase in power in all frequency bands after the inducement of ischemia (triangles = expt.II) as compared with the bandpower before ischemia (circles = expt.I). In two animals (F and G) there was an increase in power in the lower frequencies but some decrease in power in the higher frequencies. In at least five animals the power in all frequency bands decreased in the period between experiment II (triangles) and experiment III (squares). This overall decrease in power is comparable with the changes seen in humans after ischemia (compare Fig. 4).

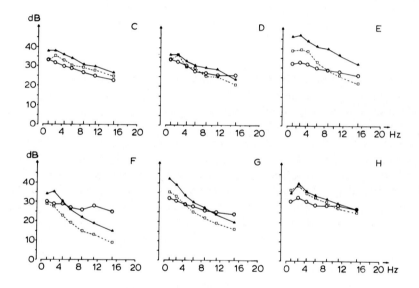

Fig. 7. Increase and decrease of power per frequency band in six monkeys (for details see section on Group results, p. 162). Expt.I = O—O, Expt.II = ▲—▲, Expt.III = □—□.

Statistical analysis was carried out to test whether the EEG power increased in all frequency bands after ischemia and subsequently decreased in the recovery period using the Wilcoxon distribution free rank test. The results are presented in Table VI. As can be seen from this Table, the trends mentioned were significant for all frequency bands for the electrodes on the ischemic side. On the non-ischemic side the trend was also significant for all frequencies as regards the increase in power in the immediate post-ischemic period. However, this was not the case for the recovery period. The EEG derived from depth electrodes in the ischemic hemisphere showed a significant trend to increase in all bands (except alpha 2) after ischemia and a significant trend to decrease in the recovery period (except for theta 1). Comparing the

164

TABLE VI

INCREASE IN POWER BETWEEN EXPT.II AND I, DECREASE IN POWER BETWEEN EXPT.III AND II.

Expt.I: mean of pre-ischemic values; Expt. II: 7–14 days after onset of ischemia; Expt.III: 24–31 days after onset of ischemia. Values (in dB) for 6 animals. Chances of misclassification as in Table II. I.H. = ischemic hemisphere, N.I.H. = non-ischemic hemisphere.

	2.1–3.3 Hz	3.6–5.4 Hz	5.6–7.2 Hz	7.5–9.9 Hz	10.2–12.3 Hz
Expt.II–Expt.I I.H.	+7.5 ***	+5.4 ***	+4.4 ***	+3.4 ***	+1.8 *
Expt.III—Expt.II I.H.	−4.2 ***	−4.4 ***	−4.4 ***	−4.8 ***	−4.7 ***
Expt.II–Expt.I N.I.H.	+4.9 ***	+5.3 ***	+5.4 ***	+5.9 ***	+6.3 ***
Expt.III–Expt.II N.I.H.	−4.4 n.s.	−4.6 n.s.	−4.7 *	−4.6 *	−4.4 *

results after 4 weeks with the EEG before ischemia it appeared that after this period there was still a significant increase in the delta 2 band.

In this analysis we have not taken into consideration the changes occurring in the delta 1 and beta bands. In human studies there is always the risk that eye-movement artefacts may influence the delta 1 band, while muscle artefacts may result in unreliable measurements in the beta bands in humans as well as in animals.

Summarizing the EEG results for this small group of animals, it appears that not only the changes in the EEG of the cortical electrodes on the ischemic hemisphere are comparable with the changes seen in humans but that comparable changes can also be seen in the EEG derived from the depth electrodes and from the cortical electrodes of the contralateral side. From the EEG data one would conclude that a diaschisis is present and is perhaps even more pronounced than in humans because the increase and subsequent decrease in power were roughly the same on both sides. A definite conclusion cannot be made at this moment because the number of electrodes over the non-ischemic hemisphere was rather small. In the period between experiment II and III all animals showed some clinical recovery, which was probably reflected in the EEG changes.

In a combination of all cortical electrodes on the ischemic side there was a significant ($p<0.0005$) trend for a decrease in rCBF (mean decrease 11.6 ml/100 g/min, original mean value 38.1 ml/100 g/min).

In the recovery period the trend for an increase in rCBF was significant ($p<0.005$) but the mean increase was extremely small (1.1 ml/100 g/min). On the non-ischemic side the CBF decrease was less (mean decrease 3.4 ml/100 g/min; $p<0.05$), the increase in the recovery period was not significant. As in humans, the overall rCBF changes in the recovery period are apparently rather limited.

Considering the correlation between rCBF and EEG we divided the measurements in two groups:

(a)   An increase in EEG power combined with a decrease in rCBF or vice versa;
(b)   An increase in EEG power combined with an increase in rCBF or a decrease in both values.

The changes occurring between the pre-ischemic period and the early post-ischemic period (days 7−14) could be classified much more frequently in group a than in group b (with a highly significant score using the chi-square test). This can be interpreted as an association between EEG and CBF results. Such an association could not be found for the superficial electrodes on the contralateral side or for the depth electrodes. Neither was such a parallelism between EEG and CBF present during the recovery period. This is probably due to the erratic behavior of the rCBF in this period, resulting in a hardly measurable mean increase in rCBF.

A more detailed analysis of all the available EEG and rCBF data from all animals is in progress.

CONCLUSION AND DISCUSSION

The aim of this study was mainly to determine whether the monkey with an artificially induced chronic ischemia could be considered as an appropriate model for spontaneous ischemia in humans and if so, what the best objective follow-up parameters would be in humans as well as in monkeys. In order to accept the monkey as a suitable model there should be at least similarities in the clinical manifestations, the pathology findings, the electrophysiological disturbances, the cerebra! blood flow changes and in pathophysiological mechanisms such as diaschisis.

In our series we could confirm that the occlusion of the MCA in monkeys results in a clinical symptomatology comparable to that seen in humans after spontaneous occlusion of the MCA. As in humans, however, the resulting neurological deficit in monkeys shows a considerable interindividual variation. The rate of recovery is also variable and hardly predictable. Acute occlusion of the MCA in monkeys may result in death within 48 h due to brain edema, a clinical course also encountered in humans.

In humans, the extent of the infarcted region as seen by CT scan or at autopsy is variable. This is probably due to the variability in existing or developing collaterals and the variable pathology of the cerebral vessels in adjacent regions. From the available autoradiograms we got the impression that in monkeys occlusion of the MCA resulted in an infarct of roughly the same size in all animals. This relatively small variability was probably caused by the fact that all animals were in an identical condition before ischemia: there were no signs of any cerebrovascular disease before the occlusion.

Considering the disturbances in electrophysiological function, we should emphasize that most patients in this study (see Table I) suffered from a mild ischemia in the region of the MCA. In the animals, we used electrodes placed around the centre of the ischemic area. In both groups we can only give a description of the effect of moderate ischemia on the EEG. The group study in humans led to an unexpected result: the ischemia did cause an increase in power in the low frequencies (as expected) but also gave rise to an increase in power in the higher frequency bands. This phenomenon, which seems to be fairly common, can easily escape detection in clinical practice for several reasons. Because even in normals the interindividual differences in absolute power values are large, an increase in power caused by ischemia can only be detected by the subsequent decrease in follow-up studies. Moreover, an increase in the alpha range can only be seen in registrations with the eyes opened because this increase in power in the alpha range can be overshadowed by an asymmetry of the alpha rhythm, which can have a lower amplitude on the diseased side. In the literature (for a review, see van Huffelen, 1980) there are indications that the activity in alpha frequencies can sometimes be larger on the affected side. In clinical practice, however, it is more common to find an increase in slow activity accompanied by a decrease in faster activities. Perhaps this is partly due to the limitations of visual inspection of the EEG.

The derivations from the cortical electrodes in the monkeys gave us the same results for the whole group as for the humans: an increase in power in all frequency bands followed by an overall decrease during the recovery period apparently was the most common result of ischemia.

It should be mentioned, however, that in both groups there were some subjects who showed the more expected changes in the spectrum: after ischemia an increase in the lower frequencies in combination with a decrease in power in the higher frequencies. A combination of both types of changes also occurred: an increase in slow activity with almost no change in the alpha band. At the moment, we are unable to decide if these three types of spectral changes indicate different prognoses.

One might presume that evoked-response studies during the course of ischemia could be at least as informative as the spontaneous EEG. A comparative study of humans and animals after ischemia ought to be undertaken.

The results of the flow studies in humans and monkeys are not contradictory, despite the differences in technique. The most important similarity is the lack of increase in CBF values during the recovery period. In monkeys, it could be shown that the occlusion of the MCA resulted in a decrease in flow in all measured regions. Comparison with humans is hardly possible because in humans the flow values before the development of ischemia are seldom known.

The effect of a local brain lesion on distant not-involved structures (diaschisis) is well known. Høedt Rasmussen and Skinhøj (1964) were the first to measure a reduced flow on both sides in patients with a one-sided lesion. This finding was confirmed by Meyer et al. (1970) and Slater et al. (1977) in stroke patients, while a bilaterally disturbed vasoregulation after a one-sided lesion was found by Paulson et al. (1972) and Melamed et al. (1975b). A flow diaschisis was found by Melamed et al. (1975a) in 16 out of 22 patients. In the same group only six patients also showed a contralateral decrease of mean EEG frequency. Signs of diaschisis in animals were found by Kempinski (1958), Waltz (1967), Ginsberg (1977) and Kanaya et al. (1983), among others.

Diaschisis for the EEG was clearly demonstrated in our patient group. Comparable changes occurred over both hemispheres but were less pronounced on the non-ischemic side. There was probably an important CBF diaschisis as well. Most patients showed relatively low flow values, a significant asymmetry was present only in a few cases (see Meyer et al., 1970). It could be proven in another patient series that this lack of asymmetry in ischemic patients was not due to faulty instrumentation.

In the animals, both the EEG and CBF showed disturbances on both sides, less pronounced on the non-ischemic side. EEG and CBF diaschisis thus seemed to occur in both groups. We cannot confirm that CBF diaschisis is less common in monkeys than it is in man (Meyer et al., 1970), nor can we confirm that EEG diaschisis occurs less frequently than CBF diaschisis (Melamed et al., 1975a).

In summary, we conclude that the animal model fulfills all the criteria stated at the beginning of this section. The rhesus monkey studied before and after occlusion of the MCA seems to be the optimal model now available for studies of human ischemia.

Regarding the suitability of the EEG and CBF parameters for follow-up studies, we want to limit ourselves to a few aspects of this complex matter. The mean regional blood flow as measured in humans with the inhalation method may have some diagnostic and prognostic value. We could not, however, establish that this measurement is of any value for follow-up during the recovery. The same applies to the regional cerebral blood flow measurements in the monkeys. It cannot be excluded that improvement of the flow may take a longer time than the intervals used in this study.

The EEG and especially the absolute power values showed deterioration after ischemia and often a continuous improvement during the recovery. Thus at the moment the quantified EEG seems a more promising method for follow-up studies than the CBF. Some restrictions must, however, be made. There was no clear correlation between the EEG results and the clinical condition and/or prognosis. This is partly due to the fact that small deep lesions may give rise to impressive clinical symptoms not accompanied by changes in the EEG. Moreover, one should realize that a correlation between clinical signs and EEG is also difficult because even the best clinical scales are inherently nonlinear.

The EEG measures found to be most useful for follow-up studies (absolute band powers) are useless for diagnostic purposes. For the diagnoses of minor ischemic disorders one has to rely on other EEG parameters, such as those described by Pfurtscheller et al. and van Huffelen et al. in this volume.

SUMMARY

This study deals with the follow-up of EEG and CBF in 25 patients with strokes in the territory of the MCA. The results are compared with those of six rhesus monkeys studied before and after occlusion of the MCA. The ischemia in humans gave rise to an increase in EEG power in the higher frequencies as well as in the lower frequencies with a subsequent decrease in power in the recovery period. The same results were obtained from the cortical electrodes in the monkeys. Changes in the power spectrum on the non-affected side could be observed in humans as well as in monkeys (EEG diaschisis). The measurements of mean rCBF (xenon inhalation) in humans gave only a limited information: the CBF values after the (minor) strokes were low but hardly asymmetrical. No consistent increase in CBF occurred in the first 3 months after the stroke. In monkeys (hydrogen clearance method) a decrease in mean 1CBF could be demonstrated after occlusion of the MCA. As in humans there was hardly any increase in mean 1CBF in the recovery period. Neurological signs were comparable in humans and monkeys. From the neurophysiological point of view, the rhesus monkey studied before and after occlusion of the MCA, seems the optimal model now available for studies of human ischemia.

ACKNOWLEDGEMENT

This work was funded in part through a grant of the Dutch Heart Foundation.

168

REFERENCES

Astrup, J., Siesjo, B.K. and Symon L. (1981) Thresholds in cerebral ischemia – The ischemic penumbra. *Stroke*, 12: 723–725.

Aukland, K., Bower, B.F. and Berliner, R.W. (1964) Measurement of local blood flow with hydrogen gas. *Circulat. Res.*, XIV: 164–187.

Binnie, C.D., Batchelor, B.G., Bowring, P.A., Darby, C.E., Herbert, L.L., Lloyd, D.S.L., Smith, D.M., Smith, G.F. and Smith M. (1978) Computer-assisted interpretation of clinical EEGs. *Electroenceph. clin. Neurophysiol.*, 44: 575–585.

Branston, N.M., Symon, L., Crockard, H.A. and Pasztor, E. (1974) Relationship between the cortical evoked potential and local cortical blood flow following acute middle cerebral artery occlusion in the baboon. *Exp. Neurology*, 45: 195–208.

Branston N.M., Symon, L. and Crockard H.A. (1976) Recovery of the cortical evoked response following temporary middle cerebral artery occlusion in baboons: relation to local blood flow and PO2. *Stroke*, 7: 151–157.

Branston, N.M., Ladds, A., Wang, A.D. and Symon, L. (1983) Critical flow thresholds for evoked potentials in thalamus and brainstem. *J. Cereb. Blood Flow Metab.*, 3, Suppl. 1: s397–398.

Chiappa, K.H., Burke, S.R. and Young R.R. (1979) Results of electroencephalographic monitoring during 367 carotid endarterectomies. *Stroke*, 10: 381–388.

Cohen, B.A., Bravo-Fernandez, E.J. and Sances, A. (1976) Quantification of computer analyzed serial EEGs from stroke patients. *Electroenceph. clin. Neurophysiol.*, 41: 379–386.

Date, H., Shima, T. and Hossmann K-A. (1983) Relationship between local cerebral perfusion pressure, blood flow, and electro-physiological function during middle cerebral artery constriction in cats. *J. Cereb. Blood Flow Metab.*, 3, Suppl. 1: s357–358.

Demeurisse, G., Verhas, M., Capon, A. and Paternot, J. (1983) Lack of evolution of the cerebral blood flow during clinical recovery of a stroke. *Stroke*, 14: 77–81.

De Weerd, A.W., Veering, M.M., Mosmans, P.C.M., van Huffelen, A.C., Tulleken, C.A.F. and Jonkman, E.J. (1982) Effect of extra-intracranial (STA–MCA) arterial anastomosis on EEG and cerebral blood flow. *Stroke*, 13: 674–679.

Doyle, T.F., Martins, A.N. and Kobrine, A.I. (1975) Estimating total cerebral blood flow from the initial slope of hydrogen washout. *Stroke*, 6: 149–152.

Drayer, B.P., Wolfson, S.K., Reinmuth, O.M., Dujovny, M., Boehnke, M. and Cooke, E.E. (1978) Xenon enhanced CT for analysis of cerebral integrity, perfusion and blood flow. *Stroke*, 9: 123–130.

Gasser, T. and Mocks, J. (1983) Graphical representation of multidimensional EEG data and classifactory aspects. *Electroenceph. clin. Neurophysiol.*, 55: 609–612.

Gasser, T., Bacher, P. and Mocks, J. (1982) Transformations towards the normal distribution of broad band spectral parameters of the EEG. *Electroenceph. clin. Neurophysiol.*, 52: 119–124.

Ginsberg, M.D., Reivich, M., Giandomenico, A. and Greenberg, J.H. (1977) Local glucose utilisation in acute focal cerebral ischemia:local dysmetabolism and diaschisis. *Neurology (Minneap.)*, 27: 1042–1048.

Gotman, J., Gloor, P. and Ray, W.F. (1975) A quantitative comparison of traditional reading of the EEG and interpretation of computer extracted features in patients with supratentorial brain lesions. *Electroenceph. clin. Neurophysiol.*, 38: 623–639.

Halsey, J.H., Capra, N.F. and McFarland, R.S. (1977) Use of hydrogen for measurement of regional cerebral blood flow. *Stroke*, 8: 351–357.

Halsey, J.H., Nakai, K. and Wariyar, B. (1981) Sensitivity of rCBF to focal lesions. *Stroke*, 12: 631–635.

Halsey, J.H., Morawetz, R.B. and Blauenstein, U.W. (1982) The haemodynamic effect of STA–MCA bypass. *Stroke*, 13: 163–167.

Heiss, W.D. and Traupe, H. (1981) Comparison between hydrogen clearance and microsphere technique for rCBF measurement. *Stroke*, 12: 161–167.

Hjorth, B. (1970) EEG analysis based on time domain properties. *Electroenceph. clin. Neurophysiol.*, 29: 306–310.

Hjorth, B. (1973) The physical significance of time domain descriptors in EEG analysis. *Electroenceph. clin. Neurophysiol.*, 34: 321–325.

Høedt-Rasmussen, K. and Skinhøj, E. (1964) Transneural depression of the cerebral hemispheric metabolism in man. *Acta Neurol. Scand.*, 40: 41–46.

Hossman, K.A. and Schuier, F.J. (1980) Experimental brain infarcts in cats. I. Pathophysiological observations. *Stroke*, 11: 538–592.

Ingvar, D.H. (1975) Invasive versus noninvasive techniques for measurement of rCBF. In W. Langfitt, L.C. McHenry, jr, M. Reivich and H. Wollman (Eds.), *Cerebral Circulation and Metabolism*, Springer-Verlag, Berlin–Heidelberg–New York, pp. 556–559.

Ingvar, D.H. and Sulg. I.A. (1969) Regional cerebral blood flow and EEG frequency content in man. *Scand. J. clin. Lab. Invest.*, Suppl. 43: 46,42–73.

Ingvar, D.H., Sjolund, B. and Ardo. A. (1976) Correlation between dominant EEG frequency, cerebral oxygen uptake and blood flow. *Electroenceph. clin. Neurophysiol.*, 41: 268–276.

Ishihara, Y., Gotoh, F., Tachibana, H., Ishikawa, Y. and Gomi, S. (1983) The effect of unilateral cerebral infarction on cerebral blood flow and glucose metabolism of the contralateral hemisphere in gerbils. *J. Cereb. Blood Flow Metab.*, 3. Suppl. 1: s321–322.

John, E.R. (1981) Neurometric evaluation of brain dysfunction related to learning disorders. *Acta Neurol. Scand.*, 64, Suppl. 89: 87–100.

Jonkman, E.J., Mosmans, P.C.M., van der Drift, J.H.A. and Magnus, O. (1970) Problems concerning the correlation of rCBF and EEG. In R.W. Ross Russell (Ed.), *Brain and Blood Flow*, Pitman, London, pp. 150–154.

Kanaya, H., Endo, H., Sugiyama, T. and Kuroda, K. (1983) "Crossed cerebellar diaschisis" in patients with putaminal hemorrhage. *J. Cereb. Blood Flow Metab.*, 3, Suppl. 1: s27–28.

Kayser-Gatchalian, M.C. and Neundorfer, B. (1980) The prognostic value of EEG in ischaemic cerebral insults. *Electroenceph. clin. Neurophysiol.*, 49: 608–617.

Kempinksy, W.H. (1958) Experimental study of distant effects of acute focal brain injury. *Arch. Neurol.* 79: 376–389.

Lassen, N.A. (1981) Regional cerebral blood flow measurements in stroke: the necessity of a tomographic approach. *J. Cereb. Blood Flow Metab.*, 1: 141–142.

Lesnick, J.E., Michele, J.A. DeFeo, S., Welsh, F.A. and Simeone, F.A. (1983) The somatosensory evoked potential (SEP), CBF, and metabolism in global ischemia. *J. Cereb. Blood Flow Metab.*, 3, Suppl. 1: s270–271.

Lopes da Silva F.H. (1982) EEG analysis: theory and practice. In E. Niedermeyer and F.H. Lopes da Silva (Eds.), *Electroencephalography*, Urban and Schwarzenberg, Baltimore–Munich, pp. 685–712.

Martins, A.N., Kobrine, A.I., Doyle, T.F. and Ramirez, A. (1974) Total cerebral blood flow in the monkey measured by hydrogen clearance. *Stroke*, 5: 512–517.

Melamed, E., Lavy, S., Portnoy, Z., Sadan, S. and Carmon, A. (1975a) Correlation between regional cerebral blood flow and EEG frequency in the contralateral hemisphere in acute cerebral infarction. *J. Neurol. Sci.*, 26: 21–27.

Melamed, E., Lavy, S. and Portnoy, Z. (1975b) Regional cerebral blood flow response to hypocapnia in the contralateral hemisphere of patients with acute cerebral infarction. *Stroke*, 6: 503–509.

Meyer, J.S. (1978) Improved method for noninvasive measurement of regional cerebral blood flow by 133 Xenon inhalation. II. Measurements in health and disease. *Stroke*, 9: 205–210.

Meyer, J.S., Shinohara, Y., Kanda, T., Fukuuchi, Y., Ericsson, A.D. and Kok, N.K. (1970) Diaschisis resulting from acute unilateral cerebral infarction. *Arch. Neurol.*, 23: 241–247.

Meyer, J.S. Hayman, L.A., Amano, T., Nakajima, S., Shaw, T., Lauzon, P., Derman, S., Karacan, I. and Harati, Y. (1981) Mapping local blood flow of human brain by CT scanning during stable Xenon inhalation. *Stroke*, 12: 426–436.

Meyer, J.S. Nakajima, S., Okabe, T., Amano, T., Centeno, R., Lee, Y.Y., Levine, J., Levinthal, R. and Rose, J. (1982) Redistribution of cerebral blood flow following STA–MCA by-pass in patients with hemispheric ischemia. *Stroke*, 13: 774–784.

Morawetz, R.B., DeGirolami, U., Ojemann, R.G., Marcoux, F.W. and Crowell, R.M. (1978) Cerebral blood flow determined by hydrogen clearance during middle cerebral artery occlusion in unanesthetized monkeys. *Stroke*, 9: 143–149.

Mosmans, P.C.M. (1974) *Regional Cerebral Blood Flow In Neurological Patients* (Thesis), Utrecht University, van Gorcum & Comp. B.V., Assen.

Mosmans, P.C.M., Veering, M.M., de Weerd, A.W. and Jonkman E.J. (1982) Some remarks on the influence of the detector position on the CBF flow values in the Xenon inhalation method. *CBF Bull.*, 4: 64–67.

Mosmans, P.C.M., Jonkman, E.J. and Veering M.M. (1983) CBF measured by the Xenon-133 inhalation technique and quantified EEG investigations in patients with unilateral internal carotid artery occlusion. *Clin. Neurol. Neurosurg.*, 85: 155–164.

Obrist, W.D., Thompson, H.K., Wang, H.S. and Wilkinson, W.E. (1975) Regional cerebral blood flow estimated by 133 Xenon inhalation. *Stroke*, 6: 245–256.

170

Pasztor, E., Symon, L., Dorsch, N.W.C. and Branston, N.M. (1973) The hydrogen clearance method in assessment of the blood flow in cortex, white matter and deep nuclei of baboons. *Stroke*, 4: 556–567.

Paulson, O.B., Olesen, J. and Stig Christensen, M. (1972) Restoration of autoregulation of cerebral blood flow by hypocapnia. *Neurology (Minneap.)*, 22: 286–293.

Pfurtscheller, G. and Auer, L.M. (1983) Frequency changes of sensorimotor EEG rhythm after revascularisation surgery. *Electroenceph. clin. Neurophysiol.*, 55: 381–387.

Pfurtscheller, G., Sager, W. and Wege, W. (1981) Correlations between CT scan and sensorimotor EEG rhythms in patients with cerebrovascular disorders. *Electroenceph. clin. Neurophysiol.*, 52: 473–485.

Pronk, R.A.F. (1982) *EEG processing in cardiac surgery*, Institute of Medical Physics, TNO Utrecht.

Risberg, J. Ali, Z., Wilson, E.M., Willis, E.L. and Halsey, J.H. (1975) Regional cerebral blood flow by 133 Xenon inhalation. *Stroke*, 6: 142–148.

Roseman, E. Schmidt, R.P. and Foltz E.L. (1951) Serial electroencephalography in vascular lesions of the brain. Neurology (Minneap.), 2: 311–334.

Shinohara, Y., Meyer, J.S. Kitamura, A., Toyoda, M. and Ryu, T. (1969) Measurement of cerebral hemispheric blood flow by intracarotid injection of hydrogen gas. *Circulat. Res.*, XXV: 735–745.

Silverman, D. (1960) Serial electroencephalography in brain tumors and cerebrovascular accidents. *Arch. Neurol.*, 2: 122–129.

Slater, R., Reivich, M., Goldberg, H. Banka, R. and Greenberg, J. (1977) Diaschisis with cerebral infarction. *Stroke*, 8: 684–690.

Strong, A.J., Goodhardt, M.J., Branston, N.M. and Symon, L. (1977) A comparison of the effects of ischaemia on tissue flow, electrical activity and extracellular potassium ion concentration in cerebral cortex of baboons. *Biochem. Soc. Trans.*, 5: 158–160.

Sulg, I.A. and Ingvar, D.H. (1968) Regional cerebral blood flow and EEG in occlusions of the middle cerebral artery. *Scand. J. clin. Lab. Invest.*, Suppl. 102, sect. XVI: D.

Sundt, T.M., Sharbrough, F.W., Anderson, R.E. and Michenfelder, J.D. (1974) Cerebral blood flow measurements and electroencephalograms during carotid endarterectomy. *J. Neurosurg.*, 41: 310–320.

Symon, L. (1975) Experimental model of stroke in the baboon. In B.S. Meldrum and C.D. Marsden (Eds.), *Advances in Neurology, Vol. 10*, Raven Press, New York, pp. 199–211.

Symon, L., Pasztor, E. and Branston, N.M. (1974) The distribution and density of reduced cerebral blood flow following acute middle cerebral artery occlusion: an experimental study by the technique of hydrogen clearance in baboons. *Stroke*, 5: 355–364.

Symon, L., Crockard, H.A., Dorsch, N.W.C., Branston, N.M. and Juhasz, J. (1975) Local cerebral blood flow and vascular reactivity in a chronic stable stroke in baboons. *Stroke*, 6: 482–492.

Symon, L., Branston, N.M. and Chikovani, O. (1979) Ischemic brain edema following middle cerebral artery occlusion in baboons: relationship between regional cerebral water content and blood flow at 1 to 2 hours. *Stroke*, 10: 184–191.

Tolonen, U. and Sulg, I.A. (1981) Comparison of quantitative EEG parameters from four different analysis techniques in evaluation of relationships between EEG and CBF in brain infarction. *Electroenceph. clin. Neurophysiol.*, 51: 177–185.

Tolonen U., Ahonen, A., Sulg, A., Kuikka, J., Kallanranta, T., Koskinnen, M. and Hokkanen E. (1981) Serial measurements of quantitative EEG and cerebral blood flow and circulation time after brain infarction. *Acta Neurol. Scand.*, 63: 145–155.

Trojaborg, W. and Boysen, G. (1973) Relation between EEG, regional cerebral blood flow and internal carotid pressure during carotid endarterectomy. *Electroenceph. clin. Neurophysiol.*, 34: 61–69.

Tulleken, C.A.F., van Dieren, A., ten Veen, J. and Lopes da Silva, F.H. (1978) *Changes in local EEG, local cerebral blood flow and flow in the distal stump of the middle cerebral artery in cats with an occlusion of the middle cerebral artery*. In "Progress Report Inst. Med. Phys. TNO. Utrecht" 6, 102–108.

Tulleken, C.A.F., van Dieren, A., ten Veen, J. and Lopes da Silva, F.H. (1982) Changes in local cerebral blood flow, local EEG, and flow in the distal stump of the middle cerebral artery in cats with occlusion of the middle cerebral artery. *Acta Neurochir.*, 61: 227–240.

Valdimarsson, E., Bergvall, U. and Samuelsson, K. (1982) Prognostic significance of cerebral computed tomography results in supratentorial infarction. *Acta Neurol. Scand.*, 65: 133–145.

Van Huffelen, A.C. (1980) *Quantitative electroencephalography in cerebral ischemia*, TNO research unit for clinical neurophysiology, The Hague.

Van Huffelen, A.C., Poortvliet, D.C.J., van der Wulp, C.J.M. and Magnus, O. (1980) Quantitative EEG in cerebral ischemia. Parameters valuable for follow-up of patients with acute unilateral cerebral ischemia. (A.U.C.I.) In. H. Lechner and A.Aranibar (Eds.), *EEG and Clinical Neurophysiology*, Excerpta Medica, Amsterdam, pp. 131–136.

Veering, M.M., Mosmans, P.C.M., de Weerd, A.W. and Jonkman, E.J. (1983) Effect of STA–MCA anastomosis (EC–IC bypass) and carotid endarterectomy on rCBF. *J. Cereb. Blood Flow Metab.*, 3, Suppl. 1: s604–605.

Waltz, A.G. (1967) Cortical blood flow of opposite hemisphere after occlusion of middle cerebral artery. *Trans. Amer. Neurol. Ass.*, 92: 293–294.

Waltz, A.G. (1979) Clinical relevance of models of cerebral ischemia. *Stroke*, 10: 211–213.

Watanabe, O., Bremer, A.M. and West, C.R. (1977) Experimental regional cerebral ischemia in the middle cerebral artery territory in primates. *Stroke*, 8: 61–70.

Experimental Models of Ischemia

Brain Ischemia: Quantitative EEG and Imaging Techniques, Progress in Brain Research, Vol. 62, edited by
G. Pfurtscheller, E.J. Jonkman and F.H. Lopes da Silva
©*1984 Elsevier Science Publishers B.V.*

Quantitative EEG and Evoked Potentials after Experimental Brain Ischemia in the Rat; Correlation with Cerebral Metabolism and Blood Flow

INGMAR ROSÉN[1], MAJ-LIS SMITH[2] and STIG REHNCRONA[3]

Departments of [1]Clinical Neurophysiology, [2]Experimental Brain Research and [3]Neurosurgery, University Hospital, S-221 85 Lund (Sweden)

INTRODUCTION

Cerebral ischemia is probably the most important pathological condition encountered in neurology and neurosurgery and is a common and often fatal complication to heart failure and shock of varying etiology. Sudden energy failure in brain tissue produced by ischemia leads to an almost immediate blockade of neuronal synaptic function as revealed by cessation of spontaneous electroencephalographic activity and disappearance of evoked responses (Meldrum and Brierley, 1969). Membrane failure occurs later with a sudden increase in extracellular potassium ion concentrations (Astrup et al., 1977). The degree of functional recovery after the ischemic insult will depend on a number of pathophysiological factors during the ischemic period as well as during recirculation (Hossmann, 1977; Siesjö, 1978). Furthermore, the final cell damage following ischemia seems to "mature" over hours and days (Ito et al., 1975; Pulsinelli et al., 1982). It is well established clinically that the brain can withstand only limited periods of pronounced ischemia with full return of normal neurological function. However, extensive recovery of cerebral energy metabolism and also some electrophysiological functions have been observed even following prolonged periods (30–60 min) of experimentally produced complete ischemia (Hossman and Kleihues, 1973; Hossmann and Zimmermann, 1974; Kleihues et al., 1975; Nordström et al., 1978a; Rehncrona et al., 1979a). One possible explanation of this discrepancy is a detrimental effect of a trickling blood flow during the ischemic period leading to an excessive tissue lactacidosis during severe incomplete ischemia (Rehncrona et al., 1980, 1981). Although extensive information is available concerning the cerebral metabolism and local distribution of cerebral blood flow during the early restitution phase after experimental ischemia (Rehncrona, 1980; Kågström, 1982), in clinical practice only neurological and electrophysiological features are usually available for the prognostic evaluation. It is therefore highly relevant to relate electrophysiological features to cerebral metabolism and blood flow in the restitution period following experimental ischemia. This paper discusses the results of different degrees of experimental ischemia as well as different degrees of brain tissue lactacidosis during the ischemic period. More detailed information is available elsewhere (Rehncrona et al., 1981, 1984).

176

METHODS

Male Wistar rats (350–400 g) were initially anesthetized with halothane, tracheotomized, paralyzed with tubocurarine and artificially ventilated. Femoral arterial and venous cannulas were inserted for continuous blood pressure recording, blood sampling and infusions. A midline incision of the scalp was made to fit a plastic funnel for later freezing of the brain in situ at the end of the experiment. In some animals the carotid arteries were dissected and in others the atlantooccipital membrane was exposed. The halothane was then discontinued and the animal kept on $N_2O + O_2$ (75% + 25%). All animals were heparinized and the rectal temperature kept at 37°C by external heating.

Compression ischemia was induced according to Neely and Youmans (1963) as modified by Ljunggren et al. (1974). A double-lumen needle was introduced into the cisterna magna for infusion of artificial CSF at 37°C and measurement of intracranial pressure (ICP). ICP was momentarily increased to and kept at A/40 mm Hg above the systolic blood pressure (*complete compression ischemia*), B/ at 5 mm Hg, or C/ 20 mm Hg below the mean arterial blood pressure (*incomplete compression ischemia*). The ischemic period was 15 min.

Incomplete hypovolemic ischemia was induced, as described by Nordström et al. (1978b). Both carotid arteries were occluded by small arterial clamps and the mean arterial blood pressure decreased to a constant level of 50 mm Hg by bleeding the animal. After 15-min ischemia, the cerebral perfusion pressure was restored by removal of the clamps and reinfusion of the blood (kept at 37°C). Systemic pH changes were prevented by sodium bicarbonate infusions.

In order to vary the *lactate accumulation* in the brain tissue during the period of *incomplete hypovolemic ischemia*, one group of animals (A) was fed normally prior to the experiment, whereas a second group (B) fasted for 24 h before the experiment. A third group (C) fasted before the experiment and was given an infusion of 2 ml of 50% glucose solution for 15 min before induction of ischemia.

Arterial blood was sampled for determination of pO_2 and glucose. The brains were frozen in situ with liquid nitrogen at the end of the ischemic period or at 90 min postischemia and then stored at −80°C until extraction for analysis of metabolites. Concentrations of glucose, lactate, phosphocreatinine (PCr), adenosine tri-, di-, and monophosphate (ATP, ADP and AMP) were determined with specific enzymatic fluorometric methods (Lowry and Passonneau, 1972) as described by Folbergrovà et al. (1972a,b). The energy charge of the adenine nucleotide pool (EC) was calculated as:

$$\frac{[ATP] + 0.5\,[ADP]}{[ATP] + [ADP] + [AMP]}$$

according to Atkinson (1968).

A pair of gold-plated copper bolts was inserted into each side of the skull; the tips were in extradural position with one prefrontal reference electrode and one active electrode over the parietal surface. On one side the integrated EEG activity was continuously quantified by a cerebral function monitor (CFM Devices Limited) and written out on a slow time base on a semilogarithmic scale (Prior, 1979). On the other side, conventional EEG was continuously recorded (frequency range 0.5–30 Hz) on an Elema Mingograph. The same channel was also used intermittently for recording of somatosensory evoked responses (SER) to electrical stimulation of the contralateral nose area through subcutaneously placed needle electrodes (frequency range of SER recording: 0.5 Hz–1 kHz; stimulus: 0.2 ms pulses of 4 mA at 5 Hz or trains of 10 stimuli at 500 Hz from a constant current stimulator. Sixty-four single sweeps were averaged in each test. For single shock stimulation the analysis time was 50 ms and for "train stimulation" 1 sec. Single shock stimulation did not cause any shifts in blood pressure and "train stimulation" was only used postischemically if no early latency SER could be elicited.

There were no gross differences between the groups in body temperature, blood pressure or blood-gas parameters. Blood glucose concentrations differed between fed and fasted animals subjected to incomplete hypovolemic ischemia. Thus in fed animals blood glucose increased from 8.9 ± 0.8 $\mu mol \cdot ml^{-1}$ to 17.6 ± 2.4 ($n = 6$) during 15-min ischemia, while the corresponding values for fasted animals were 6.6 ± 0.2 and 4.3 ± 0.9 $\mu mol \cdot ml^{-1}$. The increase in blood glucose in fed animals in this situation is most probably due to mobilization of glucose from body stores of glycogen caused by sympathoadrenal activation related to a hemorrhagic shock situation. Glucose pretreatment markedly elevated the blood glucose concentration (25–35 $\mu mol \cdot ml^{-1}$) during ischemia and these animals remained hyperglycemic during the recirculation period.

RESULTS

All animals subjected to complete and incomplete compression ischemia with perfusion pressure (PP of 5 mm Hg) as well as the groups subjected to incomplete hypovolemic ischemia, showed flat EEG and total disappearance of SER during the ischemic period. In these animals there was a total deterioration of the cerebral energy state with an energy charge (EC) of less than 0.26. However, in the group of animals with cerebral perfusion pressure decreased to only 20 mm Hg some EEG activity remained, characterized by a low-amplitude slow-wave pattern. In this group the cerebral energy state was much better preserved with an EC of 0.879 ± 0.018, which is significantly less than the non-ischemic controls (EC: 0.946 ± 0.002). The levels of accumulated lactate in the ischemic tissue varied between the groups. Thus, complete ischemia and incomplete compression ischemia with PP=20 mm Hg, only showed an increase in tissue lactate concentration to 12 and 11 $\mu mol \cdot g^{-1}$, respectively. The lactate value for incomplete compression ischemia PP 5 mm Hg was 17.7 ± 1.3 $\mu mol \cdot g^{-1}$. The degree of lactic acidosis varied in the groups of animals subjected to incomplete hypovolemic ischemia as shown in Fig. 3.

The neurophysiological features during recovery after the ischemic period were described in the same terms as are commonly used in a clinical neurophysiological context, i.e. (a) recovery of the background activity quantitatively and qualitatively; (b) time lapse between start of recirculation and the first appearance of EEG activity; (c) occurrence of epileptogenic activity and time lapse from the start of recirculation to its appearance; (d) reappearance of SER, its amplitude in relation to the preischemic value and the change of latency of the initial positive peak (normal value 6.8 ± 0.18 ms) and the following negative peak (normal value 11.8 ± 0.53 ms) of the main response complex; (e) in cases of no reappearance of early SER, the occurrence of late responses to train stimulation of the nose were recorded.

One experiment with severe incomplete compression ischemia (PP 5 mm Hg) is illustrated in Fig. 1. The onset of ischemia is followed by an almost immediate elimination of EEG as shown in the CFM record. After recirculation (indicated by *), EEG activity started to appear after 17 min and epileptogenic activity after 21 min. Early latency SER did not reappear during the observation period but late negative responses to train stimulation could be elicited with a peak latency about 300 ms.

The comparison of neurophysiological and metabolic recovery after recirculation and different degrees of ischemia lasting 15 min, is illustrated in Fig. 2. As shown at the top, all groups of animals showed complete or almost complete restoration of the energy charge. However, large differences between groups were found concerning the neurophysiological features after a 90-min recovery. Animals with severe incomplete ischemia, either by compression or hypovolemia, showed a better neurophysiological recovery than animals with the same period of complete compression ischemia. The entire group of animals with a moderate compression ischemia (PP 20 mm Hg) returned to background EEG-activity of almost normal amplitude shortly after recirculation. It is noteworthy, however, that only half of the animals recovered early SER within 90 min.

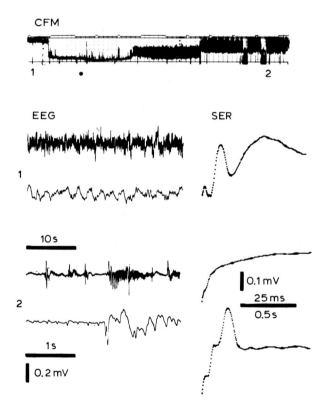

Fig. 1. Neurophysiological monitoring of an experiment with 15 min of severe incomplete compression ischemia (PP 5 mm Hg) followed by 90 min of recirculation. Start of recirculation indicated by * in CFM record. Time scale for CFM record 10 min. Full scale of CFM record 100 μV. The moments for EEG and SER samples are indicated by corresponding numbers below the CFM record. Note display of EEG on two different time scales.

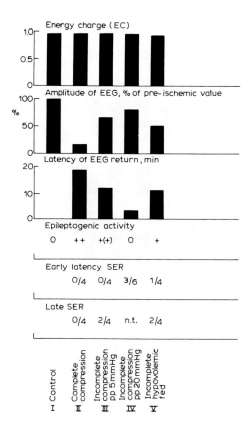

Fig. 2. Summary of metabolic and neurophysiological recovery after 90 min of recirculation following 15 min of ischemia. I: Controls without ischemia ($n = 6$), II: complete compression ischemia ($n = 4$), III: severe incomplete compression ischemia (PP 5 mm Hg) ($n = 4$), IV: moderate incomplete compression ischemia (PP 20 mm Hg) ($n = 6$), V: severe incomplete hypovolemic ischemia ($n = 4$). For explanation see text, p. 178.

The significance of the tissue lactacidosis developed in the brain during the ische-mic period for the immediate postischemic recovery is summarized in Fig. 3. As previously described, hyperglycemic rats showed an almost complete failure of neurophysiological restitution and lingering energy metabolic failure after 30 min of severe hypovolemic ischemia, whereas fasted animals showed a significant recovery of EEG, SER and energy metabolism (Rehncrona et al., 1981). After 15 min of severe hypovolemic ischemia, both starved and normally fed animals recovered their energy charge, whereas half of the hyperglycemic animals showed a lingering energy failure after 90 min of recovery. The last group also showed delayed return of low amplitude EEG and almost no recovery of evoked potentials. Fasted animals all recovered early SER, although at a reduced amplitude and with prolonged latency. Normally fed animals showed a recovery intermediate between the other two groups.

180

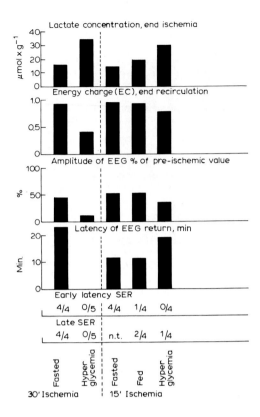

Fig. 3. Summary of metabolic and neurophysiological recovery after 90 min of recirculation following 30 min or 15 min of severe incomplete hypovolemic ischemia. The degree of brain tissue lactacidosis developed during ischemia in the different groups of animals is shown at the top. The lactate value for the hyperglyce-mic group with 15 min ischemia has been extrapolated from the data of Rehncrona et al. (1981). Number of animals in each group = 4, except hyperglycemia + 30 min ischemia, = 5 (see text, p. 178).

DISCUSSION

Three main conclusions can be drawn from these studies. First, there may be great differences in recovery of EEG and evoked potentials, despite similar metabolic recovery. Second, postischemic restoration of neurophysiological parameters was clearly superior following severe imcomplete ischemia induced either with hypovole-mia combined with carotid ligation or in the compresion model as compared with complete compression ischemia. One possible explanation for the deficient functional recovery in complete compression ischemia might be the occurrence of the wide-spread no-reflow phenomenon leaving large subcortical areas without perfusion fol-lowing recirculation (Rehncrona et al., 1979b; Kågström et al., 1983). The severe hypovolemic model of ischemia reduces the CBF to near-zero values in all cerebral cortical areas, in the caudo-putamen and in the hippocampus with less marked reduc-tion of flow rates in a number of subcortical structures (Kågström et al., 1983). The no-reflow phenomenon after recirculation is much less pronounced in this model than in complete compression ischemia.

In the incomplete ischemic models the remaining trickling blood flow will deliver glucose to brain tissue during the ischemic period. This is the reason for the excessive values of tissue lactacidosis reached in this model, which is closely similar to the situation encountered clinically in regional or global cortical ischemia. The third conclusion that can be drawn from our studies is that an increased accumulation of lactic acid during ischemia seems to impair neurophysiological recovery, even if levels critical for restitution of energy metabolism are not reached. It would seem that even a moderate lactic acidosis, i.e. lactate values between 15 and 20 $\mu mol \cdot g^{-1}$ reached during a relatively short ischemic period, may be critical for at least the immediate and probably also for the eventual recovery. The hypovolemic ischemia model has recently been adopted for long-term recovery studies (Smith et al., 1984). Starved animals exposed to 15 min of ischemia did not regain consciousness for 4–8 h and 75% of the animals developed progressive seizures leading to death. Animals exposed to 10 min of ischemia showed EEG and some late SER activity within the immediate recovery period, return to consciousness, and abnormal motor behavior. However, histopathological analysis demonstrated extensive cell damage in hippocampus, caudo-putamen and neocortex (Smith et al., in preparation). Taken together, it would seem that a flat or almost flat EEG in combination with complete absence of evoked responses 90 min after an ischemic insult in the rat is indicative of widespread cortical necrosis and a deficient recovery of energy metabolism. Recovery of EEG amplitudes to about 50% of the preischemic value, in combination with some late SER responses, is indicative of an immediate recovery of energy metabolism, although with a defective neurological recovery and quite widespread cell death within vulnerable regions. It is hypothesized that only a significant return of early evoked potentials in combination with recovery of EEG amplitude to levels above 50% of the preischemic level within the immediate postischemic period is an indication of full recovery of neurological functions at the behavioral level, as well as at the level of cortical neuronal circuits.

SUMMARY

The effects of different degrees of brain ischemia upon the short-term recovery of neurophysiological parameters were studied and compared with metabolic and CBF data.

Rats were exposed to 15 min of ischemia, either complete ischemia by a sudden increase of ICP to a level above the BP or incomplete ischemia by adjusting the perfusion pressure to 5 mm Hg or 20 mm Hg. A fourth group of animals was subjected to profound incomplete ischemia by carotid artery occlusion and lowering of BP to 50 mm Hg for 15 min. All animals recovered their brain energy metabolism within 90 min as judged by the energy charge index. The immediate neurophysiological recovery within 90 min as judged by recovery of background EEG activity, time lapse of EEG return from the start of recirculation, amount of epileptogenic activity, reappearance of early and late components of SER, however, showed great differences between groups. Neurophysiological recovery was much more incomplete after complete ischemia as compared with incomplete ischemia, possibly due to no reflow in subcortical areas. Groups of animals with high levels of lactacidosis showed less recovery than animals with a low level of lactacidosis during ischemia, confirming earlier results with 30 min duration of ischemia. It is suggested that quantitative neurophysiological recovery in the postischemic period provides more detailed prognostic information than brain energy metabolism in indicating the extent of brain cell damage and death developing later.

REFERENCES

Astrup, J., Symon, L., Branston, N. M. and Lassen, N. A. (1977) Cortical evoked potential and extracellular K$^+$ and H$^+$ at critical levels of brain ischemia. *Stroke*, 8: 51–57.

Atkinson, D. E. (1968) The energy charge of the adenylate pool as a regulatory parameter. Interaction with feedback modifiers. *Biochemistry*, 7: 4030–4034.

Folbergrovà, J., MacMillan, U. and Siesjö, B. K. (1972a) The effect of moderate and marked hypercapnia upon the energy state and upon the cytoplasmic NADH/NAD$^+$ ratio of the rat brain. *J. Neurochem.*, 19: 2497–2505.

Folbergrovà, J., MacMillan, U. and Siesjö, B.K. (1972b) The effect of hypercapnic acidosis upon some glycolytic and Krebs cycle-associated intermediates in the rat brain. *J. Neurochem.*, 19: 2507–2517.

Hossmann, K. A. (1977) Total ischemia of the brain. In K. J. Zülch, W. Kaufmann, K. A. Hossmann and V. Hossmann (Eds.), *Brain and Heart Infarct*, Springer-Verlag, pp. 107-124.

Hossmann, K. A. and Kleihues, P. (1973) Reversibility of ischemic brain damage. *Arch. Neurol. (Chic.)* 29: 375–382.

Hossmann, K. A. and Zimmerman, V. (1974) Resuscitation of the monkey brain after 1 hour's complete ischemia. I. Physiological and morphological observations. *Brain Res.*, 81: 59–74.

Ito, U., Spatz, M., Walker, J. T. and Klatzo, I. (1975) Experimental cerebral ischemia in mongolian gerbils. I. Light microscopic observations. *Acta Neuropath. (Berl.)*, 32: 209–223.

Kleihues, P., Hossmann, K. A., Pegg, A. E., Kobayashi, K. and Zimmermann, V. (1975) Resuscitation of the monkey brain after 1 hour complete ischemia. III. Indications of metabolic recovery. *Brain Res.*, 95: 61–73.

Kågström, E., Smith, M.-L. and Siesjö, B. K. (1983) Local cerebral blood flow in the recovery period *cerebral ischemia. An experimental study in rats*. Thesis. Lund.

Kågström, E., Smith, M. -L. and Siesjö, B. K. (1983) Local cerebral blood flow in the recovery period following complete ischemia in the rat. *J. Cereb. Blood Flow Metab.*, 3: 170–182.

Ljunggren, B., Ratcheson, R. A. and Siesjö, B. K. (1974) Cerebral metabolic state following compression ischemia. *Brain Res.*, 73: 291–307.

Lowry, O. H. and Passoneau, J. V. (1972) *A Flexible System of Enzymatic Analysis*, Academic Press, New York.

Meldrum, B. S. and Brierley, J. B. (1969) Brain damage in the rhesus monkey resulting from profound arterial hypotension. II. Changes in the spontaneous and evoked electrical activity of the neocortex. *Brain Res.*, 13: 101–118.

Neely, W. A. and Youmans, R. J. (1963) Anoxia of canine brain without damage. *J. Amer. Med. Ass.*, (1978a) 183: 1085–1087.

Nordström, C.-H., Rehncrona, S. and Siesjö, B. K. (1978a) Restitution of cerebral energy state, as well as of glycolytic metabolites, citric acid cycle intermediates and associated amino acids after 30 min of complete ischemia in rats anaesthetized with nitrous oxide or phenobarbital. *J. Neurochem.* 30: 479–486.

Nordström, C.-H., Rehncrona, S. and Siesjö, B. K. (1978b) Effects of phenobarbital in cerebral ischemia. II. Restitution of cerebral energy state, as well as of glycolytic metabolites, citric acid cycle intermediates and associated amino acids after pronounced incomplete ischemia. *Stroke*, 9: 335–343.

Prior, P. (1979) *Monitoring Cerebral Function – Long Term Recordings of Cerebral Electrical Activity*, Elsevier/North-Holland Biomedical Press, Amsterdam.

Pulsinelli, W. A., Brierly, I. B. and Plum, F. (1982) Temporal profile of neuronal damage in a model of transient forebrain ischemia. *Ann. Neurol.*, 11: 491–498.

Rehncrona, S. (1980) *Studies on biochemical mechanisms of irreversible cell damage in brain ischemia*. Thesis, Lund.

Rehncrona, S., Mela, L. and Siesjö, B. K. (1979a) Recovery of brain mitochondrial function in the rat after complete and incomplete cerebral ischemia. *Stroke*, 10: 437–446.

Rehncrona, S., Abdul-Rahman, A. and Siesjö, B. K. (1979b) Local cerebral blood flow in the postischemic period. *Acta Neurol. Scand.*, 60, Suppl. 72: 294–295.

Rehncrona, S., Rosén, I. and Siesjö, B. K. (1980) Excessive cellular acidosis: An important mechanism of neuronal damage in the brain? *Acta Physiol. Scand.*, 110: 435–437.

Rehncrona, S., Rosén, I. and Siesjö, B. K. (1981) Brain lactic acidosis and ischemic cell damage. I. Biochemistry and neurophysiology. *J. Cereb. Blood Flow Metab.*, 1: 297–311.

Rehncrona, S., Rosén, I. and Smith, M-L, (1984) The effect of different degrees of brain ischemia upon the short term recovery of neurophysiological and metabolical parameters, submitted for publication.

Siesjö, B. K. (1978) *Brain Energy Metabolism*, John Wiley & Son, Chichester.

Smith, M-L, Bendek, G., Dahlgren, N., Rosén, I., Wieloch, T. and Siesjö, B. K. (1984) Model for studying long-term recovery following forebrain ischemia in the rat. II. A two vessel occlusion model, submitted for publication.

Brain Ischemia: Quantitative EEG and Imaging Techniques, Progress in Brain Research, Vol. 62, edited by G. Pfurtscheller, E.J. Jonkman and F.H. Lopes da Silva
©1984 Elsevier Science Publishers B.V.

Somatosensory Evoked Potentials in Experimental Brain Ischemia

NEIL M. BRANSTON, AMANDA LADDS, LINDSAY SYMON, ALEXANDER D. WANG and JANOS VAJDA*

The Gough-Cooper Department of Neurological Surgery, Institute of Neurology, and the National Hospital, Queen Square, London WC1 3BG (U.K.)

INTRODUCTION

The amplitude and latency of components of the somatosensory evoked potential (SEP) recorded from the scalp may be affected by lesions at any stage of the sensory pathway. Consequently, the correct interpretation of changes in the SEP seen in routine clinical practice or during surgery (Desmedt and Noël, 1973; Hume and Cant, 1978; Symon et al., 1979a, 1983; Chiappa et al., 1980; Halliday, 1982; Wang et al., 1982; Grundy et al., 1983) depends on how well the anatomical origins of these components can be identified. In cases where the lesions are ischemic, interpretation must also rely upon a knowledge of the relative sensitivities to ischemia of the different stages in the afferent pathway, particularly when there may be loss of the normal capacity of the cerebral circulation to autoregulate blood flow in the face of reduced perfusion pressure.

In the cerebral cortex, it has been shown experimentally that if local cerebral blood flow (CBF) is reduced from normal to about 18 ml/100 g/min, there is attenuation of SEP amplitude recorded at the surface, and below about 12 ml/100 g/min, the SEP is abolished (Branston et al., 1974). This threshold relationship of SEP amplitude to local flow is illustrated in Fig. 1. Corresponding clinical observations on the electro-corticogram are in broad agreement (Sharbrough et al., 1973; Trojaborg and Boysen, 1973). These experimental studies have been almost exclusively confined to cortex, however, because of its accessibility. In this chapter we describe experiments which were designed to clarify the question of the relative ischemic sensitivities between regions, extending our earlier work to measure SEPs and CBF in thalamus and brainstem.

---

*Present address: National Institute of Neurosurgery, Amerikai 57, Budapest, 1145 Hungary.

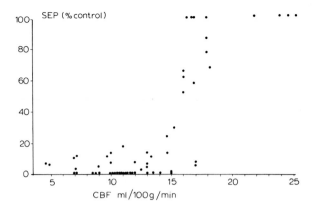

Fig. 1. The relationship between steady-state amplitude of the cortical SEP, expressed as a percentage of control value, and local CBF following MCA occlusion and further reduction in flow by controlled exsanguination. Data were recorded from the postcentral region in 19 previous experiments using a similar protocol.

METHODS

The general technique was to establish relationships between, on the one hand, the amplitude of SEP components generated in thalamus (ventral postero-lateral nucleus, VPL), brainstem (medial lemniscus, ML), and cerebral cortex and, on the other hand, local CBF or mean systemic blood pressure (MSBP) as independent variables. These relationships were then compared with that already established for cortex (Fig. 1).

Flow was measured using the hydrogen clearance method (Pasztor et al., 1973). Data were obtained from 11 baboons maintained under chloralose anesthesia. This restricted our observations on SEPs to the early components, up to 25 ms latency in the monkey; however, it is just these components which are of major utility clinically. We also studied changes in latency of the principal peaks of the SEP. These were measured relative to the onset of activity in the high cervical region, the data on central conduction time (CCT) thus obtained being related to flow and the changes with ischemia compared with corresponding clinical data (Hume and Cant, 1978; Symon et al., 1979a, 1983).

Preparation

The animals, in the weight range 7–10 kg, were intubated under light thiopentone anesthesia and the femoral vessels cannulated, prior to administration of alpha-chloralose (60 mg/kg, i.v.). Arterial $PaCO_2$ was maintained in the normal range during electrode placements and recording and controlled by pump ventilation with O_2 at appropriate stroke volume. Arterial PaO_2, pH, hematocrit and core temperature were measured and adjusted as necessary. MSBP was continuously recorded.

The skull was exposed and an SEP reference electrode of sintered Ag/AgCl was placed epidurally at Fpz. A silver-ball electrode was inserted under the spinous process of C2 in the midline, and stimulating electrodes placed over the median nerve at

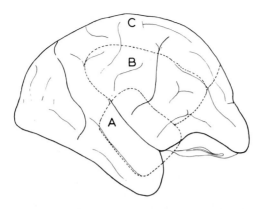

Fig. 2. Diagram of lateral view of the baboon brain, indicating principal areas of the hemisphere studied in earlier work. In the present study, only areas B and C were used.

each wrist; the stimulus voltage was adjusted to give a thumb twitch with pulse width of 0.2 ms. Then the animal's head was fixed in a stereotactic frame and two regions, one containing the SEP cortical focus (in area B; see Fig. 2) and the other situated parasagittally near Cz (in area C), were marked out on the skull bilaterally and the dura exposed through small (about 1 cm^2) craniectomies. The dura was then removed at the area C sites and electrodes inserted vertically into the VPL and ML bilaterally, the final position being determined using the averaged SEP as a guide. The dura over the area B sites was then removed, silver-ball electrodes placed on the postcentral gyrus, and additional flow electrodes (Pt/Ir wire, 125 microns diameter, exposed tip 1 mm) inserted into the cortex in all four regions before all electrodes were secured in the skull by acrylic cement. A large Ag/AgCl electrode was placed in the animal's mouth to act as common mode reference and as the reference for the hydrogen clearance system.

The animal was then removed from the frame and a transorbital dissection performed to expose the right middle cerebral artery (MCA) for its subsequent occlusion with a Scoville clip.

Experimental protocol and SEP recording

At least two control measurements of flow and SEP were made from all electrodes after the stability of the hydrogen electrode baselines and PaCO$_2$ was confirmed. The MCA was then occluded and the measurements repeated immediately in short runs (usually 64 sweeps) of SEP averages to follow any changes in the SEP until a stable waveform was obtained. The MSBP was then progressively reduced in stages of 10 or 20 torr by careful withdrawal of arterial blood in a heparinized syringe and held steady at each stage while further SEP and flow measurements were taken. Our objective was to produce a stepwise reduction in CBF. On the right side, the initial ischemic effect of the MCA occlusion on the cortical SEP would be followed by a progressive flow reduction due to loss of autoregulation; on the left, the ischemia would result almost entirely from the hypotension.

This procedure was continued until, generally, only the neck and lemniscal responses remained, following which the animal was fixation-perfused with saline/for-

188

malin so that the brain could later be removed to confirm the positions of deep electrodes by histology.

Electrodes for measurement of flow and SEP were placed in pairs in the VPL at AP 10 and in the ML at about AP 7. While the lemniscal response was quite focal and characteristic of a fiber tract, the correct placement of electrodes in the VPL required preliminary searches using voltage gradient techniques, as mentioned below. The electrodes were constructed from 0.8 mm diameter stainless steel tubing terminated at the lower end by a piece of Pt wire, the whole electrode (except for the tip) being insulated with epoxy varnish. A PDP-11 interactive system was programmed to sample up to 32 SEP channels at a sample rate of 10 kHz for each channel for 256 points per sweep to form averaged SEPs, which could be displayed, filed on disk and analyzed off-line. Averaged SEPs were smoothed (once only) before analysis using a zero phase shift digital filter with effective 3 db point of 1,300 Hz. The system also sampled up to 16 hydrogen electrode outputs, displayed the clearances, computed the flows on-line if required, and filed the clearances on disk.

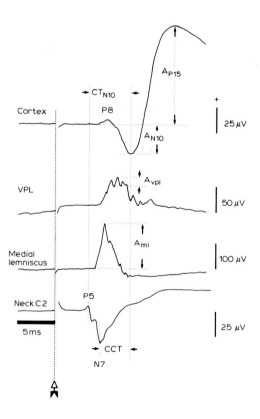

Fig. 3. Illustration of averaged SEPs recorded in the normal, anesthetized baboon from post-central cortex, VPL nuclear complex, medial lemniscus, and over the cervical cord at C2. The arrow denotes the stimulus, and the component amplitudes measured in this study are indicated. Conduction time (CT) was defined relative to the P5 peak of the neck response.

RESULTS – CONTROL PHASE

Waveforms

Figure 3 illustrates typical SEP waveforms recorded from cortex, thalamus, lemniscus and neck. The overall timing of the various peaks is given in Table I. Since the initial peak P5 of the neck response was more consistent in timing between animals than N7, we decided to use the time of occurrence of P5 as the reference event from which all events in the brain evoked by the same stimulus would be measured and designate each such measurement as the conduction time (CT). The most likely origin of P5 is the cervical cord (Sances et al., 1978; Arezzo et al., 1979). The average increase in latency of N7 measured with respect to P5 was less than 0.1 ms up to the point of failure of the cortical response, so changes in CT and CCT (which is measured from N7) were essentially the same; however, to avoid confusion, we reserve the term CCT for the N14-N20 interval in man or its homologue N7-N10 in the monkey.

TABLE I

CONDUCTION TIME (CT) OF SEP COMPONENTS IN BRAIN-STEM, THALAMUS AND CORTEX MEASURED IN THE CONTROL PHASE

Average latency from stimulus is obtained by adding the latency of P5 (neck reference marker for CT), i.e. 5.32 ± 0.80 ms. Data from 10 animals

Region	CT (ms)	
	Mean	S.D.
ML: Onset	0.92	0.20
1st peak	1.63	0.14
2nd peak	2.59	0.25
VPL: Onset	0.98	0.21
Central peak	3.47	0.46
Cortex: P8 Onset	1.27	0.38
P8 peak	2.57	0.23
N10 peak	5.32	0.49
P15 peak	11.18	1.81

Onset of the VPL response was just after, and slower than, that of the ML. A prominent feature of the VPL response was a set of oscillatory wavelets that appeared superimposed upon an overall positive or positive/negative component. Voltage gradient studies indicated that the highest, at least, of these wavelets was very likely of local origin and, further, the average CT of this wavelet (3.5 ms) was considerably longer than that of either component of the lemniscal response (Table I), so this wavelet was taken to represent the VPL response proper and its peak-to-peak amplitude and peak latency (CT) measured accordingly. This assumption was further justified by data obtained following the establishment of a selective ischemic lesion in the thalamus (Fig. 4), in which the wavelets, but not the positive wave upon which they appeared superimposed, were abolished in dense thalamic ischemia.

190

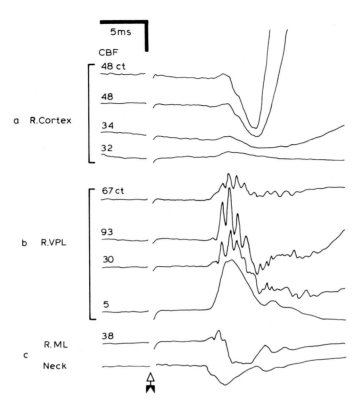

5ms

CBF

a R.Cortex
48 ct
48
34
32

b R.VPL
67 ct
93
30
5

c R.ML
Neck
38

Fig. 4. SEPs recorded in one animal with stimulus to left median nerve (at arrow) illustrating the effect of producing selective ischemia in the thalamus. In this animal, the major arteries supplying the thalamus were occluded instead of the MCA. a: Top trace: control (MSBP = 107 torr). The later cortical component P15 is off the top of the picture due to the high gain needed to show N10. Second trace: after VPL lesion but before bleeding (MSBP = 102 torr). The amplitude is marginally reduced, but local flow is not. Third trace: after reduction of MSBP to 68 torr. The cortical component has disappeared, due to subcortical ischemia since local flow is well above threshold of 18 ml/100 g/min associated with MCA occlusion. Fourth trace: MSBP reduced to 47 torr. b: Corresponding waveforms recorded in VPL, at the same stages shown in a. Note the increase in local flow and amplitude of the higher frequency components, immediately following VPL lesion (second trace). With dense local ischemia (fourth trace), these components are abolished. c: Waveform recorded in lemniscus (ML) and at the neck (C2) at the stage of dense VPL ischemia (MSBP = 47 torr). The vertical calibration bar corresponds to 12.5, 50, 50, and 25 μv in cortex, VPL, ML and neck recordings, respectively. Positive is upward.

The structure of the waveform of the early cortical SEP in the baboon is similar to that recorded in man, but to about half the time scale. The initial positive peak P8 is almost certainly of subcortical origin since it remains following focal cortical ischemia, and probably corresponds to P15 as recorded (Wang et al., 1982) in man. The subsequent negative component N10 corresponds to N20 in man and is certainly of cortical origin: it appears focal with surface exploration. Only N10 and the subsequent cortical positive wave P15 were measured in this study. P15 inverts as an exploring electrode passes through the cortex. It was followed by a variable negative wave and together these comprise the positive/negative primary cortical response referred to in our earlier work (Branston et al., 1974).

Blood flow in ML, VPL and cortex

Flow and SEP data were obtained from 31 electrodes in the ML and 30 in VPL. Table II shows the average flows recorded in all regions. Control flows were not significantly different between the two sides in any region, but those in lemniscus tended to be lower than those in VPL. Cortical flows agreed closely in value with those obtained in other series (e.g. Symon et al., 1979b) in which the closed (reconstituted) skull preparation was used, and were lower, on average, than flows recorded subcortically.

TABLE II

CONTROL BLOOD FLOWS IN THE REGIONS STUDIED AND THE CHANGES IMMEDIATELY FOLLOWING MCA OCCLUSION

Paired *t*-tests (10 animals)

| | Local CBF (initial), ml/100 g/min | | | |
| | Control | | After occlusion | |
Region	Mean	S.D.	Mean	S.D.
R. ML	52.3	35.1	48.3	37.6
L. ML	45.3	26.3	41.9	26.9
R. VPL	58.0	40.0	52.1	42.1
L. VPL	62.1	23.1	50.1	17.0, $p<0.02$
R. Cortex B	42.4	20.6	20.9	22.1, $p<0.001$
L. Cortex B	45.3	5.0	44.5	2.1
R. Cortex C	47.8	25.1	37.9	23.1
L. Cortex C	43.8	13.6	36.8	11.6

Biexponential clearances were seen at 11 electrodes in the ML and at 15 in VPL. Figure 5 shows the distribution in flow of the monoexponential clearances. No monoexponential flows below 20 ml/100 g/min were observed and, generally, the lemniscal flows were lower than those in VPL, as would be expected from tissue with a relatively higher fraction of white matter.

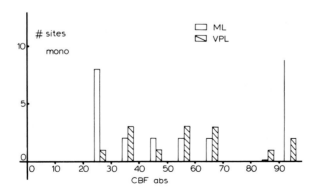

Fig. 5. Distribution of control flow values for the monoexponential hydrogen clearances recorded in the medial lemniscus (ML) and thalamus (VPL) of 11 animals.

RESULTS – ISCHEMIC PHASE

Effects of MCA occlusion alone

Table II also shows the flows remaining in the steady state immediately after occlusion of the right MCA, that is, prior to any induced hypotension. The associated change in MSBP was insignificant, from an average of 130 torr to one of 127 torr.

All regions showed some reduction in flow from control. In area B of the cortex on the right side, flow decreased to less than half on average from 42.4 to 20.9 ml/100 g/min, highly significant as expected in MCA territory. The reduction in flow in right side area C averaged about 20%, but was not significant; however, those reductions in area C of left cortex and in left VPL were significant. Their mechanism is unknown. They were caused by the MCA occlusion and not by the passage of time alone, as was confirmed by checking that corresponding changes in flow measured over an equivalent period (averaging about 26 min) during the control phase were much smaller and not significant. Paired *t*-tests were used throughout.

When MCA occlusion alone was sufficient to reduce ipsilateral local cortical (area B) flow to below the SEP threshold, the early components of responses recorded in the VPL and ML on that side were unaffected; only the later slow component (which reflects the cortical component P15) was abolished.

Occlusion plus hypotension – SEP amplitude changes

Figure 6 illustrates the effect of right MCA occlusion followed by hypotension produced by graded exsanguination. In this procedure, all SEPs were recorded in the left hemisphere so that the effect of hypotension alone could be studied. Although flow was substantially reduced throughout the brain, in contrast to the focal ischemia produced by the initial occlusion, again only the cortical components were abolished.

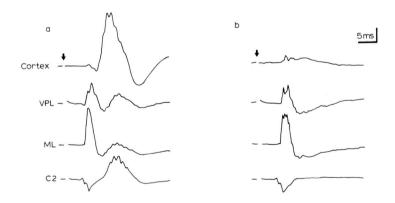

Fig. 6. Recordings from the left side before (a) and after (b) right MCA occlusion and reduction in MSBP, in one animal. Although flow was substantially reduced throughout the brain by the hypotension (to 28 torr), only the cortical components N10 and P15 were abolished. Local cortical flow was then 9 ml/100 g/min. Note the preservation of P8, the earliest positive component of the cortical response, which is probably a far-field derivation of part of the thalamic response. Vertical bar corresponds to 40 and 10 μv for the cortical responses in (a) and (b), respectively, to 20 μv for ML responses throughout, and to 10 μv for VPL and neck responses throughout. Positive is upward.

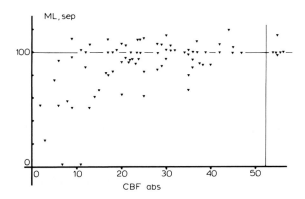

Fig. 7. Relationship between SEP amplitude (expressed as a percentage of control amplitude) and local blood flow (ml/100 g/min) in the medial lemniscus following MCA occlusion and added hypotension in 11 animals. Control points are omitted; those to the right of the vertical line correspond to flows greater than 50 ml/100 g/min.

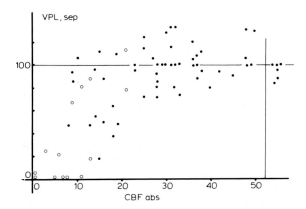

Fig. 8. Relationship between SEP amplitude (percent control) and local flow (ml/100 g/min) in the VPL following MCA occlusion and added hypotension in 11 animals. Control points are omitted; those to the right of the vertical line correspond to flows greater than 50 ml/100 g/min. Points shown as open circles represent measurements made in VPL when the amplitude of the corresponding ML response was reduced from its control value; their ordinates may therefore be underestimated.

Additional hypotension, however, reduced and finally abolished the VPL response and, ultimately, that in the ML.

To analyze the above effects systematically, we have characterized the changes in SEP amplitude in two ways: as functions of local CBF and of MSBP. In each case, a threshold relationship was sought but the different regions were compared either on the basis of a global variable (MSBP) or, alternatively, in terms of local tissue perfusion. Figure 7 shows a plot of the SEP in the lemniscus in relation to absolute local flow, and it is clear that the response is sustained down to at least 10 ml/100 g/min, in contrast to the situation in cerebral cortex which is characterized by a flow threshold of about 18 ml/100 g/min (Fig. 1). With the corresponding VPL plot (Fig. 8), the contrast with cortex is not so great as with that of the ML, but there are nevertheless several data points well above the zero level in the region of 10 ml/100 g/min.

194

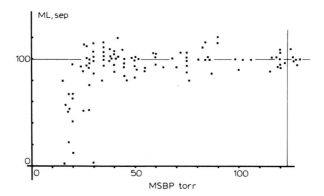

Fig. 9. Relationship between SEP amplitude (percent control) and MSBP in the ML in 11 animals. Points to the right of the vertical line were recorded at pressures greater than 120 torr. Control points are omitted.

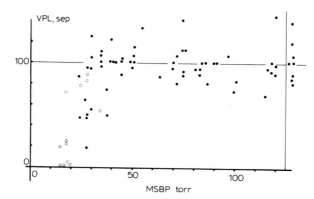

Fig. 10. Relationship between SEP amplitude (percent control) and MSBP in the VPL in 11 animals. Points to the right of the vertical line were recorded at pressures greater than 120 torr. Control points are omitted; the open circles have the same meaning as in Fig. 8.

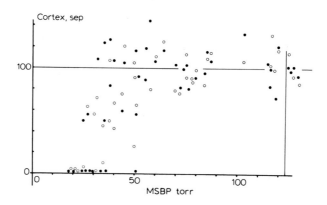

Fig. 11. Relationship between SEP amplitude (percent control) and MSBP in left cerebral cortex following (as in Figs. 9 and 10) right MCA occlusion and added hypotension in 11 animals. Points to the right of the vertical line were recorded at pressures greater than 120 torr. Control points are omitted. The open circles refer to the amplitude of P15, the closed circles to that of N10.

Figures 9, 10 and 11 show the relationships of the cortical, VPL and lemniscal responses to MSBP in hypotension. They illustrate quite clearly the preservation of the lemniscal volley down to 20–30 torr in contrast, again, to cortex and VPL.

Table III gives a statistical assessment of these graphical data. The ranges of CBF and MSBP have been divided for the purpose into bands of equal width. The cortical (P15) SEP data in this series were statistically indistinguishable from data taken from previous experiments in relation to flow (Fig. 1), so all these cortical data were combined to give the pooled data indicated for cortex in Table III. In the flow band 15–20 ml/100 g/min, the cortical SEP amplitude was significantly reduced, to an average of 73% of control (the SEP threshold of previous work), but those in VPL and lemniscus, although diminished, were not significantly below control. In the range 10–15 ml/100 g/min, the VPL response was now significantly reduced (to 46%, with the cortical response almost abolished at 10%); however, only below 10 ml/100 g/min was the lemniscal response similarly reduced.

In terms of MSBP, the left cortical SEP was first significantly reduced in the range 30–40 torr, with VPL and lemniscal responses unaffected. The VPL response was first significantly affected in the range 20–30 torr, and that in the lemniscus only at the lowest recordable pressures, below 20 torr, at which the cortical trace was invariably flat.

TABLE III

COMPARISON OF SEP AMPLITUDES IN BRAINSTEM, THALAMUS AND CORTEX IN RELATION TO LOCAL CBF AND MSBP FOLLOWING MCA OCCLUSION AND ADDED HYPOTENSION

Numbers in parentheses indicate the number of animals used (paired t-test). * $p<0.05$, ** $p<0.01$, *** $p<0.001$

Local flow (ml/100 g/min) (Initial slope)	ML		VPL		Cortex (pooled P15)	
	Mean	S.D.	Mean	S.D.	Mean	S.D.
0–5	56.5	27.6 (2)	8.3	14.4 (3)	7.9	10.3 (7) ***
5–10	72.0	28.7 (5)*	53.7	38.2 (6)*	11.3	24.8 (16)***
10–15	73.3	22.8 (6)	45.6	36.0 (7)**	9.8	22.6 (24)***
15–20	87.8	16.4 (6)	68.6	29.6 (4)	72.6	32.8 (19)**
20–25	96.4	11.0 (6)	92.5	17.3 (5)	87.0	24.4 (8)
25–30	98.4	6.5 (6)	92.0	13.6 (5)	100.0	– (4)
> 30	99.0	2.7 (7)	99.7	10.9 (8)	98.0	4.9 (10)

Mean systemic blood pressure (torr)						
10–20	48.5	8.7 (4)**	21.8	27.4 (4)**	0	– (3)***
20–30	86.1	20.0 (7)	63.9	22.4 (7)**	11.5	25.3 (6)**
30–40	96.8	11.7 (5)	91.6	26.3 (5)	27.2	21.3 (5)**
40–50	99.0	8.6 (5)	100.3	1.3 (4)	74.0	47.0 (3)
50–60	95.5	6.4 (3)	111.5	16.5 (3)	85.3	23.5 (3)
> 60	98.8	5.7 (9)	94.4	11.3 (8)	102.4	18.3 (8)

Occlusion plus hypotension – Latency changes

Changes in CT were measured for the same ML, VPL and cortical SEP components as were selected for amplitude measurements. The changes in CT with ischemia
in VPL and cortex are given in Table IV.

TABLE IV

CHANGES IN CONDUCTION TIME (CT) WITH ISCHEMIA

** $p<0.01$ (paired t-test). Numbers in parentheses indicate the number of animals used

Local flow (ml/100g/min) (Initial slope)	VPL		Cortex (N10)		Cortex (P15)	
	Mean	S.D.	Mean	S.D.	Mean	S.D.
<10	−0.20	0.55 (6)	0.38	0.50 (3)	1.17	1.68 (3)
10–15	0.15	0.16 (6)	1.55	0.21 (2)	0.64	0.86 (2)
15–20	0.23	0.40 (6)	0.28	0.59 (5)	−0.10	0.14 (2)
20–25	−0.07	0.29 (8)	0.05	0.14 (6)	0.31	0.64 (4)
>25	0.04	0.14 (11)	−0.16	0.06 (5)**	−0.26	0.45 (4)
Alternative Grouping:						
<20			0.52	0.65 (6)	0.76	1.25 (6)
>20			−0.08	0.04 (5)**	0.07	0.50 (4)

In VPL (as in the ML) no significant CT changes were seen, but in the flow range
10–20 ml/100 g/min there was an overall trend in VPL toward an increase in CT. In
cortex, there was a strong trend showing an increase in CT at local flows below 20
ml/100 g/min, especially below 15 ml/100 g/min and in both of the components N10
and P15. The alternative grouping of data in the table shows that, on average, the CT
increase of N10 below 20 ml/100 g/min was 0.52 ms and that of P15 was 0.76 ms. None
of these averages is, however, statistically significant: the effect was too variable
between animals. It is interesting that above 20 ml/100 g/min a small (0.1 ms) but
significant average decrease in the CT of N10 was observed.

DISCUSSION

The principal result of this study is the indication that as one descends the neuraxis
there is an increasing resistance of electrophysiological function to systemic hypotension, together with a decreasing threshold for local ischemia. It has been pointed out
(Gregory et al., 1979) that failure of the cortical SEP could arise from a reduction in
CBF in subcortical segments of the afferent pathway as well as in cortex. Our present
results show that (at least up to the level of the thalamus) the possibility of prior
subcortical transmission failure is unlikely in progressive hypotension; since the VPL
and lemniscus are less sensitive to ischemia than cortex, the cortically generated
components of the SEP would begin to fail while the subcortical afferent volley was
still substantially intact.

This study has also provided information on how central transmission times depend on local conditions of perfusion at various levels. Our results show that with MCA occlusion followed by a general reduction in flow due to decreased MSBP, or with hypotension alone, increases in CT recorded at cortex arise primarily in structures above the thalamus. At present the contribution of the internal capsule and thalamo-cortical radiation to CT changes, as distinct from that due to cortical failure, is unknown. The small but significant decrease in CT measured at flows above 20 ml/100 g/min, on the verge of cortical failure, may arise from a reduction in the temporal dispersion of the subcortical afferent volley, or from interaction of the cortical N10 and P15 components by superimposition within the cranial volume conductor. Such a decrease has not been seen in clinical data.

The average control CCT in this series of baboons was 3.29 ± 0.59 ms ($N = 11$ animals), whereas that in normal man is 5.4 ± 0.4 ms (Wang et al., 1982), the ratio being about 1.6. Thus, although latencies of N7 (neck) and N10 (cortex) are on average about half those of their homologues N14 and N20 recorded in man, the baboon CCT is appreciably greater than the value of half the human CCT that is suggested by this twofold change of scale. The discrepancy may arise because although the delay attributable to conduction along central fibers is less in the monkey, due to the size difference between the species, the overall synaptic delay is the same. Nevertheless, it is reasonable to apply a scale factor of 1.6 to the baboon CCT in comparing the changes in CT measured in both species, and if this is done, the average increase of 0.52 ms observed in the present study of cortical flows below 20 ml/100 g/min (Table IV) becomes 0.8 ms. This value is close to that commonly measured in the affected hemisphere of grade 4 subarachnoid hemorrhage patients, in which CCT increases on average to 6.4 ms (Wang et al., 1983). It is greater than the CCT increase observed for patients in grades 1 through 3, or seen during induction for surgery, where increases to less than 6.0 ms are encountered and are not statistically abnormal. It is, however, less than the increase to about 6.7 ms observed during surgery using halothane concentrations of up to 2% (Symon et al., 1983), and considerably less than the increases observed intra-operatively while arteries are temporarily clipped or the brain retracted, as illustrated in Fig. 12. This disparity in CCT changes during ischemia could be due to a species difference, but is more likely to arise from the use of different anesthetics in the experimental and clinical conditions.

SUMMARY

This paper presents recent experimental data from primates on the relationships between features of early (<25 ms latency) components of the SEP generated in brainstem, thalamus and cerebral cortex, and the local CBF in these regions. Quantitative evidence is given indicating that the electrophysiological responses in brainstem and thalamic stages of the somatosensory afferent pathway are relatively resistant to ischemia in comparison to those originating in cortex. The threshold of local CBF below which SEP amplitude is significantly reduced lies below the range 10–15 ml/100 g/min in the medial lemniscus, whereas in cortex the threshold, as we have demonstrated in previous work using the same anesthetic (alpha-chloralose), is in the range 15–20 ml/100 g/min. A similar gradient of SEP sensitivity along the afferent pathway is present in terms of a reduction in systemic blood pressure; the lemniscal SEP ampli-

198

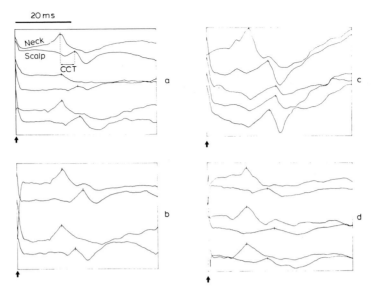

Fig. 12. Effects of brain retraction and temporary arterial occlusion on the scalp-recorded SEP in man during surgery. The reference electrode was at the nasion. Positive is downward. a: Top trace pair: control neck and scalp recordings. Second pair: before retraction (MSBP = 87). Third pair: retraction caused an increase of CCT in the operated hemisphere from 6.6 to 7.4 ms (MSBP = 85). b: Upper pair: recordings from affected hemisphere during the same retraction procedure as in a. Lower pair: recordings from unaffected hemisphere. The interhemispheric difference in CCT is 1.6 ms. c: Effect of internal carotid occlusion for 10 min during surgery for a giant internal carotid ophthalmic artery aneurysm. Top trace: neck recording. Second trace: scalp recording prior to occlusion. Third and fourth traces: scalp recording 1 and 8 min after occlusion (CCT = 10 ms). Bottom trace: 2 min after release of arterial clips, showing recovery of CCT. Patient made full recovery without hemispheral deficit. d: Top pair: control recordings in one patient during surgery for left MCA aneurysm (CCT = 7.8 ms). Second pair: CCT increased to 10 ms following clipping of the aneurysm. The MSBP did not change (55 torr). Third pair: improvement in CCT to 8 ms (MSBP = 67) following repositioning of the clip, which had been occluding an opercular branch of MCA. No detectable neurological deficit ensued postoperatively.

tude is only reduced significantly below 20 torr, the response in thalamic VPL below 30 torr, but the cortical response threshold is in the range 30–40 torr. The associated changes in latency of these SEP components in ischemia are described, and discussed in relation to increases in central conduction time observed in clinical or intra-operative practice.

REFERENCES

Arezzo, J. C., Legatt, A. D. and Vaughan, Jr., H. G. (1979). Topography and intracranial sources of somatosensory evoked potentials in the monkey. I. Early components. *Electroenceph. clin. Neurophysiol.*, 46: 155–172.

Branston, N. M., Symon, L., Crockard, H. A. and Pasztor, E. (1974) Relationship between the cortical evoked potential and local cortical blood flow following acute middle cerebral artery occlusion in the baboon. *Expt. Neurol.*, 45: 195–208.

Chiappa, K. H., Choi, S. K. and Young, R. R. (1980) Short-latency somatosensory evoked potentials following median nerve stimulation in patients with neurological lesions. In J. E. Desmedt (Ed.), *Clinical Uses of Cerebral, Brainstem and Spinal Somatosensory Evoked Potentials*, Karger, Basel, pp.264–281.

Desmedt, J. E., and Noël, P. (1973) Average cerebral evoked potentials in the evaluation of lesions of the sensory nerves and of the central somatosensory pathway. In J. E. Desmedt (Ed.), *New Developments in Electromyography and Clinical Neurophysiology, Vol. 2*, Karger, Basel, pp.352–371.

Gregory, P. C., McGeorge, A. P., Fitch, W., Graham, D. I., MacKenzie, E. T. and Harper, A. M. (1979) Effects of hemorrhagic hypotension on the cerebral circulation. II. Electrocortical function. *Stroke*, 10: 719–723.

Grundy, B. L. (1983) Intraoperative monitoring of sensory-evoked potentials. *Anesthesiology*, 58: 72–87.

Halliday, A. M. (Ed.) (1982) *Evoked Potentials in Clinical Testing*, Churchill Livingstone, New York.

Hume, A. L. and Cant, B. R. (1978) Conduction time in central somatosensory pathways in man. *Electroenceph. clin. neurophysiol.*, 45: 361–375.

Pasztor, E., Symon, L., Dorsch, N. W. C. and Branston, N. M. (1973) The hydrogen clearance method in assessment of blood flow in cortex, white matter and deep nuclei of baboons. *Stroke*, 4: 556–567.

Sances, Jr., A., Larson, S. J., Cusick, J. F., Myklebust, J., Ewing, C. L., Jodat, R., Ackmann, J. J. and Walsh, P. (1978) Early somatosensory evoked potentials. *Electroenceph. clin. Neurophysiol.*, 45: 505–514.

Sharbrough, F. W., Messick, J. M. and Sundt, Jr., T. M. (1973) Correlations of continuous electroencephalograms with cerebral blood flow measurements during carotid endarterectomy. *Stroke*, 4: 674–683.

Symon, L., Hargadine, J. R., Zawirski, M. and Branston, N. M. (1979a) Central conduction time as an index of ischaemia in subarachnoid haemorrhage. *J. Neurol. Sci.*, 44: 95–103.

Symon, L., Branston, N. M. and Chikovani, O. (1979b) Ischemic brain edema following middle cerebral artery occlusion in baboons: relationship between regional cerebral water content and blood flow at 1 to 2 hours. *Stroke*, 10: 184–191.

Symon, L., Wang, A. D., Costa E. Silva, I. E. and Gentili, F. (1983) Per-operative use of somatosensory evoked responses in aneurysm surgery. *J. Neurosurg.*, 60: 269–275.

Trojaborg, W. and Boysen, G. (1973) Relation between EEG, regional cerebral blood flow and internal carotid stump pressure during carotid endarterectomy. *Electroencephalogr. clin. Neurophysiol.*, 34: 61–69.

Wang, A. D., Symon, L. and Gentili, F. (1982) Conduction of sensory action potentials across the posterior fossa in infratentorial space-occupying lesions in man. *J. Neurol. Neurosurg. Psychiat.*, 45: 440–445.

Wang, A. D., Cone, J., Symon, L., Costa E. Silva, I. E. (1983) Monitoring of somatosensory evoked potentials during the management of subarachnoid haemorrhage from intracranial aneurysm. *J. Neurosurg.*, 60: 264–268.

Brain Ischemia: Quantitative EEG and Imaging Techniques, Progress in Brain Research, Vol. 62, edited by
G. Pfurtscheller, E.J. Jonkman and F.H. Lopes da Silva
©1984 Elsevier Science Publishers B.V.

Cortical and Thalamic Somatosensory Evoked Potentials in Brain Ischemia in the Monkey

F. H. LOPES DA SILVA[1], A. M. TIELEN[2,†], A. VAN DIEREN[2], E. J. JONKMAN[3] and
C. A. F. TULLEKEN[4]

[1]*Section Animal Physiology, Department of Zoology, University of Amsterdam, Kruislaan 320,*
1098 SM Amsterdam., [2]*Institute of Medical Physics, TNO, Da Costakade 45, Utrecht.,*
[3]*Workgroup Clinical Neurophysiology, TNO, Westeinde Hospital, Westeinde, 's Gravenhage and*
[4]*Department of Neurosurgery, Academic Hospital, Nicolaas Beetsstraat, Utrecht (The Netherlands)*

INTRODUCTION

Physiological changes occurring in experimentally induced ischemic areas of the brain in monkeys have been investigated by measuring cerebral blood flow (CBF) and by recording the spontaneous EEG or the field potentials (EPs) evoked by peripheral stimulation, as reviewed by Meyer and Marx (1972). In most early studies the experimentally induced ischemia was total and measurements were performed acutely, immediately after a massive decrease in CBF with the animals under anesthesia (Branston et al., 1974, 1976, 1983; Tulleken et al., 1978; Hossman and Schmier, 1980; Lesnick et al., 1983). However, in a clinical situation one is usually confronted with a partial ischemia, the extent and depth of which change in the course of time. As a part of an investigation into the effects of microsurgery in brain ischemia, namely of surgical interventions aimed at obtaining a revascularization of an infarcted brain area, we were interested in an experimental model of chronic brain ischemia. In order to follow the evolution of this process it is necessary to use physiological measures that may give reliable information on the activity of neuronal populations of the infarcted area. The experimental model used was the monkey in whom the middle cerebral artery (MCA) was occluded in the waking state. It was essential to this model to follow the animals in the course of weeks after the occlusion. The main questions we addressed here concern the physiological measures which should be used to assess the evolution of an infarct; two main questions were the following:

a) can the somatosensory evoked potential (SSEP) be used as a reliable measure for the evolution of a brain infarct, and

(b) which characteristics of the SSEPs provide information on the area involved and/or on the degree of the ischemia.

In another investigation, cortical SSEPs were shown to be reduced when local CBF (lCBF) falls to the range 15–20 ml/100 g/min and were abolished at flows below 12 ml/100 g/min (Branston et al., 1983) but those recorded from the thalamus (ventro-postero-lateral nucleus, VPL) were not significantly below control values in the flow

---

†A. M. Tielen deceased in December 1983

range 15–20 ml/100 g/min. In order to verify these results in the chronic model of ischemia we measured not only cortical SSEPs but also those of the VPL.

Both clinical and experimental neurophysiological studies have shown that unilateral brain ischemia can produce an alteration in the lCBF or the EEG recorded from the contralateral hemisphere, i.e. the phenomenon of diaschisis (Kempinski, 1958; Waltz, 1967; Paulson et al., 1972; Melamed et al., 1975; Ginsberg et al., 1977; Kanaya et al., 1983). It has been claimed that CBF diaschisis is not common in monkeys (Meyer et al., 1972) and that EEG diaschisis occurs less frequently than CBF diaschisis (Melamed et al., 1975). We also attempted to check these suggestions in our experimental animals measuring SSEPs bilaterally along with local CBFs.

MATERIAL AND METHODS

For this study, eight female monkeys (*Maccaca mulatta*) weighing 5–7 kg were used. At first the animals were trained to sit in a monkey chair and were intensively handled in order to accustom them to the recording conditions. Under halothane anesthesia the animals were provided with chronically indwelling electrodes of different types.

(a) Several bundles consisting, usually, of three stainless steel electrodes (bare tip 200 μm) and one platinum electrode (bare tip 200 μm) each were placed in the frontal, parietal and occipital cortex of the hemisphere where the MCA was occluded, one bundle was in the contralateral parietal cortex and a few bundles were implanted in the caudate nucleus and thalamus (VPL) under stereotaxic guidance;

(b) stainless steel pins (diameter 1 mm) were placed in the parietal bone overlying the pre- and post-central sulcus on both sides for epidural recordings.

The platinum electrodes were used for measuring local CBF (lCBF) from hydrogen (H_2) clearance curves according to the formula $lCBF = L.69.31/T_{1/2}$, in which $L = 1$ since H_2 was used and $T_{1/2}$ (in min) is the time taken by the H_2 concentration to decay to one half. All electrodes were attached to a plug which was fixed to the skull with acrylic resin.

After this initial operation the animals were allowed to recover. Thereafter control values of EEG, SSEPs and lCBF were measured over a period of a few weeks with the animal sitting in a monkey chair. When sufficient control data had been collected the animals were anesthetized and the MCA was approached by the transorbital route (Hudgins and Garcia, 1970). In four animals the artery was occluded directly resulting in the death of three animals, probably owing to massive brain edema. In the remaining four animals a ligature was placed around the MCA. The animals recovered from the operation; their behavior was carefully observed for signs of neurological impairment. Control EEG, SSEPs and lCBF recordings were made in the course of 1–2 weeks. Thereafter, the MCA was ligated yielding a brain ischemic area. The animals were again carefully observed and physiological records taken over a period of at least 2 weeks.

Recordings

Both EEG recordings and H_2 clearance measurements were made against a reference electrode placed on the occipital bone. The electrodes were connected to a multichannel isolation amplifier, the output of which was recorded by means of a Brush ink writer and fed into an Ampex 14-channel instrumentation recorder (frequency band up to 450 Hz, -3 dB); the signals were digitized at 1000 samples per second and fed into a PDP 11-40 computer for further analysis. Power spectra were computed as described by Jonkman et al. (this volume).

Evoked potentials

Somatosensory evoked potentials were elicited by square pulses, 200 μsec in duration, delivered through surface electrodes overlying the median nerve, with the anode about 1 cm above the wrist on the ventral surface of the forearm and the cathode located at 2 cm in the proximal direction. The intensity of the stimulus was such that it produced a small twitch of the thumb.

Bypass operation

In all monkeys a bypass operation, i.e. an anastomosis between one branch of the MCA and a branch of the superficial temporal artery, was carried out a few weeks after the occlusion of the MCA as described in detail by Tulleken et al. (this volume). Most of the experimental findings described here concern the period before the bypass operation.

Histology

In three monkeys 30 to 45 min before the termination of the experiment 2-deoxy-D-[^{14}C]glucose (or [^{14}C]DG) was administered intraveneously (50 μCi/kg). After killing the animal with an overdose of a barbiturate, the brain was removed and frozen at $-55°$C as described by Sokoloff et al. (1978). Coronal sections were cut in a cryostat and used for autoradiography and/or for histological determination of the electrode sites. In the two other monkeys the brains were simply perfused first with saline and then with formalin with added potassium ferrocyanide so that the position of the electrodes could be verified by the Prussian blue reaction.

RESULTS

In all animals both the cortical and the VPL SSEPs elicited by stimulation of the contralateral median nerve had the same general waveform during the control period as shown in Fig. 1. In the present study very fast components (e.g. about 1000 c/sec or higher) were not recorded and thus the SSEPs were rather smooth. The initial component of the SSEP recorded from the VPL contralateral to the median nerve being stimulated, consisted of a positive deflection peaking at about 6 msec followed in general by a negative wave. The initial components of the SSEP recorded over the precentral gyrus and over the anterior part of the postcentral gyrus were characterized by a positive deflection peaking at about 9–11 msec followed by a negative wave and a second positive peak with the maximum at about 20–22 msec. This deflection was followed by slower late components. As also described in previous studies (Arezzo et al., 1981), the VPL SSEP was critically dependent on the location of the electrodes

204

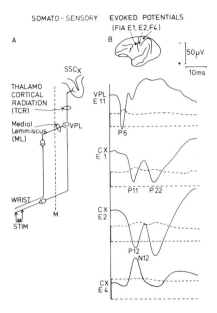

SOMATO - SENSORY   EVOKED   POTENTIALS
(FIA E1, E2,F4)

Fig. 1. A: Diagram of the pathways involved in eliciting Somatosensory Evoked Potentials (SSEPs); VPL= ventro-postero lateral nucleus of the thalamus; SSCx = somatosensory cortex. B: Examples of SSEPs recorded from the VPL (E11) and the cortex, E1 from the pre-central gyrus, E2 from the post-central gyrus and E4 from the superior parietal gyrus. Note the main positive peak at 6 msec (P6) in VPL and the positive peaks at 11 msec (P11) in E1, at 12 msec in E2 and the late positive peaks at 22 msec (P22). On E4 there is a potential reversal.

within the VPL. Cortical SSEPs could be recorded over relatively large areas of the pre- and post-central cortex, but the waveforms were characteristic of the recorded area. Thus SSEPs recorded from electrodes overlying the central sulcus showed a dominant P10-P11 component, whereas those recorded from the posterior part of the post-central gyrus had a dominant P12 component (Fig. 1). Over more posterior regions, namely the superior parietal gyrus, a reversal of polarity of this component was observed (Fig. 1). In general terms the morphology and timing of these components of the cortical SSEPs agree with the detailed description of Arezzo et al. (1981) although in this study the very early and other fast components were not studied.

In the following sections we will describe the successive changes in SSEPs from the cortex and VPL, ipsilaterally and contralaterally to the side of the occluded MCA. A summary of the main results is presented in Table I. The measurements of SSEPs, both amplitudes and latencies, and of lCBF were tested statistically using the nonparametric Mann–Whitney U test; significant differences and corresponding probability levels refer to comparisons between measurements obtained in the control period and those obtained after occlusion of the MCA.

Changes in cortical SSEPs ipsilaterally to the ischemic area

In four out of the five monkeys a significant decrease in the amplitude of the P10 or P12 component followed the occlusion of the MCA. This decrease coincided with the appearance of hemiplegia in three monkeys. One of the cases may be taken as example (Herma); this is shown in Fig. 2. A decrease of the amplitude of both P10 and P22

TABLE I

			Monkey				
			Herma	Erica	Dora	Ina	Fia
Ipsilateral to occluded MCA	Cortex	Amplitudes P10	< p<.001	< (P20)[1]	< p<.036	< p<.018	*2
		Latencies P10	> p<.004	> p<.033	ns	ns	*2
		CBF	< p<.005	< p<.015	< p<.001	ns	< p<.006
	VPL	Amplitudes P6	< p<.001	ns	ns	ns	< p<.05
		Latencies P6	< p<.025	ns	ns	ns	ns
		CBF	ns	ns	–	ns	< p<.047
Contralateral to occluded MCA	Cortex	Amplitudes	< p<.032	ns	–	ns	ns
		Latencies P10	> p<.009	ns	–	ns	ns
		CBF	ns	ns	ns	ns	ns
	VPL	Amplitudes P6	< p<.005	ns	–	ns	–
		Latencies P6	ns	ns	–	ns	–
		CBF	ns	ns	–	ns	–

Statistical analysis of the SSEPs and lCBF from the central region and VPL ipsilateral and contralateral to the occluded MCA. In case a significant increase (>) or decrease (<) between pre- and post-occlusion MCA of the component indicated on the left (P10, P6) or in lCBF was found, the probability level is indicated. In the other cases ns (nonsignificant) is indicated (statistics were done using the Mann–Whitney U test). [1]The significant changes were found not in component P10 but in P20. [2]The change in waveform was so radical that no specific component could be detected after occlusion.

can be seen; the latter disappeared almost completely during the first week post-occlusion; the former decreased significantly in amplitude ($p < 0.001$) during the first 26 days. On the 24th day a bypass operation was carried out. Thereafter an increase in amplitude could be seen (4th day after bypass, or day 30 in Fig. 2) but the early positive component peaked not at 10 msec but at 12 msec. In Fig. 2 the relation between the change in SSEPs and the EEG power in the delta-2 band (2.1–3.3 Hz) can be seen. It appears that the decrease in amplitude of the SSEPs takes place at the same time as the increase of delta-2 power but that at the end of the observation period the relative recovery of the SSEP amplitude is not accompanied by a decrease in delta-2 power. Figure 2 also illustrates the change in lCBF accompanying the decrease in SSEP amplitude. The question of the relationship between these two variables was further analysed as shown in Fig. 3A. It should be noted that the two parameters – SSEP P10 amplitude and lCBF – were not measured exactly from the same site, since the SSEP was recorded epidurally and the lCBF was measured intra-cortically. Nevertheless, a significant correlation was obtained (Spearman Rank Cor-

206

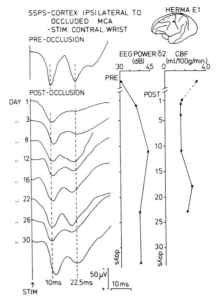

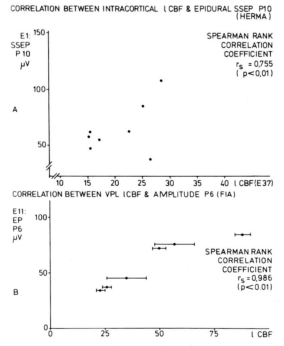

Fig. 2. Left side: SSEP recorded from the spot indicated in the inset, in the pre-occlusion period and at different days after occlusion: day 1 up to day 30. The stimulus to the contralateral median nerve was given at the start of the recording. Note the decrease in amplitude and the change in latency. Right side: plots of the power in the delta-2 band of the cortical EEG and of the lCBF measured along the same time scale. Note that not all measurements were made on the same days. From day 1 onwards there is an increase in delta-2 power and a decrease in lCBF.

Fig. 3. A: Plot of the relationship between lCBF (in ml/100 g/min) and the amplitude of the P10 component of the cortical SSEP with the corresponding statistical data. B: The same for the relationship between lCBF and the amplitude of the P6 component of the VPL SSEP. Note that both correlation coefficients are significant at $p<0.01$.

relation coefficient $r_s = 0.755$, $p<0.01$). In addition to the decrease in amplitude of the SSEP components, ischemia was also accompanied by a small, although significant, increase ($p<0.004$) in peak latency of the first positive peak.

In monkey Dora the same general pattern of SSEP changes was encountered as in Herma. In this case, however, the second positive peak (P22) disappeared completely after occlusion of the MCA. In this monkey there was also a significant decrease of lCBF measured in the pre-central gyrus, but the lowest flow after occlusion was only 31.3 ml/100 g/min (64% of controls) whereas in monkey Herma values as low as 15.4 ml/100 g/min (50% of controls) were measured (Fig. 3A). The same general pattern was also found in monkey Ina. A significant decrease in amplitude of the P11 component after MCA occlusion was noted ($p<0.018$) which was, however, slighter than in Herma. In this case a change in latency of P11 was not apparent but the latency of the second positive peak appeared to increase slightly from 21 to 23 msec; however, this difference was not significant ($p<0.133$), probably due to the relatively small number of observations available. The lCBF in the same region decreased only slightly, and the changes were not significant. In this monkey no clear hemiplegia was observed. In another monkey (Fia) there was a dramatic change in SSEP recorded over the pre-central gyrus. The characteristic waveform with the two positive peaks (P11 and P22) changed radically as shown in Fig. 4; it was replaced by a rather slow positive wave. It

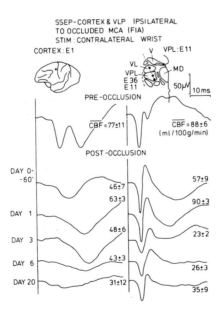

Fig. 4. Left side: cortical SSEPs before and after occlusion recorded from the precentral gyrus as indicated in the inset. Note the change in the waveform at different days after occlusion and the accompanying decrease in lCBF indicated by the number on each recording. Right side: data recorded simultaneously from the VPL showing the decrease in amplitude of component P6, the change in the late negative wave and the decrease in lCBF. The SSEP was recorded from electrode E11 and the lCBF from E36 as indicated in the inset.

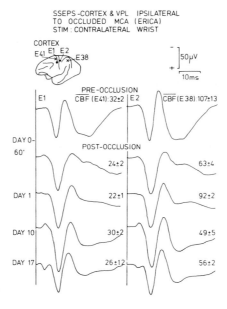

Fig. 5. SSEPs recorded from two sites E1 and E2 as shown in the inset. The corresponding lCBF values are indicated on the recordings; these data were obtained from electrodes placed on the spots indicated by crosses. Note that the change in lCBF (in ml/100 g/min) is more pronounced in the posterior site. The change in SSEP is mostly apparent in the second positive peak.

may be noted that from day 6 onwards this wave becomes less clear and the SSEP almost submerges in the background noise. Immediately after the occlusion the animal became hemiplegic. There was a clear decrease of lCBF within the pre-central gyrus reaching values of 65% of the control period (absolute measurements indicated in Fig. 4). It should be noted that the change in SSEPs was much more pronounced than the change in lCBF, suggesting that the ischemic area must be very localized around the central sulcus.

In one monkey (Erica) the SSEPs behaved differently from those described above; in this case a significant increase of the amplitude of the P10 component, recorded from the pre-central gyrus, and of the P11, recorded post-centrally, were found. The corresponding waveforms are shown in Fig. 5. This case is particularly interesting not only because of this unexpected result but also because in contrast with P10 or P11 the second positive component (P20) was strongly affected by the occlusion; immediately after (60' and day 1) it practically disappeared, to return at a later date, (day 10, day 17) in a rather disturbed form. The increase in amplitude of the P10 or P11 components recorded from the two cortical sites was accompanied by a significant increase in latency (see Table 1) in both cases from a value of 10.8 ± 0.5 to 11.4 ± 0.4 msec. In this context it should be noted that there were significant changes in lCBF after MCA occlusion measured in the pre-central gyrus ($p < 0.015$) and in the inferior parietal gyrus ($p < 0.01$). In the former case the lCBF after occlusion became 80% of the control values; in the latter it reached 62%.

Changes in VPL SSEPs ipsilaterally to the ischemic area

In all five monkeys electrodes were placed in the VPL ipsilaterally to the side of the occluded MCA. However, only in two were there significant changes in the SSEPs elicited by stimulation of the contralateral median nerve. These two cases are illustrated in Figs. 4 and 6. Figure 4 (monkey Fia) shows a slight but significant ($p<0.05$) decrease of the amplitude of P6 component accompanied by a change in the late negative slow wave which reversed polarity. Simultaneously, a clear decrease in lCBF in the VPL was noted ($p<0.047$) which reached, after occlusion, 26% of control values (88 ± 6 ml/100 g/min). Figure 6 (monkey Herma) also shows a significant decrease in amplitude of the component P6 ($p<0.001$); simultaneously a decrease in peak latency from 7.8 ± 0.3 to 7.2 ± 0.4, significant at the level $p<0.025$, was found. In the same figure the decrease in peak amplitude of component P6 recorded from another VPL site in the same animal has been plotted as function of time. An interesting additional observation was that the lCBF in the VPL showed also a slight decrease from a control value of 58.8 ± 15.6 to a value as low as 38.9 ± 10.2 ml/100 g/min, but this decrease did not reach a significant level ($p<0.123$).

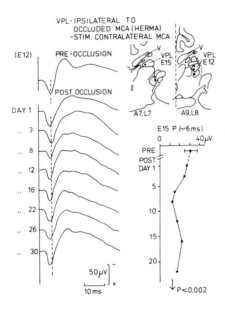

Fig. 6. Changes in two VPL SSEPs recorded from electrodes E12 and E15; the former is shown as the series of curves on the left-hand side; the latter is represented by the plot of the amplitude of P6 on the right-hand side. The difference between pre- and post-occlusion values was very significant as indicated by $p<0.002$.

The relationship between amplitudes of the P6 component in the VPL and lCBF was studied in the monkeys that presented significant decreases of these measures after MCA occlusion. In Herma the electrodes from which the SSEPs and the lCBF were measured were separated by a distance of 2.3 mm. The Spearman correlation coefficient between both sets of data was $r_s = 0.572$, which was not significant ($p>0.05$). In this case the lowest lCBF measured was 22.0 ml/100 g/min, corresponding to an amplitude of P6 of 27.5 μV. In Fia the VPL electrodes were closer to each other and only 1 mm apart. In this case the correlation coefficient $r_s = 0.986$ was highly significant ($p<0.01$) (Fig. 3B). Here the lowest lCBF value was 23 ± 2 ml/100 g/min, corresponding to an amplitude of 35 μV of component P6.

Changes in cortical and VPL SSEPs contralaterally to the ischemic area

In four monkeys cortical electrodes were placed symmetrically on both hemispheres and in three electrodes were also placed bilaterally in the VPL. However, in only one monkey (Herma) were there significant changes in the amplitude of both cortical and VPL SSEPs on the side contralateral to the occluded MCA (Table I). In these cases SSEPs were also elicited by stimulation of the contralateral median nerve. In the cortical SSEP there was a significant decrease in the peak amplitude of component P12.5 ($p<0.032$) and a significant increase in peak latency which rose from 12.5 ± 0.6 to 14.0 ± 0.8 ($p<0.009$). In the VPL there was a significant decrease in the amplitude of component P7 ($p<0.005$) but no change in latency. It is of interest to note that neither in the cortical area nor in the VPL were there significant decreases in lCBF accompanying the decreases in amplitude of the SSEPs.

In all other monkeys investigated no significant changes in SSEPs and in lCBF over the contralateral hemisphere were encountered.

Clinical observations and the uptake of [^{14}C]DG

It was of particular interest to test whether clear differences in the extent of the ischemic area, as revealed by the uptake of [^{14}C]DG, could be found between monkeys showing different types of changes in SSEPs. This was only possible in three monkeys: Herma, Erica and Ina. As regards neurological deficits, Herma and Erica became hemiplegic immediately after the occlusion of the MCA, whereas Ina did not present any immediate clinical signs. Contrast angiography was performed to see if the MCA had indeed been effectively occluded in the latter monkey. This revealed an occluded MCA in spite of the lack of clinical signs. A bypass operation was attempted in all these monkeys. In Herma and in Erica no important changes in the animals motor behavior took place but a slight improvement was noted. On the other hand, in Ina the bypass operation precipitated a clear hemiplegia. The two first-named animals were allowed to recover from the bypass attempt for a period of about 3 months in order to study the development of their state. Therefore in these animals the injection of [^{14}C]DG took place after a relatively long time after the occlusion. In contrast, in Ina the final experiment with [^{14}C]DG took place 2 weeks after the operation since the animal had become hemiplegic.

The autoradiograms from Herma showed that the uptake of [^{14}C]DG was slightly less in the cortex of the right hemisphere than on the left side with a relatively good contrast between white and gray matter. On the side of the occluded MCA there were large necrotic areas in the nucleus caudatus, putamen and capsula interna reaching caudally to the anterior thalamus. An example of a section at the level of the central sulcus, around the area from which SSEPs and lCBF measurements were made, is shown in Fig. 7. In Erica a different picture was obtained: although in this case there were also relatively large necrotic areas in the caudatus and putamen reaching the level of the thalamus, the uptake of [^{14}C]DG in the cortex was strongly asymmetric.

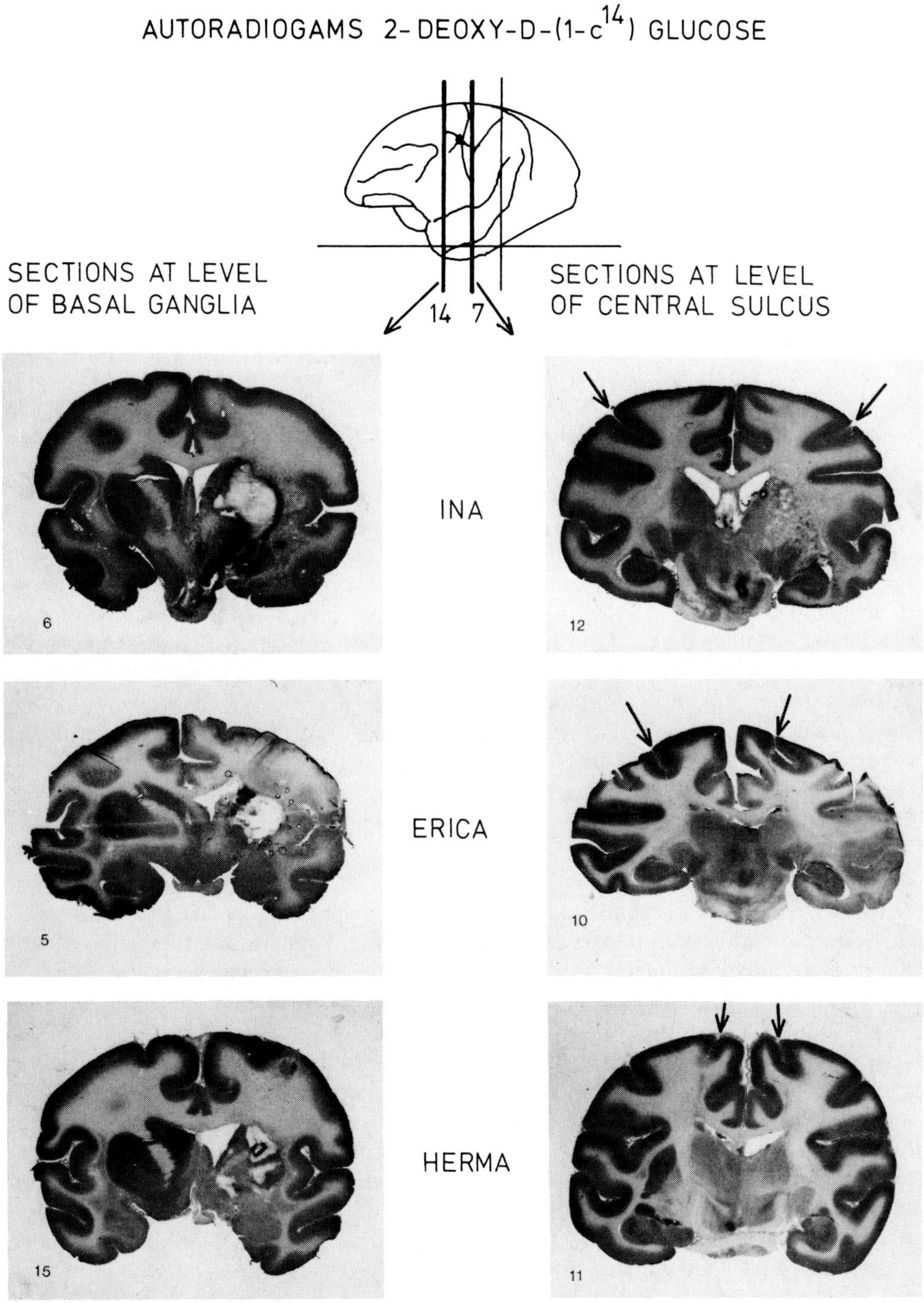

AUTORADIOGAMS 2-DEOXY-D-(1-c^{14}) GLUCOSE

SECTIONS AT LEVEL
OF BASAL GANGLIA

14 7

SECTIONS AT LEVEL
OF CENTRAL SULCUS

INA

ERICA

HERMA

Fig. 7. Examples of autoradiograms obtained from three monkeys: Ina, Erica and Herma. For each monkey, sections taken on two frontal planes are shown, one at the level of the caudatus-putamen and the other of the caudal part of the central sulcus. Note in all monkeys the necrotic areas in the basal ganglia. As regards the cortical areas, a clear asymmetry in the uptake of [^{14}C]DG is seen in Erica around the central sulcus (CS) although not for the pre-central gyrus. Ina and Herma also show an asymmetry but this is less pronounced than in Erica.

There was a clear reduction over the occluded hemisphere. This decreased uptake was evident laterally and posteriorly to the sulcus centralis, involving the post-central and temporal gyri. An example is shown in Fig. 7. In Ina the picture obtained approached that of Herma. In this case there were also necrotic areas in the striatum extending caudally to the thalamus; as regards the cortical uptake of [^{14}C]DG there was a reduction over the occluded side including the pre- and post-central and the temporal gyri, as illustrated in Fig. 7.

DISCUSSION

This study demonstrates that the occlusion of the MCA in the monkey constitutes a useful experimental model of chronic brain ischemia; it also provides a clear demonstration that the effects of MCA occlusion vary appreciably from monkey to monkey, mainly in the extent to which the thalamus (VPL) and the hand projection area around the central sulcus may become ischemic. A number of new findings have been put forward. We may consider these aspects in terms of the three questions formulated in the introduction.

(a) The first question, whether the SSEP can be used as a reliable measure for the evaluation of brain activity in the course of brain infarction, can be answered positively. It should be emphasized that this applies to the SSEP elicited by stimulation of the contralateral median nerve at the level of the wrist. We found that an improvement of the condition of the brain, revealed by an improvement in clinical state, was clearly accompanied by a gradual return of the SSEP waveform to the pattern encountered in the control period. In monkey Herma it even appeared that the SSEP was more sensitive in this respect than the EEG power or the lCBF. In contrast, in monkey Fia (Fig. 4) cortical SSEPs became almost indistinguishable from background noise in the course of time. This suggests that brain ischemia may worsen in the course of days after MCA occlusion. This may reflect what Kirino (1982) called the delayed neuronal death.

(b) As regards the second question, which characteristics of the SSEP provide reliable information on the extent and degree of the infarct, we should mention that the most sensitive parameter was the amplitude of component P10 of the cortical SSEP. Only in one monkey did this component not decrease in amplitude; in this case, rather, the second positive component P22 decreased significantly in amplitude. It appears that whether the first or the second positive component, or both, change in amplitude depends upon the extent of the cortical area infarcted. We should keep in mind that P10 is generated over the pre-central gyrus whereas P20-22 is generated over the post-central gyrus (Arezzo et al., 1981). Therefore, an ischemia which does not extend as far as the medial part of the pre-central gyrus may lead to a change in component P20-22 without impairing P10. This is what probably happened in monkey Erica, as also suggested by the [^{14}C]DG autoradiograms (Fig. 7). Thus we may conclude that different components of the cortical SSEP may provide useful information on the localization of the infarcted cortical area. A second finding is that the amplitude of the VPL SSEP may also change significantly after the occlusion of the MCA. However, the impairment of the VPL SSEP is less likely to occur than that of the cortical SSEP; this has also been shown by Branston et al. (1983). These authors found in the acute preparation that the VPL SSEP was only significantly reduced if the mean systemic blood pressure decreased appreciably; they only found a VPL SSEP with a reduced amplitude at very low levels of lCBF (10–15 ml/100 g/min). The fact that we, on the contrary, found significant reductions of VPL SSEP amplitude at higher levels of lCBF (Table I and Fig. 4) suggests that differences in hemodynamic factors between experimental conditions may play a role in this respect. A third finding concerns the change in latency of cortical SSEP after MCA occlusion. The most salient change, although seen only in two monkeys, was an increase in latency of the first positive peak (P10). This component is considered (Arezzo et al., 1981) to reflect the activity of cortical neurons due to inputs conducted by large fibers of the medial lemniscus and thalamo-cortical radiation (cutaneous and group Ia muscle spindle afferents); the cortical activity causing a positive peak at 12 msec is mainly due to a combination of cutaneous and kinesthetic inputs conducted along slower conducting pathways including the dorsolateral funiculus. In the light of these data it may be concluded that the increase in latency of the first positive peak of the cortical SSEP reflects the fact that the large fibers of the medial lemniscus and thalamo-cortical radiation are more readily impaired in this experimental model of ischemia than the slower conducting fibers.

(c) The third question, whether diaschisis may be revealed by way of SSEP recordings, can also be answered positively, although this was only clearly encountered in one animal.

Another point for discussion concerns the relationship between SSEP amplitude and lCBF. In our experiments, extremely low values of lCBF were not present, probably because we did not reduce the mean blood pressure. Nevertheless, we were able to find that cortical SSEP could be clearly measured, down to lCBF values of 15 ml/100 g/min. It should be noted, however, that the lCBF was measured intracortically, whereas the SSEPs were recorded epidurally. Therefore the latter may represent the activity of a larger area than that being reflected in the lCBF measurement. In our experience both the cortical and the VPL SSEPs are closely related to the lCBF. It is interesting to emphasize that in the VPL a strong correlation between SSEP amplitude and lCBF ($r_s = 0.986$) could be found on the condition that the two measurements be taken from very closely spaced electrodes. In other studies (Branston et al., 1974,1983), it has been remarked that the amplitude of the cortical SSEP changes with a decrease in lCBF according to a threshold-type relationship; amplitude reductions would occur only at or below lCBF values of 16–22 ml/100 g/min (Leswick et al., 1983). In our experience, however, the relationship between these two variables is approximately linear at least in the range from about 60 ml/100 g/min to 15 ml/100 g/min. There are, of course, methodological differences between those studies and ours. Whereas in our experiments the measurements were obtained in the waking monkey on different days, in the other studies quoted above they were taken during the acute ischemic phase with the animals under anesthesia. Whether these methodological differences explain the somewhat different results is a matter for further experimental investigation.

In conclusion, thalamic (VPL) and cortical SSEPs elicited by stimulation of the contralateral median nerve can be reliably used to determine the extent, the degree and the evolution of a chronic brain infarct induced by occlusion of the MCA in the monkey. However, these electrophysiological measurements reveal only the state of neural activity over a relatively small part of the infarcted area. Therefore for a more complete assessment of the brain condition such measurements should be complemented by others particularly directed to recording the activity of the temporal gyri and of the basal ganglia.

SUMMARY

Physiological changes occurring in experimentally induced ischemic areas of the brain in monkeys have been investigated by measuring cerebral blood flow (CBF) and recording somatosensory evoked potentials (SSEPs) to median nerve stimulation in the cortex and thalamus (ventro-postero-lateral nucleus, VPL). Ischemia was produced by occlusion of the middle cerebral artery (MCA). SSEPs were shown to be reliable indicators of brain activity in the course of brain infarction. The most sensitive parameter was found to be the amplitude of component P10 of the cortical SSEP, generated over the pre-central gyrus.

Different components of the cortical SSEP provide useful information on the localization of the infarcted cortical area. In addition, the amplitude of the VPL SSEP may also change significantly after the occlusion of the MCA. Evidence for the phenomenon of diaschisis was also found.

The study of the relationship between CBF and SSEPs showed that cortical SSEPs could be measured at local CBF levels as low as 15 ml/100 g/min. The relationship between local cerebral blood flow (lCBF) and SSEP amplitude was approximately linear in the range from about 15 ml/100 g/min to 60 ml/100 g/min.

REFERENCES

Arezzo, J. C., Vaughan, H. G. and Legatt, A. D. (1981) Topography and intracranial sources of somatosensory evoked potentials in the monkey. II. Cortical components. *Electroenceph. clin. Neurophysiol.*, 51: 1–18.

Branston, N. M., Symon, L., Crockard, H. A. and Pasztor, E. (1974) Relationship between the cortical evoked potential and local cortical blood flow following acute middle cerebral artery occlusion in the baboon. *Exp. Neurol.*, 45: 195–208.

Branston, N. M., Symon, L. and Crockard, H. A. (1976) Recovery of the cortical evoked response following temporary middle cerebral artery occlusion in baboons: relation to local blood flow and PO2. *Stroke*, 7: 151–157.

Branston, N. M., Ladds, A., Wang, A. D. and Symon, L. (1983) Critical flow thresholds for evoked potentials in thalamus and brainstem. *J. Cereb. Blood Flow Metab.*, 3, Suppl. 1: 397–398.

Ginsberg, M. D., Reivich, M., Giandomenico, A. and Greenberg, J. H. (1977) Local glucose utilisation in acute focal cerebral ischemia: local dysmetabolism and diaschisis. *Neurology (Minneap)*, 27: 1042–1048.

Hossman, K. A. and Schmier, F. J. (1980) Experimental brain infarcts in cats. I. Pathophysiological observations. *Stroke*, 11: 583–592.

Hudgins, W. R. and Garcia, J. H. (1970) Transorbital approach to the middle cerebral artery of the squirrel monkey; a technique for experimental cerebral infarction applicable to metastructural studies. *Stroke* 1: 107–111.

Kanaya, H., Endo, H., Sugiyama, T. and Kuroda, K. (1983) 'Crossed cerebellar diaschisis' in patients with putaminal hemorrhage. *J. Cereb. Blood Flow Metab.*, 3, Suppl. 1: 27–28.

Kempinski, W. H. (1958) Experimental study of distant effects of acute focal brain injury, *Arch. Neurol.*, 79: 376–389.

Kirino, T. (1982) Delayed neuronal death in the gerbil hippocampus following ischemia. *Brain Res.*, 57: 239–257.

Lesnick, J. E., Michele, J. A., DeFeo, S., Welsh, F. A. and Simeone, F. A. (1983) The somatosensory evoked potential (SEP), CBF and metabolism in global ischemia. *J. Cereb. Blood Flow Metab.*, 3: Suppl. 1: 270–271.

Melamed, E., Lavy, S. and Portnoy, Z. (1975) Regional cerebral blood flow response to hypocapnia in the contralateral hemisphere of patients with acute cerebral infarction. *Stroke*, 6: 503–509.

Meyer, J. S. and Marx, P. (1972)The pathogenesis of EEG changes during cerebral anoxia. In A. Remond (Ed.), *Handbook of EEG and Clinical Neurophysiology, Vol. 14A*, Elsevier, Amsterdam, pp. 5–11.

Meyer, J. S., Shinohara, Y., Kanda, T., Fukuuchi, Y., Ericsson, A. D. and Kok, N. K. (1970) Diaschisis resulting from acute unilateral cerebral infarction. *Arch. Neurol.* 23: 241–247.

Paulson, O. B., Olesen, J. and Stig Christensen, M. (1972) Restoration of autoregulation of cerebral blood flow by hypocapnia. *Neurol. (Minneap.)*, 22: 286–293.

Sokoloff, L. (1978) Mapping cerebral functional activity with radio-active deoxyglucose. *Trends Neurosc.*, 1: 75–79.

Tulleken, C. A. F., van Dieren, A., ten Veen, J. and Lopes da Silva, F. H. (1978) Changes in local EEG, local cerebral blood flow and flow in the distal stump of the middle cerebral artery in cats with an occlusion of the middle cerebral artery. *Progr. Report Inst. Med. Phys. TNO Utrecht*, 6: 102–108.

Waltz, A. G. (1967) Cortical blood flow of opposite hemisphere after occlusion of middle cerebral artery. *Trans. Amer. Neurol. Ass.*, 92: 293–294.

Brain Ischemia: Quantitative EEG and Imaging Techniques, Progress in Brain Research, Vol. 62, edited by
G. Pfurtscheller, E.J. Jonkman and F.H. Lopes da Silva

Global Incomplete Ischemia in Dogs Assessed by Quantitative EEG Analysis. Effects of Hypnotics and Flunarizine

A. WAUQUIER, G. CLINCKE, W. A. E. VAN DEN BROECK, C. HERMANS, W. MELIS
and J. VAN LOON

Department of Neuropharmacology, Janssen Pharmaceutica, B-2340 Beerse (Belgium)

INTRODUCTION

Paradoxically the induction of incomplete ischemia appears more harmful than complete ischemia (Hossmann and Zimmermann, 1974; Nordström et al., 1978a, b). This suggestion was put into question by Steen et al. (1979) who found a better outcome after incomplete than after complete ischemia. Siesjö (1981) emphasized that the latter is true provided that the animals are hypoglycemic and that ischemia is short-lasting.

However, a poorer outcome is expected if incomplete ischemia is severe and prolonged. When the cerebral energy state is disrupted to such an extent that it leads to excessive cellular acidosis, incomplete ischemia may be more deleterious for the cells (Rehncrona et al., 1981).

In the present experiments, incomplete ischemia in dogs was produced by two different methods. In the first experiment, oligaemic ischemia was produced by blood withdrawal. The effect of etomidate was compared with pentobarbital and thiopental. In the second experiment, ischemia was produced by vessel clamping and effects of flunarizine, a calcium entry blocker, were assessed.

OLIGAEMIC ISCHEMIA

Hemorrhagic shock was experimentally induced by withdrawing blood in non-premedicated and non-anesthetized animals (François et al., 1979; De Bie et al., 1980). In contrast to other studies, the design allowed to approach the clinical situation because treatment started after the hemorrhage. A follow-up permitted further evaluation of survival and general behavioral state of the dogs, following the interventions. The present study was carried out to assess the effects of etomidate in comparison with two barbiturates: the long-acting hypnotic pentobarbital and the short-acting hypnotic thiopental and saline.

Materials and methods

Twenty healthy mongrel dogs (10 females and 10 males) of mean ($\pm$ S.E.M.) weight of 15.1 kg ($\pm$ 0.63) were selected. The dogs were quarantined for at least 2 weeks and treated against infectious diseases; hematology showed normal values.

Two weeks before the experiments, the animals were anesthetized (5 ml of pento-barbital sodium 60 mg/ml given i.v., after a s.c. premedication of 10 mg/kg of Hyp-norm), artificially ventilated and implanted with eight cortical stainless steel screw electrodes, which were connected to a plug fixed with dental cement on the skull. The electrodes were placed in the left and the right frontal, temporal, central and occipital part of the skull. The procedure of surgery has been described in detail previously (Wauquier et al., 1978a).

For the experiments, the dogs were partially restrained in a basket. One silastic catheter was inserted in the femoral artery and a second in the vena saphena under local anesthesia (Xylocaine 2%). Heparine 500 U.I./kg was given to keep the lumen of the inserted catheters open. After a control recording of at least 15 min, hypovole-mia–hypotension was initiated by withdrawing arterial blood in equal volumes of 50 mg/min until a mean arterial blood-pressure (BP) of 40–45 mm Hg was recorded.

After the BP had been stabilized at that low level for 15 min, a bolus injection of saline (1 ml/2 kg), 1 mg/kg of etomidate (clinical solution of 2 mg/ml), 3 mg/kg of pentobarbital or 10 mg/kg of thiopental was given i.v. Five minutes and 30 sec after the start of the bolus, an intravenous infusion commenced with 1 ml/min of saline, 0.1 mg/kg/min of etomidate (clinical solution 125 mg/ml), 0.3 mg/kg/min of pentobarbital or 1 mg/kg/min of thiopental, for 90 min. Continuous recording lasted for 240 min following the bolus injection. Thereafter, the femoral artery was repaired, the wound closed and the dogs treated with Dicastrepton® i.m. before being returned to their quarters; the withdrawn blood was not re-infused. The animals were examined daily and the time of death (or survival if > 2 weeks) was noted.

During the experiment, the arterial blood pressure, the ECG, respiration and EEG were continuously recorded on an Elema–Schönander mingograph.

The following eight cortical bipolar derivations were taken: frontal left (F_L), frontal right (F_R), occipital left (O_L), occipital right (O_R), temporal left (T_L), temporal right (T_R), central left (C_L), central right (C_R), frontal-occipital left and right hemisphere, temporal-central left and right hemisphere. The filters were set at 30 Hz and the time constants at 0.3. A continuous paper-recording was taken at a speed of 15 mm/sec for 6 h from the start of the experiment.

Tape-recordings were taken of the EEGs and subsequently analyzed with a pro-gram designed for sleep–wakefulness analysis (Wauquier et al., 1979). The power contained in the delta- (0.5–3.5 c/sec), theta- (3.5–7.5 c/sec), alpha- (7.5–13.5 c/sec) and beta-band (13.5–25.0 c/sec) was calculated and a special algorithms detected the amount of spindles (10.5–14.5 c/sec band) of the frontal-occipital derivation (F_3–O_1) each 30 sec epoch.

An on-line computer analysis was made of the F_L–F_R, O_L–O_R, T_R–C_R derivations for 6 min 15 sec periods (4 1/2 min effective EEG analyzed and calculation and printing time). The time schedule and the analysis is the same as that used for the EEG analysis of the effects of etomidate in normovolemic dogs (Wauquier et al., 1978b). Schematically the analysis of the 6 min 15 sec periods was as follows: 2 control periods before the induction of hypovolemia; 15 min after hypovolemia; bolus injec-tion: 1 period; infusion: 15 periods taken consecutively; post-infusion: 10 periods taken consecutively and 8 periods taken each 15 min.

An off-line computer analysis was carried out to calculate the relative power. The relative contribution of the power contained in seven pre-defined frequency bands to the total power (total band width 0.5–40.0 c/sec) equalized at 100 at each time period, was calculated. This was done for four derivations: F_L-F_R, O_L-O_R, T_L-C_L and T_R-C_R and is visualized in Fig. 3. It has to be taken into account that a decreased (or increased) contribution of power in one band to the total power, does not implicate that the actual power decreased (or increased) only that its relative contribution decreased (or increased).

Results

Hemodynamic and behavioral variables

After the mean pressure stabilized at 40–45 mm Hg for 15 min, dogs were treated with saline or drug. In *control dogs* there was a very slight rise in mean BP to a maximum of 56, but an increased heart rate following the bolus and infusion of saline to a maximum of 179 beats/min. One dog died during the infusion. Following infusion, two other dogs died and in the two remaining dogs, there was an augmentation of tachycardia and in one of them, a slight increase in mean BP.

Following a bolus injection of 1 mg/kg of *etomidate*, the mean BP increased from 47 to 64 mm Hg, the heart rate decreased from 139 to 106 beats/min and the respiratory rate increased from 30 to 43/min.

During an infusion of 0.1 mg/kg/min of etomidate, the mean BP further increased to reach 94 mm Hg at the end; the respiratory rate decreased from 33 to 28 waves/min and the heart rate increased to 128 beats/min.

After infusion of etomidate, the mean BP remained at about 90 mm Hg, the heart rate increased further to 160 beats/min, whereas the respiratory rate moderately decreased from 30 to 20–25 waves/min.

Following a bolus injection of 10 mg/kg of *thiopental*, the mean BP dropped to 36 mm Hg. The heart rate increased to 177 beats/min. None of the dogs continued to respire spontaneously and all were artificially ventilated within the first minutes following the bolus injection, with a mixture of 25% oxygen and room air.

During infusion of 1 mg/kg/min of thiopental, three dogs died. The mean BP gradually decreased to 15 mm Hg. The heart rate initially increased to more than 180 beats/min and then decreased to 97 beats/min. After infusion the two remaining dogs died, which was preceded by a further decrease of mean BP.

Following a bolus injection of 3 mg/kg of *pentobarbital*, the mean BP dropped immediately from 46 to 25 mm Hg. The heart rate remained high. Only one out of five dogs continued to respire spontaneously. Four dogs were intubated and artificially ventilated. During infusion of 0.3 mg/kg/min of pentobarbital, one dog died. In the other four dogs, the mean BP gradually increased to a maximum of 54 mm Hg. The heart rate remained at the same high level.

After infusion of pentobarbital, the mean BP increased to a maximum of 65 mm Hg at 90 min. Concurrently, the heart rate was increased to 180–185 beats/min and the spontaneous respiration started again. Another dog died during the post-infusion period.

In the 24 h following the experiment, the two remaining control dogs, two of the three pentobarbital-treated dogs and two of the five etomidate-treated dogs died. Survival for more than 2 weeks occurred in one pentobarbital- and in three etomidate-treated dogs (Table I).

TABLE I

SURVIVAL TIME OF MONGREL DOGS ($n = 5$ PER GROUP) FOLLOWING 15 MIN OF HYPO-
VOLEMIA–HYPOTENSION AND TREATMENT WITH SALINE, ETOMIDATE, THIOPENTAL
OR PENTOBARBITAL

Dog	Compound Bolus Infusion	Saline 0.5 ml/kg 0.05 ml/kg/min	Etomidate 1 mg/kg 0.1 mg/kg/min	Thiopental 10 mg/kg 1 mg/kg/min	Pentobarbital 3 mg/kg 0.3 mg/kg/min
1		200 min	22 h	88 min	18 min
2		170 min	24 h	7 min	15 min
3		25 min	> 2 weeks	96 min	16 h
4		8 h	> 2 weeks	185 min	20 h
5		13 h	> 2 weeks	140 min	> 2 weeks

At autopsy, in the non-surviving dogs, it was clear that all dogs had hemorrhages at the splanchnic level, these were especially severe in the thiopental-treated group.

Changes in the EEG and power spectral analysis

Saline-treated dogs (Fig. 1). Following hypovolemia, there was only a slight increase in the amplitude and a slight decrease of the frequency of the EEG. During infusion of saline, there were mainly irregular low amplitude fluctuations. However, there were short periods of high amplitude slow waves, during which fast frequencies disappeared. In some dogs, as illustrated, high voltage slow waves occurred followed by isoelectric activity. The very slow waves are reflected by a high increase in power in all frequency bands followed by a gradual decrease in the alpha- and beta-bands and a sudden drop of the power in the delta- and theta-band.

Etomidate-treated dogs (Fig. 2). During hypovolemia, there was a slight decreased frequency, best seen in the central region. Following induction of etomidate, high amplitude biphasic waves were observed. During infusion there was a predominant activity in the theta- and alpha-frequency domain. High amplitude sharp waves on a

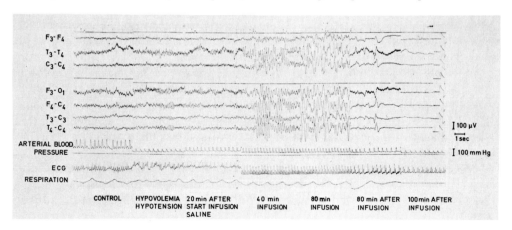

Fig. 1. Parts of an actual EEG recording of one dog during control, a bolus injection of 1 ml/2 kg, infusion of saline (1 ml/min) and following infusion. Abbreviations: F_3: frontal left, F_4: frontal right, T_3: temporal left, T_4: temporal right, O_1: occipital left, O_2: occipital right, C_3: central left, C_4: central right, ECG: electrocardiogram.

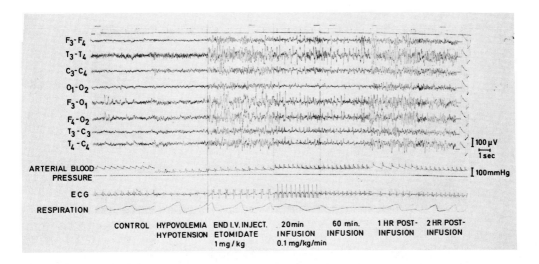

Fig. 2. Parts of an actual EEG recording of one dog during control, injection of 1 mg/kg of etomidate, infusion of 0.1 mg/kg/min of etomidate (1 ml/min over 90 min). Abbreviations are the same as in Fig. 1.

fast activity background were mainly seen in the frontal and temporal region of the cortex.

The computer analysis of the frontal-occipital derivation, showed a predominant increase of the power in the theta-, alpha- and beta-bands, but only a slight increase in the delta-power. Following infusion the power increased in all frequency bands and was most pronounced in the theta- and alpha-bands.

Thiopental-treated dogs. During hypovolemia, there was a slight decrease in the frequency and an increased amplitude of the EEG. Following induction of thiopental, very high amplitude slow waves in the delta- and theta-frequency domain were seen. This continued for a short time following infusion of thiopental. However, burst suppressions occurred shortly after the start of the infusion, which was followed by isoelectric activity and cerebral death.

The computer analysis demonstrates a very high increase in the power of the various frequency bands, which then gradually decreased to zero level.

Pentobarbital-treated dogs. There were few changes on the EEG following hypovolemia. After the induction of pentobarbital, there was an increase of high amplitude fast activity even in the F–O derivations. During infusion of pentobarbital, high amplitude slow waves and high amplitude bursts of negative sharp waves in the beta-frequency domain (mainly in the frontal and temporal cortex) occurred. Burst suppressions occurred during infusion. The effects seen during the infusion persisted up to the end of the recording.

Following induction and infusion, the power in the various frequency bands increased dramatically. This was then followed by a decrease to a very low level, associated with burst suppressions. Thereafter, a gradual increase in power was again observed.

Relative power

The relative power is the percentage contribution of the power contained in various frequency bands, to the total power equalized at 100 (Fig. 3).

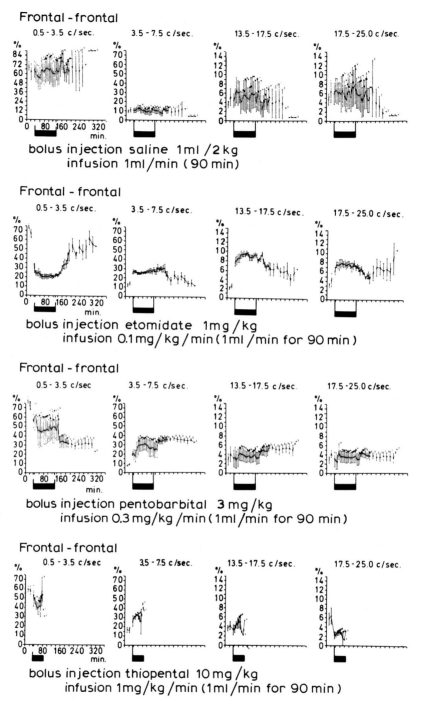

Fig. 3. Relative contribution of the power in various frequency bands (indicated in top) to the total power (frequency range 0.5–40.0 c/sec) equalized at 100 at each time period, in frontal left–right cortex, calculated for 6 min 15-sec periods: 2 before inducing hypovolemia–hypotension, 1 period 15 min thereafter at the time of the bolus injection of saline (1 ml/2 kg), 15 periods during infusion of 1 ml/min of saline for 90 min, and for 10 consecutive periods and 8 periods taken each 15 min following infusion.

Saline-treated dogs. In all cortical structures derived, there is a relatively high contribution of the delta-power (0.5–3.5 c/sec band) and a low contribution of the power in the other frequency bands. The power in the various bands show large fluctuations. Following infusion, there is a gradually increased contribution of the delta-power and a decreased contribution of the power in the other frequency bands. The individual variability is very pronounced.

Etomidate-treated dogs. In the F–F derivation, there is a decreased contribution of the delta-power, an increased contribution of the power in the frequency range 3.5–25.0 c/sec and a tendency to a decreased contribution of the power in the high frequency band 25.0–40.0 c/sec, during infusion of etomidate. Thereafter, there is a gradual normalization in the frequency range 0.5–17.5 c/sec, but an increased contribution of the power in the frequency range 17.5–40.0 c/sec. In the O–O derivation, during control there is a lower contribution of the delta-power and a higher contribution of the power in the other frequency bands than in the F–F derivation. During infusion, there is a decrease in the contribution of the delta-power and of the power in the frequency range 17.5–40.0 c/sec; there is an increased contribution of the power in the frequency range 3.5–13.5 c/sec; the contribution of the power in the frequency band 13.5–17.5 c/sec is not changed. After the infusion, there is a gradual normalization of the power in the frequency range 0.5–13.5 and 25.0–40.0, but an increased contribution of the power in the frequency range 13.5–25.0 c/sec. In the T–C derivations, the effects are similar to those seen in the O–O derivation. In addition, there is no difference between the left and right T–C derivations.

Thiopental-treated dogs. Since in all dogs isoelectric activity was seen during infusion and all dogs died within 3 h after the start of the bolus injection, only the initial changes can be described. In the F–F and O–O derivation, there is a decreased contribution of the delta-power and the power in the high frequency range 17.5–40.0 c/sec, and an increase of the power in the other frequency bands.

In the T–C derivations (left and right are similar) there is a decreased contribution of the power in the frequency range 0.5–7.5 c/sec and 25.0–45.0 c/sec, an increased contribution of the power in the frequency range 13.5–25.0 c/sec and no change in the 7.5–13.5 c/sec bands.

Pentobarbital-treated dogs. In general, the individual variability is very pronounced. In the F–F derivation, there is a decreased contribution of the power in the delta-band and high frequency range 25.0–40.0 c/sec, an increased contribution of the power in the frequency range 3.5–13.5 c/sec and no change in the contribution of the power in the frequency range 13.5–25.0 c/sec. After the infusion, the effects seen persisted in the surviving dogs.

In the O–O derivation, there is a decreased contribution of the power in the delta-band and in the frequency range 13.5–40.0 c/sec, the contribution of the power in the frequency range 3.5–13.5 c/sec fluctuated. After infusion there is some increase of the power in the frequency range 17.5–25.0 c/sec.

In the T–C derivations (left and right hemisphere) there is an increased contribution of the power in the 3.5–7.5 c/sec band and a decreased contribution of power in the 17.5–40.0 c/sec range. The effects persisted during the post-infusion period.

Discussion

The conditions in this experiment are comparable to the clinical situation in that drug treatment started *after* blood loss; they differ in that there was no volume replacement. In conventional shock therapy, volume is replaced to prevent venous collapse due to a decrease in the tangential wall tension.

The treatment with pentobarbital was not very successful, in spite of the reported efficacy of post-ischemic barbiturate loading (e.g. Mitchenfelder et al., 1976). The total dose given in our experiments was 30 mg/kg which is somewhat lower than those used in experiments dealing with focal ischemia produced by occlusion of the middle cerebral artery in the dog (Smith et al., 1974; Mitchenfelder and Milde, 1975; Corkill et al., 1976). However, in preliminary experiments we found that higher doses were lethal.

The treatment with thiopental was extremely deleterious since all animals died within a period of 3 h. None of the animals was able to restore its blood pressure. We conceive the dose to be appropriate at least as based on those used in dogs in which the medial cerebral artery was occluded (Smith et al., 1974). Further, this dose induced sleep of a similar duration as etomidate (in normal animals).

This raises the question of whether barbiturates are really able to protect against brain ischemia. Though the answer might be yes (Safar et al., 1978), the significant cardiorespiratory-depressant action appears to suggest that the safety of barbiturates in a clinical situation is not assured (Hoff, 1974).

The efficacy of etomidate in the present study demonstrates that pharmacological treatment is able to prevent the circulatory arrest, the end result of hemorrhagic shock. The pressure-restoring capacity of etomidate is quite unexpected since in normovolemic dogs etomidate, if anything, slightly decreases the pressure. Further investigation is required to elucidate its mode of action.

This study demonstrated that the EEG changes following various treatments in hypovolemic–hypotensive dogs are a sensitive index of the functional state of the brain and that a deterioration of the brain activity precedes a complete hemodynamic collapse. A long duration of hypotension induced paroxysmal slow activity of the EEG and isoelectric activity even when the ECG and heart frequency appear normal. Thus hypovolemia–hypotension also involves cerebral ischemia. Since the arterial pressure did not build up after thiopental treatment, cerebral death occurred, before failure of the heart occurred. In some pentobarbital-treated dogs, periods of burst-suppressions and isoelectric activity were followed by a short-lasting restoration of the EEG activity. However, also in four out of the five dogs, these periods were followed by cerebral death and heart failure.

The EEG changes during the development of brain ischemia due to hypovolemia–hypotension probably reflect reduced blood supply to the brain leading to a deficient oxygen supply especially involving the cerebral cortex. The bloodflow to the brain can be normal even when the bloodpressure is as low as 50 mm Hg. However, at this borderline and below this level, "autoregulation" which serves to compensate for the low perfusion pressure fails. The autoregulation involves a dilatation of the precapillary arterioles which then decreases the vascular resistance. When the perfusion pressure decreases, no further dilatation of the arterioles can take place and as a consequence, the cerebral bloodflow further decreases. The decreased perfusion pressure is, in addition, associated with an increased intracranial pressure, which further tends to decrease the cerebral bloodflow, finally inducing brain ischemia and infarction.

In hypovolemic–hypotensive dogs, etomidate has a beneficial and thiopental and pentobarbital a deleterious effect. It is evident that brain ischemia ensued from the

cardiohemodynamic-respiratory depressant effects caused by thiopental and pentobarbital.

GLOBAL INCOMPLETE ISCHEMIA INDUCED BY VESSEL CLAMPING IN DOGS

Cell toxicity is suggested to be due to an excessive Ca^{2+}-influx (Siesjö, 1981; Wauquier et al., 1981), whereas the finding that particular brain regions are selectively vulnerable to hypoxia-ischemia, is suggested to be due to neuronal hyperexcitability, associated with excessively raised intracellular Ca^{2+} (Meldrum et al., 1982).

In view of this, drugs which prevent excessive Ca^{2+}-entry may be of interest in protecting the brain against ischemia. Flunarizine is a selective Ca^{2+}-entry blocker: as shown in vitro by Van Nueten et al. (1978, 1982) in peripheral and cerebral vessels, it prevents vasoconstriction induced by Ca^{2+}, endogenous vasoactive substances or by hypoxia, without having an effect on spontaneous myogenic activity. Flunarizine has been shown to be effective against cerebral hypoxia and ischemia in a large number of tests (for survey see Wauquier, 1984; Wauquier et al., 1983). Recently, White et al. (1982) demonstrated that a very low dose of flunarizine (6 μg/kg) given i.v. following resuscitation from cardiac arrest in dogs, resulted in a return of cerebral blood flow (CBF) equal to pre-arrest flow.

In the present study, the efficacy of i.v. flunarizine is assessed by the EEG and CBF, using cortical brain temperature as a qualitative measure of tissue perfusion, in dogs where ischemia was produced by vessel ligation.

Materials and methods

The subjects were 14 adult male mongrel dogs of about 20 kg body weight, which were fasted overnight before the experiment.

Dogs were anesthetized with 0.16 mg/kg of alfentanil, muscle relaxation was achieved with succinylcholine (5 mg/h), they were intubated and ventilated with an air/oxygen mixture (50/50%) (Servo ventilator 900, Siemens) adjusted as to obtain normal blood gases (pO_2, pCO_2) and pH values. A femoral vein was cannulated for drug application and the femoral artery for monitoring blood pressure. Four screws were placed in the left (L) and right (R) frontal (F) and occipital (O) cortex allowing to derive the EEG. A temperature probe was stereotaxically positioned in the sensory cortex (at the level of the gyrus sigmoideus posterior). A needle inserted into the cisterna magna served to derive intracranial pressure. After opening the thorax, the intercostal arteries (usually nine) descending along the aorta were ligated.

Following parameters were continuously monitored during the experiment and recorded on a mingograph (Elema–Schönander, Siemens): arterial blood pressure (BP) via a Statham transducer, ECG via electrodes placed on thorax and paw; cortical, rectal and thoracic temperature; intracranial pressure and the EEG (four derivations F_L–F_R, O_L–O_R, F_L–O_L, F_R–O_R).

After stabilization of the various parameters, both the left subclavian and brachiocephalic artery were occluded as close as possible to the aortic arch for 20-min periods, with an interval of 72.5 min between each occlusion, repeated maximally three times.

226

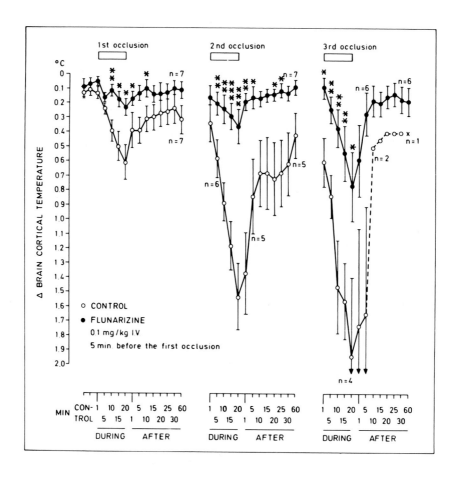

Fig. 4. Difference between brain cortical and thorax temperature preceding, during and following 20-min occlusions of the left subclavian and brachiocephalic artery after previous ligation of intercostal arteries in dogs ($n = 7$ in each group), treated i.v. with solvent ($\bigcirc - \bigcirc$) or 0.1 mg/kg of flunarizine ($\bullet - \bullet$) 5 min before the first occlusion period. *$p < 0.05$, ** $p < 0.01$, *** $p < 0.001$. Student's t-test.

Dogs were given either solvent (0.05 ml/kg body weight) or 0.1 mg/kg of flunarizine (solution of 2 mg/ml of flunarizine dihydrochloride solved in water containing 25 mg of tartaric acid per ml) 5 min before the 1st occlusion period through the venous line. The catheter was then flushed with 5 ml of Ringer solution.

The various parameters recorded on paper, except for the EEG, were calculated at the following time periods: 2 times before the 1st occlusion, at 1, 5, 10, 15 and 20 min during each occlusion and at 1, 5, 10, 15, 20, 25, 30 and 60 min after the end of each occlusion. The mean and S.E.M. of each group were calculated and Student's t-test applied to assess the difference between solvent- and flunarizine-treated dogs.

The EEGs were analysed on-line for 2.5-min periods continuously (5 periods before, 8 periods during and 22 periods after each occlusion) and subsequently processed by a PDP 11/10 computer, using previously described methods (Wauquier et al., 1978b, 1979). Further, all EEGs were visually analysed.

Results

Figure 4 shows the effects on the brain cortical temperature (CT). During the successive occlusion periods, CT progressively diminished, each occlusion period resulting in a larger drop in CT, which failed to return to the base-line following reperfusion. In flunarizine-treated dogs, CT did not change following the first occlusion, decreased slightly following the second occlusion and decreased moderately following the third occlusion. There was a significant difference between CT in solvent- and flunarizine-treated dogs.

Figure 5A,B illustrate the EEG changes seen in a solvent and a flunarizine-treated dog and Fig. 6 shows part of the computer analysis carried out in both groups.

Following the onset of the first occlusion in solvent-treated dogs, the amplitude of the EEG slightly increased from 20 to 50 μV to about 100 μV and the frequency decreased to slow beta (< 17.5 c/sec) and $alpha_2$ (9.5–13.5 c/sec); this was followed during occlusion by the development of activity mainly in the theta (3.5–7.5 c/sec) frequency range of ≥ 100 μV amplitude; thereafter, for a short period (2–10 min) there was more slow activity of ≥ 100 μV, predominantly in the theta-frequency domain, whereafter the EEG almost normalized.

During the second occlusion, there was a rapid development towards slow theta- and delta- (0.5–3.5 c/sec) waves of high amplitude (100–250 μV) followed at variable intervals (10–18 min) with a progressive flattening of the EEG with very slow waves of low amplitude (about 20 μV). Following reperfusion, the EEG remained flat for about 10–15 min, whereafter slow delta-waves of ≥ 150 μV developed. However, in one dog the EEG remained flat and in another a seizure pattern was seen. Both dogs did not survive.

Following the third occlusion, the EEG went flat within 10 sec, the amplitude was 10–20 μV. One dog collapsed during the occlusion, two others after occlusion and in the remaining dog the EEG remained flat during the reperfusion period.

The computer analysis, as exemplified by the relative power in the delta- and $beta_2$-band (17.5–25.0 c/sec) illustrates the visual analysis (Fig. 6). There were small fluctuations during which the contribution of the delta-power tended to decrease during the occlusion, followed initially after the occlusion by an increase and a subsequent decrease of the delta-power associated with an increased contribution of the power in the beta-band. Following the second occlusion, the relative delta-power progressively increased and persisted thereafter, whereas the relative beta-power decreased to near zero. The third occlusion period is characterized by a predominant delta-power.

In the flunarizine-treated dogs (Figs. 5B and 6), striking differences were seen as compared to the solvent-treated dogs. Following injection of flunarizine, the EEG pattern consisting of beta-frequency waves ≥ 50 μV remained unchanged. During the first occlusion there was a waxing and waning of activity in the beta-frequency domain, with a slightly increased amplitude (≥ 100 μV). There were intervening periods of small bursts of $alpha_2$-activity of 50–75 μV. The pattern did not change after occlusion. A similar pattern was seen during and following the second and third occlusion. In two dogs, some slow activity in the theta- and delta-domain of about 100 μV was seen which persisted for about 10 min after the end of the third occlusion. The stability of the EEG activity can also be seen from the computer analysis (Fig. 6).

228

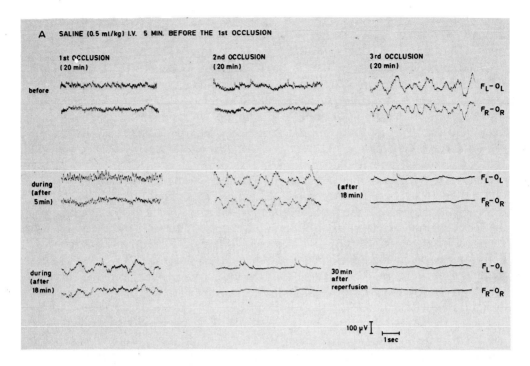

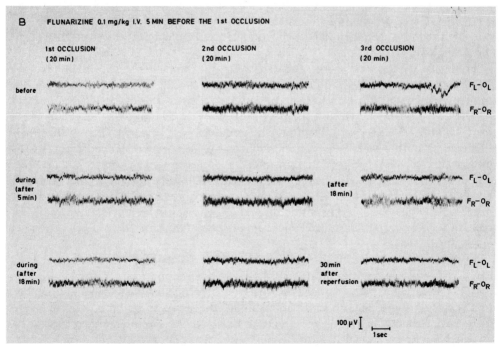

Fig. 5A. Examples from EEG recordings (frontal-occipital left hemisphere derivation) in a solvent-treated dog taken at the indicated time intervals. B: Examples from EEG recordings (frontal-occipital left hemisphere derivation) in a flunarizine-treated dog taken at the indicated time intervals.

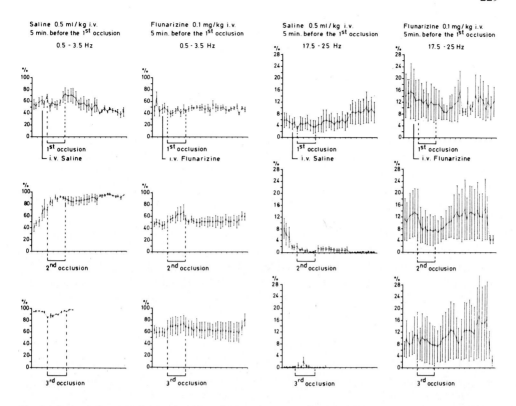

Fig. 6. Mean relative contribution (± S.E.M.) of the power in the delta- (0.5–3.5 c/sec) and beta- (17.5–25.0 c/sec) band to the total power (equalized at 100) preceding, during and following 20-min period occlusions in solvent- and flunarizine-treated dogs (*n* = 7 in each group). The EEG was sampled in consecutive periods of 2.5 min and power spectral analysis carried-out on different frequency bands, after which the relative power was calculated (see Methods and Wauquier et al., 1981).

Discussion

This part of the paper describes the effects of i.v. flunarizine preceding the induction of ischemia by vessel clamping in dogs. Flunarizine prevented a decrease in cortical temperature and preserved EEG functioning; in addition, the compound appeared to protect against cardiovascular collapse.

After ligation of the intercostal arteries, clamping the brachiocephalicus and left subclavian did result in a large reduction of the blood supply to the brain. However, ischemia was not complete. Remaining blood supply can possibly arise from, for instance, the epigastric artery which feeds into the right subclavian and from there via the carotid artery to the brain, bypassing the occlusions and possibly from the omocervical artery as well. It was evident from the EEG and brain temperature that severe ischemia was produced.

Though brain temperature is an inadequate quantitative measure of cerebral blood flow (Adams et al., 1980), it can be suggested that it provides a qualitative measure of tissue perfusion. The simultaneously recorded EEG, an adequate measure of the functional state of the brain in hypoxic-ischemic conditions (Wauquier and De Clerck, 1982), showed parallel changes to the brain cortical temperature. These findings

230

suggest that the changes in temperature are indicative of changes in brain perfusion. It has been reported that different thresholds of ischemia exist (Astrup et al., 1977): one being the critical level of cerebral blood flow resulting in electrical failure, attained at about 15 ml/100 g/min in man as well as animals (Branston et al., 1977).

The present experiments suggest that these critical levels of CBF are progressively reached during the occlusion and that flunarizine prevents the occurrence of these critical levels, in spite of a still large decrease in blood supply to the brain.

Brain perfusion is critically dependent on the systemic perfusion and the resistance at the microcirculatory level. Following occlusion of major vessels responsible for adequate brain perfusion, vasospasms may occur, due to the contractions of vascular smooth muscle cells as a consequence of raised cytoplasma Ca^{2+} concentrations or the production of endogenous vasoconstrictors such as 5-hydroxytryptamine (Vanhoutte, 1982). Cerebral vessels, in particular, are very sensitive towards Ca^2-induced contractions (Van Nueten and Vanhoutte, 1980).

Insufficient tissue perfusion leads to hypoxia and a further release of vasoactive substances, aggravating diminished tissue perfusion. This cascade of events might be antagonized by flunarizine as shown in in vitro experiments (Van Nueten and Vanhoutte, 1980; Van Nueten and De Clerck, 1982; Van Nueten et al., 1982). The contraction of peripheral and cerebral vessels, as a consequence of hypoxia in the presence of a threshold dose of a vasoactive substance is dose-relatedly prevented by flunarizine. Using a combined ischemic-hypoxic model (Levine preparation) in rats, van Reempts et al. (1983) demonstrated that flunarizine protected against coagulative necrosis (dense shrunken neurons surrounded by vacuoles) and astrocytic swelling.

Electron-microscopic studies in hypoxic-ischemic rats (Van Reempts and Borgers, 1982) showed calcium precipitation in damaged areas in the matrix of mitochondria, in the euchromatinic part of the nucleus and accumulation was found in swollen cell processes. In flunarizine-treated rats, the ultrastructure of cells was preserved and calcium distribution comparable to that seen in normal rats.

These findings suggest that flunarizine acts at both the vascular and the cellular level. Since edema is produced at a level of CBF (Crockard et al., 1980) which is also the threshold level of massive K^+ release (Astrup et al., 1977), it might be suggested that flunarizine's ability to prevent cellular necrosis and edema is due to an effect on CBF (vascular effect), without necessarily denying rheological effects and the inhibition of deleterious calcium influxes into the cells (cellular protective event).

SUMMARY

Incomplete but global ischemia was produced in dogs by two different methods. In the first experiment, hypovolemia–hypotension was initiated by withdrawing arterial blood. After stabilization of the arterial blood pressure at 40–45 mm Hg for 15 min, saline, or the hypnotics etomidate, pentobarbital or thiopental were given in a bolus followed by an infusion. Eight cortical derivations were recorded on paper, on-line analysis was done of four cortical derivations calculating the absolute power and off-line, the relative contribution of the power contained in seven pre-defined frequency bands to the total power was calculated.

In saline-treated dogs, hypotension induced paroxysmal slow activity followed by an isoelectric EEG. Treatment with etomidate prevented the circulatory arrest and as a consequence the EEG appeared not dramatically different from that seen in normotensive dogs. Survival for more than 2 weeks occurred in three out of five dogs. In pentobarbital-treated dogs, periods of burst suppressions were seen which in some cases were followed by a short-lasting restoration of the EEG activity. However, cerebral death occurred in four out of five dogs. In thiopental-treated dogs, an isoelectric EEG appeared within a short time and in spite of artificial ventilation, cerebral death occurred in all cases. This is probably due to its severe cardio-depressant effects.

In the second experiment, global incomplete ischemia was produced by ligation of major vessels supplying blood to the brain. These arteries were occluded for 20-min periods, with an interval of 72.5 min between each occlusion, repeated maximally three times. Dogs were treated with either solvent or with the calcium entry blocker flunarizine, at the dose of 0.1 mg/kg i.v., 5 min before the first occlusion or 5 min after the reperfusion following the first occlusion. The EEG was continuously monitored and quantitative analysis was done on 2.5-min periods.

Comparison of the relative power in the delta- and beta-bands clearly indicated the progressive deterioration of the EEG in conjunction with a decrease in cortical temperature (a qualitative measure of cerebral blood flow).

Flunarizine prevented the occurrence of the critical levels of CBF, which might be due to an anti-vasoconstrictive effect. The differentiation between the treated and the untreated dogs was also evident neurologically, as scored 24 h to 2 weeks after the insult.

REFERENCES

Adams, T., Heisey, S. R., Smith, M. C., Steinmetz, M. A., Hartman, J. C. and Fry, H. K. (1980) Thermodynamic technique for the quantification of regional blood flow. *Amer. J. Physiol*, 238: H682–H696.

Astrup, J., Symon, L., Branston, N. M. and Lassen N. A. (1977) Cortical evoked potential and extracellular K^+ and H^+ at critical levels of brain ischemia. *Stroke*, 8: 51–57.

Branston, N. M., Strong A. J. and Symon, L. (1977) Extracellular potassium activity, evoked potential and tissue blood flow. *J. neurol. Sci.*, 32: 305–321.

Corkill, G., Chikovani, O. K. and McLeish, I. (1976) Timing of pentobarbital administration for brain protection in experimental stroke. *Surg. Neurol.*, 5: 147–149.

Crockard, A., Jannotti, F., Hunstock, A. T., Smith, R. D., Harris R. J. and Symon, L. (1980) Cerebral blood flow and edema following carotid occlusion in the gerbil. *Stroke*, 11: 494–498.

De Bie, F. C., François, P., Hermans, C., Will, J., Loots, W., Opsteyn, M., Hörig, C. and Jageneau, A. H. M. (1980) Thalamonal, droperidol and fentanyl in induced hypovolemic shock in the conscious dog. *Anaesthesist*, 29: 78–84.

François, P., Hermans, C., Van Loon, J., Opsteyn, M., De Bie, F., Hörig, C. and Jagenau, A. (1979) *An experimental model of emergency therapy after acute hypovolemia*, Comment at the First Aid Congress, Oslo, June 19–23.

Hoff, J. T. (1978) Resuscitation in focal brain ischemia. *Crit. Care Med.* 6: 245–253.

Hossmann, K.-A. and Zimmermann, V. (1974) Resuscitation of the monkey brain after 1 h complete ischemia. I. Physiological and morphological observations. *Brain Res.*, 81: 59–74.

Meldrum, B., Griffiths, T. and Evans M. (1982) Hypoxia and neuronal hyperexcitability. A clue to mechanisms of brain protection. In A. Wauquier, M. Borgers and W. K. Amery (Eds.), *Protection of Tissues Against Hypoxia*, Elsevier Biomedical Press, Amsterdam, pp. 276–286.

Mitchenfelder, J. D. and Milde, J. (1975) Influence of anesthetics on metabolic, functional and pathological responses to regional cerebral ischemia. *Stroke*, 6: 405–410.

Mitchenfelder, J. D., Milde, J. H. and Sundt, T. M. (1976) Cerebral protection by barbiturate anesthesia. Use after MCA occlusion in Java monkeys. *Arch. Neurol.*, 33: 345–350.

Nordström, C. H., Rehncrona, J. and Siesjö, B. K. (1978a) Restitution of cerebral energy state, as well as of glycolytic metabolites, citric acid cycle intermediates and associated amino acids after 30 min of complete ischemia in rats anaesthesized with nitrous oxide or phenobarbital, *J. Neurochem.*, 30: 479–486.

Nordström, C. H., Rehncrona, J. and Siesjö, B. K. (1978b) Effects of phenobarbital in cerebral ischemia. II. Restitution of cerebral energy state, as well as of glycolytic metabolites, citric acid cycle intermediates and associated amino acids after pronounced incomplete ischemia. *Stroke*, 9: 335–343.

Rehncrona, J., Rosén, I. and Siesjö, B. K. (1981) Brain lactic acidosis and ischemic cell damage. 1. Biochemistry and neurophysiology. *J. Cereb. Blood Flow Metab.* 1: 297–311.

Safar, P., Bleyaert, A., Nemato, E. M., Moossy, J. and Snyder, J. V. (1978) Resuscitation after global brain ischemia-anoxia. *Crit. Care Med.*, 6: 215–227.

Siesjö, B. K. (1981) Cell damage in the brain: a speculative synthesis. *J. Cereb. Blood Flow Metab.*, 1: 155–183.

Smith, A. C., Hoff, J. T. and Nielsen, S. L. (1974) Barbiturate protection in acute focal cerebral ischemia. *Stroke*, 5: 1–7.

Steen, P. A., Mitchenfelder, J. D. and Milde, J. H. (1979) Incomplete versus complete cerebral ischemia: improved outcome with a minimal blood flow. *Ann. Neurol.*, 6: 389–398.

Vanhoutte, P. M. (1982) Effects of calcium entry blockers on tissue hypoxia. *J. Cereb. Blood Flow Metab.*, 2, Suppl. 1: S42–S44.

Van Nueten, J. M. and De Clerck, F. (1982) Protection against hypoxia-induced decrease in tissue blood flow. In F. Clifford-Rose and W. K. Amery (Eds.), *Hypoxia in the Pathogenesis of Migraine Attacks*, Pitman, London, pp. 176–184.

Van Nueten, J. M. and Vanhoutte, P. M. (1980) Improvement of tissue perfusion with inhibitors of calcium influx. *Biochem. Pharmacol.*, 29: 479–481.

Van Nueten, J. M., Van Beek, J. and Janssen P. A. J., (1978) Effect of flunarizine on calcium-induced responses of peripheral vascular smooth muscle. *Arch. Int. Pharmacodyn. Ther.*, 232: 42–52.

Van Nueten, J. M., De Ridder, W. and Van Beek, J. (1982) Hypoxia and spasms in the cerebral vasculature. *J. Cereb. Blood Flow Metab.*, 2, Suppl. 1: S29–S31.

Van Reempts, J. and Borgers, M. (1982). Morphological assessment of pharmacological brain protection. In A. Wauquier, M. Borgers and W. K. Amery (Eds.), *Protection of Tissues Against Hypoxia*, Elsevier Biomedical Press, Amsterdam, pp. 263–274.

Van Reempts, J., Borgers, M., Van Dael, L., Van Eyndhoven J. and Van de Ven, M. (1983) Protection with flunarizine against hypoxic-ischemic damage of the rat cerebral cortex. A quantitative morphologic approach, *Arch. Int. Pharmacodyn. Ther.*, 262: 76–88.

Wauquier, A. and De Clerck, A. C. (1982) Neurophysiology of the hypoxic brain. In A. Wauquier, M. Borgers and W. K. Amery (Eds.), *Protection of Tissues against Hypoxia*, Elsevier Biomedical Press, Amsterdam, pp. 71–86.

Wauquier, A. (1984) Effect of calcium entry blockers in models of brain hypoxia. In T. Godfraind, A. Herman and D. Wellens (Eds.), Calcium Entry Blockers in Vascular and Cerebral Dysfunctions, Martinus Nijhoff Publ., pp. 241–254.

Wauquier, A., Melis, W., Niemegeers, C. J. E. and Janssen, P. A. J. (1978a) A putative multipartite model of haloperidol interaction in apomorphine-disturbed behavior of the dog. *Psychopharmacology*, 59: 255–258.

Wauquier, A., Van den Broeck, W. A. E., Verheyen, J. L. and Janssen, P. A. J. (1978b) Electroencephalographic study of the short-acting hypnotics etomidate and methohexital in dogs. *Europ. J. Pharmacol.*, 47: 367–377.

Wauquier, A., Verheyen, J. L., Van den Broeck, W. A. E. and Janssen, P. A. J. (1979) Visual and computer-based analysis of 24 hr sleep-wake patterns in the dog. *Electroenceph. clin. Neurophysiol.*, 46: 33–48.

Wauquier, A., Clincke, G., Ashton, D. and Van Reempts, J. (1981) Considerations on models and treatment of brain hypoxia. In M. W. Van Hof and S. Mohn (Eds.), *Developments in Neuroscience, Vol. 13: Functional Recovery from Brain Damage*, Elsevier North-Holland Biomedical Press, Amsterdam, pp. 95–114.

Wauquier, A., Ashton, D., Hermans, C. and Clincke, G. (1983) Pharmacological effects in protective and resuscitative models of brain hypoxia. In K. Wiedemann and J. Hoyer (Eds.), *Brain Protection*, Springer Verlag, Berlin, pp. 100–111.

White, B. C., Gadzinski, D. S., Hochner, R. J., Krane, C., Hochner T., White J. D. and Trombley, J. H. (1982) Effect of flunarizine on canine cerebral cortical blood flow and vascular resistance post cardiac arrest. *Ann. Emerg. Med.*, 11: 119–126.

Brain Ischemia: Quantitative EEG and Imaging Techniques, Progress in Brain Research, Vol. 62, edited by
G. Pfurtscheller, E.J. Jonkman and F.H. Lopes da Silva

A New Technique for the Revascularization of a Chronic Ischemic Brain Area in Cats and Monkeys

C. A. F. TULLEKEN[1], A. VAN DIEREN[2] and E. J. JONKMAN[3]

[1]*University Hospital, Neurosurgery Department, P. O. Box 16250, 3500 CG Utrecht,*
[2]*Institute of Medical Physics, TNO, Brain Research Department, P. O. Box 5011, 3502 JA Utrecht and*
[3]*TNO Research Unit for Clinical Neurophysiology, Westeinde Hospital, 32 Lijnbaan, 2512 VA The Hague*
(The Netherlands)

INTRODUCTION

Carotid endarterectomy and extra-intracranial bypass procedures are performed for prophylactic reasons. However, the possibility that the improved perfusion of the brain induced by these operations may have a favorable effect on neuronal function in hypoperfused brain areas cannot be excluded. Experiments on cats and monkeys with focal brain ischemia induced by occlusion of the middle cerebral artery (MCA) (Symon et al., 1974; Tulleken et al., 1982; Strong et al., 1983 a,b), show that around an infarcted area in the center of the middle cerebral artery territory, a so-called penumbra exists where the cerebral blood flow (CBF) is sufficient to prevent infarction but too low for neuronal function. The existence of this penumbra is primarily demonstrated in acute and sub-acute experiments. It is very likely that this penumbra with so-called "idling neurons" is also present in the chronic stage. A beneficial influence of an increase in perfusion pressure on the function of the neurons located in this area may be hypothesized.

We got the impression that in a number of patients with a fixed neurological deficit, an improvement in neurological function occurred after an extra-intracranial bypass operation. Also, in some patients, who still showed a steady improvement in neurological function, a more rapid recovery seemed to take place after the bypass operation. It is almost impossible to prove or disprove such a phenomenon in a clinical study, since objective criteria for these mostly minor, but for the patient highly important, changes in neurological function are lacking. The only way to study the effect of improved perfusion on the function of the neurons in and around a chronic ischemic brain area is to revascularize it in a suitable experimental animal (cat or monkey). A satisfactory revascularization study, however, was not until now possible as a reliable revascularization procedure had not yet been described.

For anatomical reasons, the extra-intracranial bypass operation cannot be performed on cats. The results of the extra-intracranial bypass procedure in the monkey are also highly inconsistent, mostly for anatomical reasons. Moreover, the trephination necessary for the preparation of the cortical artery is a major intervention in the monkey and local brain edema is a frequent after effect. This makes the model useless for the study of the effect of the revascularization on parameters such as the EEG, sensory evoked potentials, CBF, metabolism and, of course, the clinical picture.

236

We attempted an extra-intracranial bypass operation in five rhesus monkeys with an average weight of 6 kg. Since the superficial temporal artery cannot be used, we took an arterial graft from the artery running along the dorsal aspect of the calf. The graft was interposed between the external carotid artery and a cortical branch of the MCA. A suitable cortical artery could be identified in only one of the five animals. A patent extra-intracranial bypass was obtained in this animal (see Figs. 1 and 2). However, in this case as well, the cortical branch of the MCA was of such a small calibre that no real increase in retrograde perfusion of the MCA, which was occluded at its origin, could be expected. In the other four cases, the cortical branches of the MCA were so small that in our opinion a bypass made no sense. In two of these cases, we found a suitable branch of the MCA deep in the sylvian fissure, and we used this artery for the bypass. This procedure, however, induced brain swelling and neither animal survived the operation. If the animals had survived the operation and the bypass had been patent, the experiment would still have been useless because the effect of revascularization would have been overshadowed by the effect of the local brain trauma.

Recently we have developed a new technique that enables us for the first time to revascularize a focal ischemic brain area in cats and monkeys. The operation is a further extension of the transorbital occlusion of the MCA, as described by Hudgins and Garcia (1970). The transorbital approach is, in our opinion, the best way to

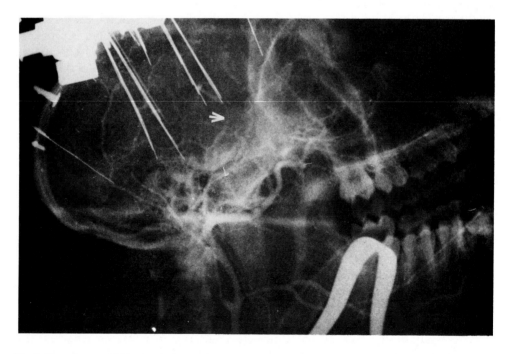

Fig. 1. Extra-intracranial bypass in a rhesus monkey, one week after the operation. The arrow indicates the bypass (arterial graft from the leg interposed between the external carotid artery and a cortical branch of MCA).

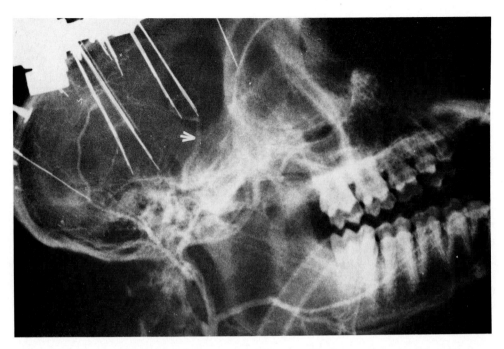

Fig. 2. Angiogram 3 weeks after the operation. The bypass has increased considerably in size.

produce focal brain ischemia. Without any retraction of brain tissue, the MCA can be occluded at its origin with a clip or ligature. A temporary occlusion can be produced by removal of the clip within 6 h after its application to the MCA. Removal of the clip after a longer period of time, however, is useless because in the meantime the proximal section of the MCA (from clip to first major branch) has become occluded with a thrombus. Therefore, revascularization can only be studied in this way for a maximum of 6 h after the occlusion.

As early as 1975 (Tulleken and Abraham), we described a variation on the method of Hudgins and Garcia. The MCA was ligated at its origin and just distal from this ligature, a fine catheter was inserted in the MCA, pointing in the distal direction. The catheter was fixed with another ligature around the MCA. The MCA stump pressure could be recorded continuously through this catheter.

Extensive use of this experimental model improved our handling of the MCA and we finally explored the possibility of a microvascular reconstruction of the proximal portion of the MCA via the transorbital route. A transorbital replacement of the thrombosed MCA segment was considered as a possibility, because in chronic experiments we always found the occlusion of the MCA to be restricted to the so-called M1 segment. In all the cases studied, the MCA remained patent distally from the point where the first branch originated. In all these cases, after excision of the thrombosed M1 portion, an excellent backflow from the MCA territory could be established. We then realized that an anastomosis between the internal carotid artery and the distal MCA was at least theoretically possible.

METHODS

The transorbital approach to the MCA (Hudgins and Garcia)

The eye is removed and, using the operating microscope, the optic foramen is enlarged at the top and on the lateral side by only a few millimeters. The opening must be as small as possible because otherwise the normal anatomical relations are disturbed afterwards by adhesions that make the revascularization operation, which is performed about one month later, much more difficult. The dura mater is opened, the MCA is dissected and a ligature is placed at its point of origin. A canula is slid over the ligature and is guided under the skin from the orbit to the opening in the skin at the vertex, where a connector for EEG, CBF and SEP electrodes is fixed. Both ends of the ligature protrude from the external opening of the canula. The enlarged optic foramen is covered with gel foam and the orbit is partly filled with acryl. The skin is closed. A week later, in the conscious animal, the ends of the ligature protruding from the canula are pulled slightly outward, causing an occlusion of the MCA at its origin. Four weeks later, under general anesthesia, the acryl is removed from the orbit. The optic foramen is further enlarged in the lateral and inferior directions. This exposes the M1 portion of the MCA and a portion of the internal carotid artery. From this moment on, the procedures in the cat and monkey differ slightly.

Monkey

After extensive exposure of the distal portion of the internal carotid artery, the M1 segment and the first branches of the MCA (Fig. 3a), the proximal portion of the anterior cerebral artery is also exposed by removing some bone in the medial direction. The anterior cerebral artery is ligated at its most proximal point. Clips are applied to the internal carotid artery, about 3 mm proximally from its bifurcation and to the MCA just distally from the thrombosed M1 segment (Fig. 3b). The thrombosed M1 segment is excised (Fig. 3c). An arterial graft (a portion of a branch of the femoral artery) 3–4 mm long is interposed between the internal carotid artery and the MCA (Fig. 3d). For both end-to-end anastomoses, 5–6 interrupted 10.0 prolene B.V. 6 sutures are used (Ethicon®). The microscope is set at a magnification of 16.

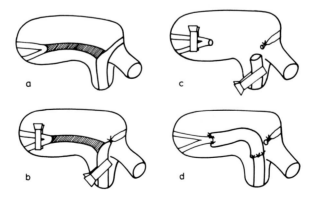

Fig. 3. The revascularization operation through the enlarged optic foramen in the monkey in four successive steps (a–d). For details see text.

Cat

The distal portion of the internal carotid artery, the M1 segment of the MCA and the proximal portion of the branches of the MCA are extensively exposed by further enlargement of the optical foramen. The proximal portion of the anterior cerebral artery is exposed by removal of some bone in the medial direction (Fig. 4a). The anterior cerebral artery is ligated at its most proximal portion. The MCA is clipped just distally from the thrombosed M1 segment and divided with microscissors between clip and thrombosed portion. A clip is then applied to the internal carotid artery as proximally as possible (Fig. 4b). The internal carotid artery is cut with microscissors at its most distal point (Fig. 4c). In the cat, it is then possible to connect the internal carotid artery and the MCA without undue tension on the vessels by one end-to-end anastomosis (Fig. 4d). For this anastomosis, 4–5 10.0 prolene B.V. 6 sutures are used.

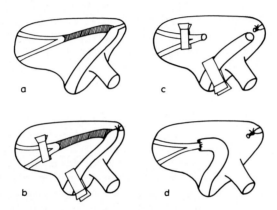

Fig. 4. The revascularization operation through the enlarged optic foramen in the cat in four successive steps (a–d). For details see text.

MATERIAL AND RESULTS

The feasibility of the method was tested in three acute experiments in monkeys and three acute experiments in cats. Despite the first author's fairly extensive experience with microvascular techniques, the end-to-end anastomosis between the small MCA and the internal carotid artery, through a rather small aperture at some depth, created several difficulties that had to be overcome. The technique was mastered as follows: in 10 experiments, the carotid artery of the rat was dissected. The skull of a monkey with an enlarged right optic foramen was then put into a fixture and placed 1–2 cm above the carotid artery of the rat. The enlarged optic foramen was centered over the carotid artery and via the enlarged optic foramen, the carotid artery was cut and a portion (0.5 cm) of the left carotid artery was interposed between the two ends of the right carotid artery, making two end-to-end anastomoses with 6 sutures, of 10.0 prolene. In the first three cases, one or both of the anastomosis sites became occluded. In the remaining seven cases, however, thanks to an improved technique, a patent anastomosis could always be made. In three monkey experiments and three cat experiments performed after this training period, we were able to perform a successful transorbital revascularization.

DISCUSSION

We were frustrated by the fact that such an important phenomenon as the effect of revascularization of a chronic ischemic brain area could not be studied in experimental animals because a reliable method of revascularizing a chronic ischemic brain area in cats and monkeys was lacking: we thus explored the possibility of a transorbital anastomosis between the internal carotid artery and the MCA after excision of the occluded M1 segment of the MCA. The anatomical feasibility of the method was tested in a number of acute experiments. In cats, it became clear that after excision of the M1 segment of the MCA, a direct anastomosis could be made between the internal carotid artery and MCA. In the monkey, it is necessary to interpose an arterial segment (we used a segment of a branch of the femoral artery) between the internal carotid artery and the MCA after excision of the occluded M1 segment. The disadvantage of the small-caliber and the very fragile wall of the cats' MCA is balanced to a certain extent by the fact that because of the particular anatomical situation in the cat, only one anastomosis has to be made between the internal carotid artery and the MCA after excision of the M1 segment, while in the monkey a graft must be used, necessitating two end-to-end anastomoses. In order to gain experience with the end-to-end anastomosis between small arteries (the MCA in the cat has a diameter of about 0.4 mm and a very fragile wall; the MCA in the monkey has a diameter of about 0.8 mm and a firm wall) via a small, rather deep hole, we practiced by performing a number of end-to-end anastomoses in the carotid artery of the rat, via the enlarged optic foramen of the monkey skull which was fixed 1–2 cm above the neck of the rat. The monkey and cat experiments performed after this training period proved that patent anastomoses can be made between the internal carotid artery and MCA after excision of the M1 segment of the MCA. In our experiments on cats and monkeys, 4 weeks after occlusion of the MCA via the transorbital route, the internal carotid artery-MCA anastomosis was performed. Using depth electrodes, the EEG, CBF (H_2 clearance) and sensory evoked potentials were recorded three times a week. At the end of the experimental period, 2-deoxy-D-[^{14}C] glucose was injected intravenously half an hour before the animal was sacrificed. Autoradiograms of the brain were made to study the brain metabolism.

We hope in due time to be able to use this work to study the dynamic changes in a chronic ischemic brain area after revascularization.

SUMMARY

Since the beginning of the '60s, a number of animal models have been described in which a focal or global ischemia of the brain can be produced. The most used focal ischemia model is Hudgin's and Garcia's: the MCA is occluded using the transorbital route. This is an excellent model in monkeys and cats and was extensively used by us since 1973. However, a reliable method to revascularize the ischemic brain area after a longer period of time is not available. When the clip is removed from the MCA after a period of 1 or 2 days, the artery is already thrombosed in its proximal segment. In the monkey the extra-intracranial bypass is a highly unreliable method for revascularization, since the caliber of the cortical branches of the MCA is too small. Moreover the trephination necessary for this procedure can produce local brain damage.

A new method is described in which the MCA territory is revascularized via the transorbital route.

ACKNOWLEDGMENT

This work was funded in part through a grant of the Dutch Heart Foundation.

REFERENCES

Hudgins, W. R. and Garcia, J. H. (1970) Transorbital approach to the middle cerebral artery of the monkey: a design for experimental cerebral infarction applicable to ultrastructural studies. *Stroke*, 1: 107–111.

Strong, A. J., Venables, G. S. and Gibson, G. (1983a) The cortical ischaemic penumbra associated with occlusion of the middle cerebral artery in the cat. I. Topography of changes in blood flow, potassium ion activity and EEG. *J. Cereb. Blood Flow Metab.*, 3: 86–96.

Strong, A. J., Tomlinson, B. E., Venables, G. S., Gibson, G. and Hardy, J. A. (1983b) The cortical ischaemic penumbra associated with occlusion of the middle cerebral artery in the cat. II. Studies of histopathology, water content and in vitro neurotransmitter uptake. *J. Cereb. Blood Flow Metab.*, 3: 97–108.

Symon, L., Pasztor, E. and Branston, N. M. (1974) The distribution and density of reduced cerebral blood flow following acute middle cerebral artery occlusion: an experimental study by the technique of hydrogen clearance in baboons. *Stroke*, 5: 355–364.

Tulleken, C. A. F. and Abraham, J. (1975) The influence of changes in arterial CO_2 and blood pressure on the collateral circulation and the regional perfusion pressure in monkeys with occlusion of the middle cerebral artery. *Acta neurochir. (Wien)*, 32: 161–173.

Tulleken, C. A. F., Van Dieren, A., Ten Veen, J. and Lopes da Silva, F. H. (1982) Changes in local cerebral blood flow, local EEG and flow in the distal stump of the middle cerebral artery in cats with occlusion of the middle cerebral artery. *Acta. neurochir. (Wien)*, 61: 227–240.

Brain Imaging Techniques

Brain Ischemia: Quantitative EEG and Imaging Techniques, Progress in Brain Research, Vol. 62, edited by
G. Pfurtscheller, E.J. Jonkman and F.H. Lopes da Silva

Regional Cerebral Blood Flow Measured by Xenon-133 and [123I]Iodo-Amphetamine in Patients with Cerebrovascular Diseases

LEIF HENRIKSEN, SISSEL VORSTRUP and OLAF B. PAULSON

Department of Neurology, Rigshospitalet, DK-2100 Copenhagen (Denmark)

INTRODUCTION

Regional cerebral blood flow (rCBF) measured by single photon emission computer tomography (SPECT) of inhaled xenon-133 has proven to be of high value for the detection of both low and high flow areas in the brain. With earlier methods, xenon-133 was injected intra-arterially and the washout of the isotope was followed by stationary detector systems with up to 254 detectors over one hemisphere (Lassen et al., 1978). Such stationary systems are hampered by poor depth resolution, and the traumatic nature of this method, requiring puncture of a neck artery, has restricted its use to patients requiring a diagnostic angiogram. Furthermore, CBF was only visualized from brain areas supplied by the artery injected. The recent development of the three-dimensional technique with computer assisted tomography of either inhaled or intravenously injected xenon-133 was a major advance, and has allowed further investigation of cerebrovascular disease (Lassen et al., 1981). Radioisotopes other than xenon-133 have been investigated for measurements of flow distribution in the brain, and [123I]iodo-isopropyl-amphetamine (IAMP-123) is a possibility (Winchell et al., 1980a, Hill et al., 1982; Lassen et al., 1983). In the normal brain, CBF reflects neuronal activity due to the close coupling between flow and metabolism. This aspect of visualizing the dynamic properties of the brain must be emphasized in contrast to transmission computerized tomography (TCT), which reflects anatomy (X-ray attenuation). Flow abnormalities have been found repeatedly in several different diseases (Henriksen, 1983; Lou et al., 1984; Vorstrup et al., 1983).

Quantitative assessment of rCBF in ischemic cerebrovascular disease represents both a clinical and technical challenge. Detection of low flow areas in the acute or chronic phase of cerebrovascular disease could either represent an area with potentially viable tissue where restoration of blood flow may re-establish cellular function (ischemic penumbra), or an area partially damaged or perhaps disconnected from adjoining brain areas, resulting in a reduced functional state with reduced metabolism and hence a low rCBF. Patients with a minor stroke and/or transient ischemic attacks (TIA) with arteriosclerotic lesions of the major neck vessels or intracranial arteries constitute the main group of patients who from a clinical point of view could benefit from rCBF studies.

The results of our recent studies of serial measurements of rCBF in patients with stroke in the acute or chronic phase, as well as CBF measurements in patients before and after reconstructive neck vessel or extracranial intracranial (EC–IC) shunt operations will be presented and illustrated by some examples.

METHOD

The instrument (Tomomatic 64, Medimatic Inc., Copenhagen) is essentially a fast-rotating four-gamma-camera system, and has been described in detail elsewhere (Stokely et al., 1980; Celcis et al., 1981; Lassen et al., 1981). Briefly, simultaneous recordings are made from three "slices" of brain tissue; each slice is 2 cm thick and the distance between slices is 2 cm. The resolution element is about 1.7 cm in the plane and 2.0 cm perpendicular to the plane, measured as full width at half maximum (FWHM).

Xenon-133 is inhaled for 1.5 min at a concentration of 20 mCi/l, giving an equilibration concentration in the lungs of about 10 mCi/l. During the 1.5-min period of xenon-133 inhalation the total counts per slice are approximately 500.000. The washout is followed during three subsequent 1-min periods and each of the four integral pictures in the three slices is used for calculating regional cerebral blood flow (Celcis et al., 1981). The arterial input of xenon-133 is assessed by a narrow collimated scintillation detector placed over the upper part of the right lung. The radioabsorbed dose for a single study, as calculated for both gamma and beta radiation, has been calculated as approximately 0.6 rad to the lungs and 0.06 to the gonads (Atkins et al., 1980).

IAMP-123 was given intravenously and a dose of 2 mCi gave approximately 300.000 counts per slice for a 5-min sampling time. The radioabsorbed dose to the lungs (target organs) and gonads has been calculated as approximately 1.0 and 0.1 rad per study, respectively. The extraction in the brain was measured following an intracarotid injection in two patients and found to be over 90%, also when CBF was increased by hypercapnia. The input curve was not recorded with IAMP-123 since that would necessitate arterial sampling and hence violate the atraumatic nature of the study. As IAMP-123 distributes itself early in proportion to flow, only the first 10 min were used for the tomographic maps. For IAMP-123, the area-to-area difference in CBF was assumed to be given by the unaltered tomograms (Lassen et al., 1983).

Fig. 1. Normal adult man studied with his eyes closed and with environmental noise reduced to a minimum. Note the symmetric flow distribution on the left and the right sides, and in the anterior to the posterior regions. *In all figures the scale of CBF is indicated on the right; maximal values are in white, minimal in dark blue.

Fig. 2. A 58-year-old woman who suffered a completed stroke of sudden onset with a left-sided hemiparalysis and a moderate non-fluent aphasia (see case 2 for details p. 248). *See legend, Fig. 1.

Fig. 3. This 33-year-old man suffered transient ischemic attacks in his right hemisphere. He was considered a candidate for an EC–IC shunt operation, and CBF tomograms were performed (A) before and (B) 3 months following surgery. Flow-distribution maps (rCBF×100/mean CBF) have been used to illustrate that no regional changes could be discerned following surgery (see case 3 for details, p. 248). *See legend, Fig. 1.

Fig. 4. A 66-year-old woman with hemiparkinsonian symptoms in her left extremities. Regional CBF showed an asymmetry with a reduced flow in the right subcortical area corresponding to the globus pallidus and the antero-ventral thalamic nuclei. Measurements were obtained with (A) xenon-133 and (B) IAMP-123. Note a better delineation of gray and white matter with IAMP-123 (see case 4 for details, p. 248). *See legend, Fig. 1.

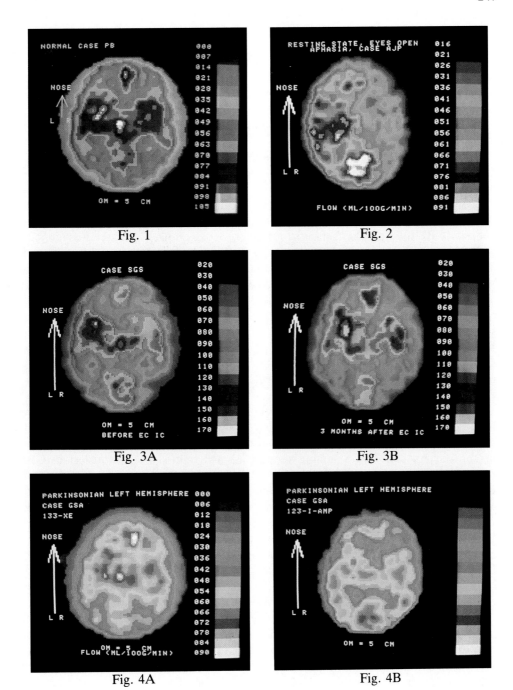

Fig. 1

Fig. 2

Fig. 3A

Fig. 3B

Fig. 4A

Fig. 4B

ILLUSTRATIVE CASES

Four cases have been selected: (1) an adult man from our material; (2) a patient with a completed stroke of sudden onset, studied in the chronic phase; (3) a patient with a stenosing middle cerebral artery who had had multiple TIAs. Measurements were obtained before and following an EC–IC shunt operation; (4) a hemiparkinsonian patient with left-sided symptoms, investigated with both xenon-133 and IAMP-123.

Case 1, Fig. 1: A 42-year-old normal adult man measured during rest with his eyes closed and with the noise level reduced to a minimum. Note the left/right and anterior/posterior symmetry.

Case 2, Fig. 2: This 58-year-old strictly right-handed woman suffered a completed stroke of sudden onset with a left-sided hemiparalysis and a moderate non-fluent aphasia. CBF tomography 2 months after the stroke showed a marked asymmetry with reduced flow in the right hemisphere. Activation studies (spontaneous speech and naming of pictures displayed on a screen) showed a normal activational pattern with increased rCBF in both of the classical speech centers (Broca's and Wernicke's areas), but failed to increase rCBF in the diseased right hemisphere. TCT showed a hypodense lesion in the right hemisphere located deep in the region of the caudate, the lenticular nucleus and the anterior part of the internal capsule. This patient might represent a rare case where the speech centers are located in both hemispheres. Comparison between the tomographic flow map and the TCT scan showed that the hypoperfused area exceeded the TCT structural changes, and included the overlying cortical areas.

Case 3, Figs. 3A and 3B: This 33-year-old man suffered TIAs with dysesthesia of his left-sided extremities of minutes' duration, and on one single occasion with a left-sided hemiparesis lasting 15 min. Angiography showed a stenosis of the right middle cerebral artery and TCT scanning showed a small right-sided frontal lesion. CBF tomography showed an asymmetry with reduced flow in the anterior part of the right middle cerebral artery territory. The clinical symptoms subsided with anticoagulant and antiplatelet therapy. The finding of a focal flow area exceeding the TCT lesion in size was considered to support the indication for a EC–IC bypass shunt operation. Surgery was uncomplicated and he recovered without any further neurological complaints. CBF tomography was performed 3 months after the surgery and was found to be unchanged as compared to the preoperative studies (Fig. 3B).

Case 4, Figs. 4A and 4B: A 66-year-old woman who had hemiparkinsonism over the last 3 years. She responded well to levodopa therapy without suffering side effects. The symptoms were strictly limited to the left extremities with rigidity, some akinesia and minimal tremor. Regional CBF showed a left/right asymmetry with a reduced flow in the right subcortical area corresponding to the globus pallidus and the anteroventral thalamic nuclei (Fig. 4A). We performed a tomographic study of this patient after intravenous injection of 2 mCi of IAMP-123 (Fig. 4B). Due to the better imaging properties of this compound the brain structures are better defined. However, the flow pattern resembles the xenon-133 flow map, showing a reduced isotope uptake in the globus pallidus and the thalamic areas (Fig. 4B).

GENERAL REMARKS

Our stroke series now comprises more than 50 patients studied in the chronic phase, i.e. 6 weeks to half a year after the ischemic event. Focal low flow areas were readily detected in areas corresponding to the clinical symptoms and the TCT lesion. In most cases the size of the low flow area exceeded the size of the hypodense lesion noted with TCT (Lassen et al., 1981). Serial measurements in acute stroke patients (less than 48 h) and follow-up studies weeks to months later have shown persistent low flow areas. However, in acute stroke there is not a steady state, as arterial occlusion may disappear and edema develop and later resolve. Therefore, rCBF may change from hypo- to hyperemia and back to low flow.

In a series of 33 TIA patients with arteriosclerotic lesions in their neck vessels, approximately 20% had hypodense areas with TCT, whereas approximately 40% showed a focal low flow on their CBF maps. These low flow areas persisted after reconstructive neck vessel surgery in all but 10% where an improvement compared to the preoperative rCBF asymmetry was noted. These latter 10% all had severely stenosing arteriosclerotic lesions probably of hemodynamic importance.

The finding of a persistent low flow in areas larger than the corresponding TCT lesion in the majority of our patients with ischemic cerebrovascular disease deserves further comments. In the absence of a vascular occlusion the low rCBF may be caused by a partial infarction of the most vulnerable cells, the neurons, or it could be the result of a lowered metabolic demand due to a neuronal disconnection caused by remote tissue damage. A reduced CBF surrounding and remote from a deep TCT lesion is illustrated by the stroke case presented (case 2), who had a deep TCT lesion and a reduced rCBF also in the overlying cortical areas and in the contralateral cerebellar hemisphere ("crossed cerebellar diaschisis", Baron et al., 1981). In the case of a vascular occlusion a third possibility exists, a hemodynamic impediment resulting in a state of "misery perfusion" (Baron et al., 1981). It is important to recognize these cases as vascular surgery is the only important rational therapy to prevent permanent ischemic damage. Resting state CBF measurements may not distinguish between the different pathogenetic mechanisms, but e.g. the occurrence of clinical symptoms related to postural changes may indicate a hemodynamic mechanism. Under these circumstances the cerebral vessels are locally dilated with a reduced perfusion pressure. Recent reports on cerebral blood volume (CBV) indicate that it may be increased, and measurements thereof may be used as an indicator of the local circulatory reserve (Gibs et al., 1983).

The EC–IC case presented here (case 3) is one of 20 consecutive patients who were studied prior to and 3 months after surgery. These patients were selected for surgery based on the following criteria: (a) clinical reasons, preferably minor stroke and/or TIAs; (b) angiographic lesions that were not accessible by conventional neck vessel surgery, i.e. occlusion of the internal carotid artery or occlusion/stenosis of the middle cerebral artery or its major branches; (c) CBF measurements showing a local low flow area in agreement with the clinical and angiographic findings, and larger than the hypodense area shown by TCT (three cases had a normal TCT scan in the hemisphere operated upon). Following surgery, an increase in rCBF was seen in four cases. The others had no definite increase in rCBF or changes of left/right asymmetry. The clinical findings in the patients with neurological deficits prior to surgery were unchanged, but the TIAs ceased in the majority (12 of 14 cases). Still, it remains to be proven that EC–IC bypass surgery reduces the incidence of future ischemic events. It is to be hoped that this will be achieved by the large multicenter study presently being carried out. However, our findings indicate that rCBF can only be improved in a few cases by an EC–IC bypass operation. Preoperative assessment may be useful to select cases who may benefit from shunting. Resting state measurements of rCBF do not seem to give sufficient information on the significance of hemodynamic mechanisms with "misery perfusion". But it may be expected that in such regions the cerebral vessels are partially or totally dilated in order to maintain a flow as normal as possible. A vasodilatory stimulus may be expected to reduce the response in such regions. Our preliminary findings with the acetazolamide test during CBF measurements and recent studies on cerebral blood volume (Gibs et al., 1983) indicate that these pathophysiological considerations may apply to the clinical situation, and allow for the preoperative recognition of patients where the low flow area is at least partially caused by a hemodynamic impediment.

Other radioisotopes than xenon-133 to map local CBF have been sought and IAMP-123 is promising. Compared to rCBF measured with either xenon-133 or labeled microspheres, good agreement had been obtained over a wide range of CBF. Quantification of IAMP-123 and the scaling between gray and white matter tissue can be performed with a xenon-133 tomogram prior to the IAMP-123 study.

The IAMP-123 tomograms offer a better resolution, especially of deeper structures (Fig. 4), mainly due to a reduction in Compton scatter. Preliminary studies with a high-resolution collimator give a resolution down to approximately 10 mm. In all cases good agreement was found between xenon-133 and IAMP-123 studies. A tendency toward a reduction in gray and white matter ratio due to redistribution of IAMP-123 with time was noted.

Other brain-seeking compounds will probably become available to image specific regions or receptors. Highly sensitive instruments are necessary to provide a reasonable resolution, i.e. below 2 cm (FWHM), a reasonably short sampling time, and an acceptable radiation exposure for the patient and personnel. These demands are not met by conventional single crystal orbiting gamma cameras.

Quantification of rCBF is possible with SPECT of inhaled xenon-133, and the method gives valid information about the distribution of rCBF. However, the quantification is hampered by Compton scatter, which results in an overestimation of flow, especially in low flow areas. Despite this precaution we have reason to believe that the level at which rCBF becomes critical for tissue viability can be established empirically from our serial measurements of patients with cerebrovascular diseases.

SUMMARY

Single-photon-emission computerized tomography (SPECT) of xenon-133 and [123I]iodo-amphetamine (IAMP-123) images regional cerebral blood flow (rCBF). The method has the potential to disclose anatomically normal but functionally abnormal brain areas in contrast to, e.g. transmission computerized tomography (TCT) which is restricted to imaging structure in terms of density. The device and method have been developed specifically for routine clinical studies of patients with cerebrovascular diseases, i.e. stroke cases, patients with transitory ischemic attacks, and candidates for an extracranial–intracranial (EC–IC) shunt operation.

The instrument consists of four gamma cameras rotating rapidly around the head (10 sec per rotation). A series of four 1-min pictures is taken during and after inhalation of xenon-133 for 1 min (10 mCi/l), and these rCBF maps are used for the flow calculations. IAMP-123 (2 mCi) was injected intravenously and the constructed image was scaled according to area-to-area difference seen with the xenon-133 technique.

Quantitative assessment of rCBF in areas of brain ischemia is a clinical challenge, and the method seems to be particularly useful for evaluating patients with cerebrovascular diseases. The hypoperfused areas in stroke cases are often more extensive than the hypodense areas noted on TCT. The same pattern was noted in a series of patients with transitory ischemic attacks, and several cases showed flow abnormalities despite a normal TCT. In recent studies we have found the method most useful for evaluating patient's suitability for EC–IC shunt operations, or the effect of endarterectomy on rCBF in patients with neck vessel disease.

REFERENCES

Atkins, H. L., Robertson, J. S., Croft, B. Y., Tsui, B., Susskind, H., Ellis, K. J., Loken, M. K. and Treves, S. (1980) Estimates of radiation absorbed doses from radioxenons in lung imaging. *J. Nucl. Med.*, 21: 459–465.

Baron, J. C., Bousser, M. G., Rey, A., Guillar, A., Comar, D. and Castaigne, P. (1981) Reversal of focal "misery perfusion syndrome" by extra-intracranial arterial bypass in hemodynamic cerebral ischemia. *Stroke*, 12: 454–459.

Celcis, P., Goldman, T., Henriksen, L. and Lassen, N. A. (1981) A method for calculating regional cerebral blood flow from emission computed tomography of inert gas concentrations. *J. Comput. Assist. Tomogr.*, 5: 641–645.

Gibs, J., Wise, R., Leenders, K. and Jones, T. (1983) The relationship of regional cerebral blood flow, blood volume, and oxygen metabolism in patients with carotid occlusions: evaluation of perfusion reserve. *J. Cereb. Blood Flow Metab.* Suppl. 1: 590–591.

Henriksen, L. (1983) Asymmetrical cerebral blood flow in hemiparkinsonian patients. Tomography of inhaled Xe-133 before and after Levodopa treatment. In: A. Hartmann and S. Hoyer (Eds.), *Cerebral Blood Flow and Metabolism Measurements*. Springer Verlag, Berlin, in press.

Hill, T. C., Homan, B. L., Lovett, R., O'Leary, D. H., Front, D., Magistretti, P., Zimmerman, R. E., Moore, S., Clouse, M. E., Wu, J. L., Lin, T. H. and Baldwin, R. M. (1982) Initial experience with SPECT (Single-Photon Emission Computerized Tomography) of the brain using N-isopropyl I-123 p-iodoamphetamine: concise communication. *J. Nucl. Med.*, 23: 191–195.

Lassen, N. A., Ingvar, D. H. and Skinhøj, E. (1978) Brain function and blood flow. *Sci. Amer.*, 239: 62–71.

Lassen, N. A., Henriksen, L. and Paulson, O. B. (1981) Regional cerebral blood flow in stroke by Xenon-133 inhalation and emission tomography. *Stroke*, 12: 384–388.

Lassen, N. A., Henriksen, L., Holm, S., Barry, D. I., Paulson, O. B., Vorstrup, S., Poncin-Lafitte, M., Moretti, J. L., Askienazy, S. and Raynaud, C. (1983) Cerebral blood-flow tomography: Xenon-133 compared with isopropyl-amphetamine-iodine-123: concise communication. *J. Nucl. Med.*, 24: 17–21.

Lou, H. C., Henriksen, L. and Bruhn, P. (1984) Focal cerebral hypoperfusion in children with dysphasia and/or attention deficit disorder. *Arch. Neurol.*, 41: 825–829.

Stokely, E. M., Sveinsdottir, E., Lassen, N. A. and Rommer, P. (1980) A single photon dynamic computer-assisted tomograph (DCAT) for imaging brain function in multiple cross-sections. *J. Comput. Assist. Tomogr.*, 4: 230–240.

Vorstrup, S., Hemmingsen, R., Henriksen, L., Lindewald, H., Engell, H. C. and Lassen, N. A. (1983) Regional cerebral blood flow in patients with transient ischemic attacks studied by Xenon-133 inhalation and emission tomography. *Stroke*, 14: 6: 903–910.

Winchell, H. S., Baldwin, R. M. and Lin, T. H. (1980a) Development of I-123-labelled amines for brain studies: Localization of I-123 iodophenylalkylamines in rat brain. *J. Nucl. Med.*, 21: 940–946.

Winchell, H. S., Horst, W. D. and Braun, L. (1980b) N-isopropyl-(123-I)p-iodoamphetamine: Single-pass brain uptake and washout; binding to brain synaptosomes; and localization in dog and monkey brain. *J. Nucl. Med.*, 21: 947–952.

Brain Ischemia: Quantitative EEG and Imaging Techniques, Progress in Brain Research, Vol. 62, edited by
G. Pfurtscheller, E.J. Jonkman and F.H. Lopes da Silva
©1984 Elsevier Science Publishers B.V.

Positron Emission Tomography Study of Regional Glucose Metabolism in Cerebral Ischemia – Topographic and Kinetic Aspects

G. PAWLIK, K. WIENHARD, K. HERHOLZ, R. WAGNER and W. -D. HEISS

Max-Planck-Institut für Neurologische Forschung, Ostmerheimer Str. 200, D-5000 Köln 91 (FRG)

INTRODUCTION

Since the development of positron emission tomography (PET) and appropriate kinetic tracer methods for non-invasive studies of local cerebral metabolism in humans (Phelps et al., 1979; Reivich et al., 1979), distant effects of brain infarcts on glucose consumption or oxygen uptake were repeatedly observed in regions appearing anatomically intact in X-ray computed tomography (XCT) (Kuhl et al., 1980; Baron et al., 1981; Lenzi et al., 1981; Metter et al., 1981; Dichiro et al., 1982; Heiss et al., 1983). As to remote deactivation, a number of explanations have been suggested, but the controversy remains whether this effect requires a large anatomical lesion (Baron et al., 1981; Lenzi et al., 1981) or a severe neurologic deficit, e.g. hemiplegia or hemianopia (Baron et al., 1981; Phelps et al., 1981; Heiss et al., 1982). Furthermore, results of animal experiments (Gjedde, 1982; Pardridge et al., 1982) and patient studies (Hawkins et al., 1981) indicate that the rate constants of the deoxyglucose model (Sokoloff et al., 1977) are significantly different in normal and ischemic brain tissue, but it is still unclear whether functional deactivation primarily affects transmembrane substrate transport (Heiss et al., 1982), hexose phosphorylation, or all kinetics of glucose use represented by those rate constants. This study thus intends to define the characteristics of an infarct – its size, localization, and the degree of the resulting neurologic deficit – associated with a decrease in glucose metabolism in non-infarcted brain regions, and to determine the differential effect of ischemia and functional deactivation on regional sets of rate constants.

METHODS

Patients

The study included 36 to 78-year-old patients with a recent ischemic stroke documented by XCT. Their neurologic deficits ranged from mild paresis or aphasia to severe disturbances including impairment of consciousness. All subjects rested in a reclining chair in a room with low ambient light and noise, eyes closed and ears unplugged. Approximately 15 min before the start of recordings, short catheters were placed into one cubital vein for injection and into a vein of the contralateral heated hand for blood sampling.

Procedure and equipment

(^{18}F)-2-fluoro-2-deoxyglucose (FDG) was synthesized according to a modification of the method of Ido et al. (1977). At the time of application, specific activity was 10–20 mCi per milligram. Each patient received a rapid intravenous bolus injection of approximately 5 mCi FDG in 5 ml sterile pyrogen-free normal saline solution. Blood was sampled and plasma glucose as well as FDG concentrations were determined as described by Phelps et al. (1979). Seven equally spaced parallel planes, from the canthomeatal line (CML) up to 81 mm above it, were simultaneously scanned with a four-ring positron camera (Scanditronix PC 384) at a spatial resolution of approximately 8 mm full width at half-maximum in 11 mm slices (Eriksson et al., 1982). Recordings were taken at consecutive intervals increasing from 1 to 5 min during a period of 40 min, starting at FDG injection.

Subsequently, another set of 7 images was obtained with the lowest section positioned at 7 or 20 mm above CML. This procedure yielded both dynamic and static information on tracer accumulation in virtually all major structures of the brain. Data from the tomographic device and from a sample changer used for plasma counting, as well as plasma glucose values, were stored in the memory of a VAX 11/780 (DEC) computer for later processing.

Data processing

Following decay correction, the activity distribution in the scanned slices was reconstructed using an edge-finding algorithm to determine the skull contour for attenuation correction (Bergström et al., 1982), a deconvolution for subtraction of the scattered radiation (Bergström et al., 1983), and a filtered backprojection algorithm. Between 10 and 30 regions of interest were outlined (Fig. 1) on each cross-sectional image representing either the infarcted area or distinct anatomical structures as demonstrated by the individual XCT. The model equation described by Sokoloff et al. (1977) was then fitted to the regional time-activity data. This model implies three compartments: FDG in plasma, precursor pool of free FDG in the tissue, and tissue FDG-6-phosphate. The time course of the total (^{18}F)-activity in the tissue, $C_i^*(t)$, and of the arterial plasma FDG concentration, $C_P^*(t)$, are related by rate constants describing the kinetics of FDG transport from plasma to brain tissue (k_1), from tissue back to plasma (k_2), and FDG phosphorylation in the tissue (k_3). From the measured concentration-time course of FDG in plasma and (^{18}F) in tissue, the best fitting set of

---

Fig. 1. Typical PET slice and topographical standard regions in a patient with an infarct of the right temporal pole and operculum (bottom view).

Fig. 2. Metabolic maps of a patient with an ischemic infarction in the left temporal opercular and insular cortex. Values on the reference color scale are in μmol/100 g/min. From left to right: horizontal (bottom view) and coronal (front view) section across the infarct, horizontal (bottom view) section across the cerebellum.

Fig. 3. Metabolic maps of a patient with an ischemic infarction in the right cerebellar hemisphere. Values on the color reference scale are in μmol/100 g/min. From left to right: horizontal and 45° angular section across the infarct, horizontal brain section at the level of the basal ganglia, all bottom view.

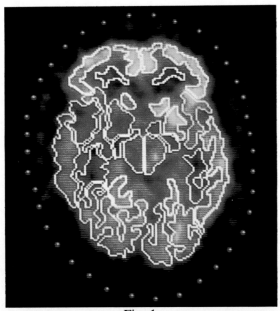

Fig. 1

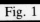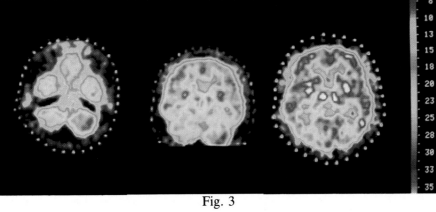

Fig. 2

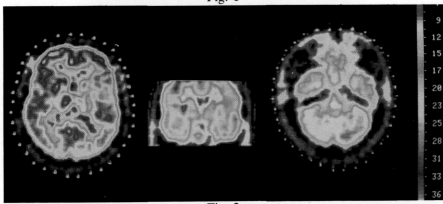

Fig. 3

parameters was determined using a fast non-linear fit algorithm. The regional cerebral metabolic rate for glucose (rCMRGlc) was estimated from these fitted rate constants and from plasma glucose concentration, C_p, according to rCMRGlc = $(C_p/LC) \times (k_1 \times k_3)/(k_2 + k_3)$, where a value of 0.42 (Huang et al., 1980) was used for the lumped constant, LC, describing differences in the behavior of FDG and glucose. In addition to this dynamic evaluation, static images recorded between 30 and 50 min after FDG injection were transformed into metabolic maps employing a model that incorporates the slow hydrolysis of FDG-6-PO_4 to FDG (Phelps et al., 1979). Slices could be reconstructed from the latter images at any thickness and angle of cut for optimal visualization of points of interest.

RESULTS AND DISCUSSION

Topographic relationships of infarcts and deactivated areas

Characteristic distant effects of focal ischemic lesions on selected non-ischemic brain regions in patients with a typical infarction in the supply territory of the middle cerebral artery are shown in Table I. Metabolic changes were most severe in the infarct proper, but glucose consumption also was significantly decreased in other ipsilateral cortical and subcortical gray matter structures, as well as in the contralateral cerebellum.

Detailed analysis of another series of stroke patients with infarcts in various brain regions provided some insight into the topographical nature of remote deactivation. Patients with cortical or subcortical lesions and a neurologic deficit consisting exclusively of neuropsychological disturbances exhibited hypometabolism not only in the infarcted, but also in related ipsilateral cortical areas, basal ganglia, thalamus, and contralateral cerebellum, suggesting ischemic disruption of connecting fiber systems in the subcortical white matter. Figure 2 gives an example of such an aphasic patient. In unilateral thalamic infarction, glucose consumption was slightly reduced both in the ipsilateral cerebral and cerebellar cortex, indicating lack of input to diverging thalamo-cortical projections and olivo-cerebellar circuits. A lesion in the cerebral peduncle

TABLE I

rCMRGlc (μmol/100 g/min) IN VARIOUS BRAIN REGIONS OF PATIENTS WITH AN ISCHEMIC STROKE

	n	rCMRGlc (μmol/100 g/min, mean ± standard deviation) ipsilateral	contralateral	Sign test p<
Infarction	17	8.2 ± 7.03	29.6 ± 11.84	0.00001
Frontal cortex	16	24.6 ± 10.49	30.0 ± 13.74	0.01
Temporal cortex	18	24.6 ± 7.89	31.5 ± 12.07	0.001
Parietal cortex	15	26.2 ± 9.27	31.9 ± 11.93	0.02
Occipital cortex	19	26.9 ± 10.68	33.2 ± 13.56	0.005
Thalamus	14	25.2 ± 7.36	31.9 ± 7.77	0.002
Striatum	14	25.6 ± 9.79	35.0 ± 11.72	0.001
Cerebellum	8	27.8 ± 9.65	21.7 ± 10.62	0.005

damaged the pyramidal tract and corticopontine fibers, and only the contralateral cerebellum was deactivated. However, in patients with a severe impairment of motor function from an ischemic brainstem lesion leaving the corticopontine projections intact, no decrease in cerebellar glucose metabolism was found. Conversely, unilateral cerebellar infarction, as demonstrated in Fig. 3, caused no focal remote deactivation. From these examples it may be concluded that distant effects on cerebral glucose metabolism are brought about primarily by intracerebral deafferentation, and not by infarct size per se or by severe neurologic disturbances.

Regional kinetics of glucose metabolism in ischemic and deactivated tissue

As first described by Hawkins et al. (1981), indiscriminate use of average rate constants obtained in young healthy adults often results in false low metabolic values, particularly in ischemic tissue. The physiological basis of this phenomenon becomes obvious when dynamic data on regional tracer accumulation are available. Under pathological conditions leading to changes in enzyme kinetics and transport mechanisms, time-activity curves assume characteristic shapes that are quite different from the normal state (Fig. 4). Therefore, it may be expected that metabolic rates based on individually fitted rate constants approximate the unknown true value more closely, although another possible source of errors, the lumped constant (LC), cannot be determined regionally in man because this would require knowledge of the regional

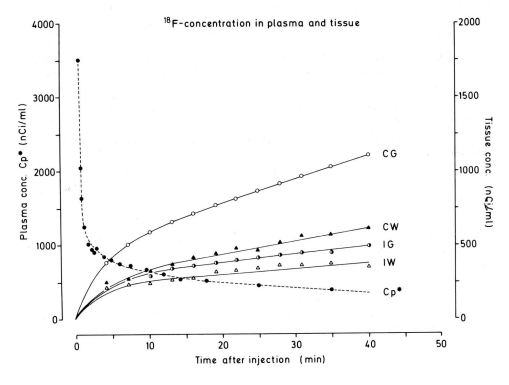

Fig. 4. Measured (^{18}F)-activity and corresponding fitted curves in plasma (C_p*), infarcted gray (IG) and white (IW) matter, and in the respective contralateral gray (CG) and white (CW) matter regions of a stroke patient, as a function of time after FDG injection.

258

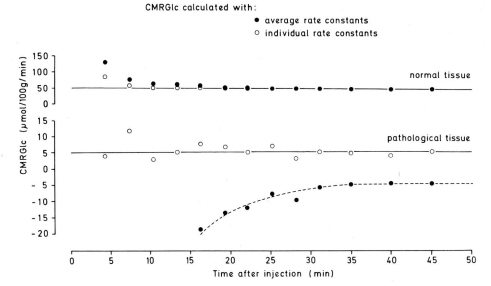

Fig. 5. Cerebral metabolic rate for glucose (CMRGlc) as computed with the Sokoloff equation from regional activity at various points in time after FDG injection, using either individually fitted or standard average rate constants determined in healthy young adults. Data were obtained from a normal (upper graph) and infarcted (lower graph) cortex region of a typical stroke patient.

brain glucose concentration (Crane et al., 1983). Despite the fact that the operational equation of the Sokoloff model tends to minimize the influence of rate constants on the resulting metabolic value, it is not entirely insensitive to violations of the basic assumptions of the model as demonstrated in Fig. 5; in normal tissue, metabolic rates computed from regional tracer activity after 20–30 min and standard rate constants approach the values obtained by the dynamic fit procedure, while in infarcted tissue even negative values may be found, no matter how long regional activity is recorded.

Correction for biased metabolic rates, however, is not the only advantage of following the time course of tracer uptake. Individually determined rate constants may yield additional insight into the mechanisms primarily affected in tissue with decreased glucose metabolism: transport, phosphorylation, or both. In the present series of stroke patients, an average reduction within the infarcted area of k_1 by 36%, and of k_3 by 38%, as compared to the respective contralateral region, was found, while k_2 showed only a slight decrease. In deactivated regions, k_2 was similar to the value in ischemic and normal tissue, but k_1 was reduced by 11%, and k_3 by 21% of the respective individual control value. In deactivated cerebellum, an even larger decrease was observed for k_1 (by 22%) and k_3 (by 32%). These results suggest that changes in the rate of phosphorylation in general are not exactly paralleled by changes in bidirectional transmembrane transport. Differences in the individual constellation of rate constants may even be of some prognostic value. Figure 6 shows predominant reduction of k_3 in 44 deactivated regions, out of a total of 101 brain regions in a stroke patient during the early stage of the disease; the outcome was poor. Figure 7, in contrast, demonstrates a rather proportional decrease of k_1 and k_3 in deactivated brain regions of a patient who later recovered almost fully from his ischemic stroke.

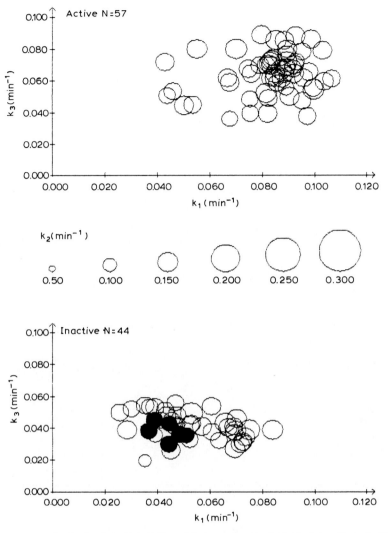

Fig. 6. Rate constants k_1, k_2, k_3 of the Sokoloff model, determined by individual data fitting in 101 distinct brain regions of a stroke patient with poor prognosis. k_2 is indicated by circle size, infarcted regions are represented by full black circles. Rate constants in normal (upper graph) and deactivated tissue (lower graph) are clearly separated.

CONCLUSIONS

Deafferentation by ischemic disruption of connecting fiber tracts seems to be the major cause of deactivation of anatomically intact remote brain regions in stroke. Dynamic recording can substantially improve the reliability of metabolic measurements in both infarcted and deactivated areas. Regional rate constants provide a sound basis for multivariate analyses of the kinetics of cerebral glucose metabolism.

260

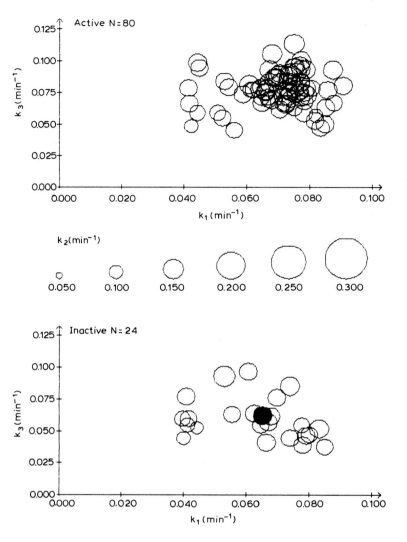

Fig. 7. Rate constants k_1, k_2, k_3 of the Sokoloff model, determined by individual data fitting in 104 distinct brain regions of a stroke patient with good prognosis. k_2 is indicated by circle size, the infarcted region is represented by a full black circle. Rate constants in normal (upper graph) and deactivated tissue (lower graph) are poorly separated.

SUMMARY

Regional metabolic rates for glucose and kinetics of (^{18}F)-2-fluoro-2-deoxy-D-glucose were determined in patients with brain infarcts of variable size and localization as documented by X-ray computed tomography, using both dynamic and static positron emission tomography with a high-resolution, 7-slice positron camera. Patients with large typical infarctions in the supply territory of either middle cerebral artery exhibited decreased glucose consumption not only within the morphological lesion but also, to a lesser degree, in other ipsilateral cortical and subcortical gray matter structures as well as in the contralateral cerebellum. Detailed topographical analysis of glucose metabolism in another group of patients with single small infarcts in various brain regions and neurologic deficits ranging from mild neuropsychological disturbances to hemiplegia, revealed that remote deactivation is caused primarily by deafferentation, i.e. by lack of excitatory input due to ischemic destruction of activating neuronal systems or disruption of connecting fiber tracts. Although the Sokoloff model is rather insensitive to changes in local rate constants, more reliable metabolic rates were obtained particularly in structurally or functionally abnormal tissue, when calculations were based on individual kinetic constants determined by fitting the operational equation to sequentially sampled regional activity data. Results indicate a differential effect on rate constants of ischemia and functional deactivation: while transport out of the tissue was hardly affected, phosphorylation usually showed a marked decrease and transport to the tissue was variable. Certain kinetic patterns appear to be characteristic of postischemic functional outcome.

REFERENCES

Baron, J. C., Bousser, M. G., Comar, D., Duquesnoy, N., Sastre, J. and Castaigne, P. (1981) Crossed cerebellar diaschisis: A remote functional depression secondary to supratentorial infarction in man. *J. Cereb. Blood Flow Metab.*, 1, Suppl. 1: S500–S501.

Bergström, M., Litton, J. Eriksson, L., Bohm, C. and Blomqvist, G. (1982) Determination of object contour from projections for attenuation correction in cranial positron emission tomography. *J. Comput. Assist. Tomogr.*, 6: 365–372.

Bergström, M., Eriksson, L., Bohm, C., Blomqvist, G. and Litton, J. (1983) Correction for scattered radiation in a ring detector positron camera by integral transformation of the projections. *J. Comput. Assist. Tomogr.*, 7: 42–50.

Crane, P. D., Pardridge, W. M., Braun, L. D. and Oldendorf, W. H. (1983) Kinetics of transport and phosphorylation of 2-fluoro-2-deoxy-D-glucose in rat brain. *J. Neurochem.*, 40: 160–167.

DiChiro, G., Paz, de la R. L., Brooks, R. A., Sokoloff, L., Kornbluth, P. L., Smith, B. H., Patronas, N. J., Kufta, C. V., Kessler, R. M., Johnston, G. S., Manning, R. G. and Wolf, A. P. (1982) Glucose utilization of cerebral gliomas measured by (^{18}F)fluorodeoxyglucose and positron emission tomography. *Neurology*, 32: 1323–1329.

Eriksson, L., Bohm, C., Kesselberg, M., Blomqvist, G., Litton, J., Widen, L., Bergström, M., Ericson, K. and Greitz, T. (1982) A four ring camera system for emission tomography of the brain. *IEEE Trans. Nucl. Sci.*, NS-29: 539–543.

Gjedde, A. (1982) Calculation of cerebral glucose phosphorylation from brain uptake of glucose analogs in vivo: A re-examination. *Brain Res. Rev.*, 4: 237–274.

Hawkins, R. A., Phelps, M. E., Huang, S. -C. and Kuhl, D. E. (1981) Effect of ischemia on quantification of local cerebral glucose metabolic rate in man. *J. Cereb. Blood Flow Metab.*, 1: 37–51.

Heiss, W. -D., Vyska, K., Kloster, G., Traupe, H., Freundlieb, C., Hoeck, A., Feinendegen, L. E. and Stoecklin, G. (1982) Demonstration of decreased functional activity of visual cortex by (^{11}C) methylglucose and positron emission tomography. *Neuroradiology*, 23: 45–47.

Heiss, W. -D., Ilsen, H. W., Wagner, R., Pawlik, G. and Wienhard, K. (1983) Remote functional depression of glucose metabolism in stroke and its alteration by activating drugs. In W. -D. Heiss and M. E. Phelps (Eds.), *Positron Emission Tomography of the Brain*, Springer-Verlag, Berlin–Heidelberg–New York, pp. 162–168.

Huang, S. -C., Phelps, M. E., Hoffman, E. J., Sideris, K., Selin, C. J. and Kuhl, D. E. (1980) Non-invasive determination of local cerebral metabolic rate of glucose in man. *Amer. J. Physiol.*, 238: E69–E82.

Ido, T., Wan, C. N., Fowler, J. S. and Wolf, A. P. (1977) Fluorination with F2, a convenient synthesis of 2-deoxy-2-fluoro-D-glucose. *J. Org. Chem.*, 42: 2341–2342.

Kuhl, D. E., Phelps, M. E., Kowell, A. P., Metter, E. J., Selin, C. J. and Winter, J. (1980) Effects of stroke on local cerebral metabolism and perfusion: Mapping by emission computed tomography of ^{18}FDG and ^{13}N$_3$. *Ann. Neurol.*, 8: 47–60.

262

Lenzi, G. L., Frackowiak, R. S. and Jones, T. (1981) Regional cerebral blood flow (CBF), oxygen utilization (CMRO$_2$), and oxygen extraction ratio (OER) in acute hemispheric stroke. *J. Cereb. Blood Flow Metab.*, 1 Suppl. 1: S504–S505.

Metter, E. J., Wasterlain, C. G., Kuhl, D. E., Hanson, W. R. and Phelps, M. E. (1981) [18]FDG-positron emission computed tomography: A study of aphasia. *Ann Neurol.*, 10: 173–183.

Pardridge, W. M., Crane, P. D., Mietus, L. J. and Oldendorf, W. H. (1982) Nomogram for 2-deoxyglucose lumped constant for rat brain cortex. *J. Cereb. Blood Flow Metab.*, 2: 197–202.

Phelps, M. E., Huang, S. -C., Hoffman, E. J., Selin, C. J., Sokoloff, L. and Kuhl, D. E. (1979) Tomographic measurement of local cerebral glucose metabolic rate in humans with (F-18)2-fluoro-2-deoxy-D-glucose: Validation of method. *Ann. Neurol.*, 6: 371–388.

Phelps, M. E., Mazziotta, J. C., Kuhl, D. E., Nuwer, M., Packwood, J., Metter, J. and Engel, Jr. J., (1981) Tomographic mapping of human cerebral metabolism: Visual stimulation and deprivation. *Neurology*, 31: 517–529.

Reivich, M., Kuhl, D., Wolf, A., Greenberg, J., Phelps, M. E., Ido, T., Casella, V., Fowler, J., Hoffman, E., Alavi, A., Som, P. and Sokoloff, L. (1979) The (^{18}F)fluorodeoxyglucose method for the measurement of local cerebral glucose utilization in man. *Circulat. Res.*, 44: 127–137.

Sokoloff, L., Reivich, M., Kennedy, C., Des Rosiers, M. H., Patlak, C. S., Pettigrew, K. D., Sakurada, O. and Shinohara, M. (1977) The (^{14}C)-deoxyglucose method for the measurement of local cerebral glucose utilization: Theory, procedure, and normal values in the conscious and anesthetized albino rat. *J. Neurochem.*, 28: 897–916.

*Brain Ischemia: Quantitative EEG and Imaging Techniques, Progress in Brain Research, Vol. 62, edited by
G. Pfurtscheller, E.J. Jonkman and F.H. Lopes da Silva
©1984 Elsevier Science Publishers B.V.*

Simultaneous Cerebral Glucography with Positron Emission Tomography and Topographic Electroencephalography

M.S. BUCHSBAUM[1], R. KESSLER[2], A. KING[3], J. JOHNSON[3] and J. CAPPELLETTI[3]

[1] *Department of Psychiatry, University of California, Irvine, CA 92717, [2]Department of Nuclear Medicine,
NIH Clinical Center, Bethesda, MD 20205 and [3]Section of Clinical Psychophysiology, NIMH, Bethesda,
MD 20205 (U.S.A.)*

INTRODUCTION

In a normal subject resting with his eyes closed, a 10 c/sec electroencephalographic (EEG) pattern appears over the posterior parietal and occipital scalp. This pattern, the alpha rhythm, is blocked when the subject opens his eyes, supporting a functional relationship to the visual areas in the cortex underneath these scalp areas. In general, with alerting and mental activity, the slower rhythms of the brain (alpha and the still slower theta and delta activity) are replaced by faster beta activity (12–20 c/sec). Since local functional activity of the brain is closely tied to the use of glucose, the major energy source of the brain (Sokoloff, 1981), one might expect relationships between EEG activity and local cerebral glucose use.

This relationship has been studied indirectly taking advantage of the close coupling of blood flow to glucose use (Sokoloff, 1981). Correlations between EEG frequency and cerebral oxygen uptake as well as blood flow assessed by the xenon clearance technique have been reported (Ingvar et al., 1976; Tolonen and Sulg, 1981). Electrical impedance rheoencephalography (REG) revealed high alpha and decreased blood flow (Jacquy et al., 1980). In these studies, individuals rested with their eyes closed without a specific mental task. In this state, considerable individual differences are seen with some individuals showing almost continuous alpha and others little or none: the correlations observed depend on this variation. These three studies did not actually assess the region by region relationships between blood flow and EEG as only a single EEG lead was recorded. Jacquy (1980) assessed left parietal temporal EEG ($T_5–P_z$) and used $T_3 T_4$ input and $T_5 T_6$ pickup for REG.

In our study we have directly measured local cerebral glucose use by positron emission tomography (PET) with simultaneous recording of EEG from 16 electrodes spaced over the left hemisphere to maximize spatial resolution.

[263]

METHODS

PET technique

The subjects were four male and two female (mean age 26) volunteers. All were right-handed and selected as controls for PET studies reported elsewhere (Buchsbaum et al., 1982b). Subjects were seated slightly reclining in an acoustically treated darkened room. Intravenous lines for injection of the radioisotope and withdrawal of blood samples were placed well in advance of the procedure and subjects were allowed to relax. At 5–10 min intervals before the 2-deoxyglucose ^{18}F injection, room lights were extinguished and subjects were asked to close their eyes and keep them closed throughout the 30–40 min post-injection period. Blood sampling, time-keeping and other activities were done by the light of a small low intensity lamp and flashlight; subjects were monitored for eye closure. Blood samples for ^{18}F-2DG and glucose were withdrawn from the left arm, which was warmed to arteriolize the venous blood; 1.5 cc samples were made at 15-sec intervals for the next 10 min and then at 10-min intervals until after the last slice was scanned. Thirty-five minutes after injection subjects were transferred to the scanner; seven to eight scans parallel to the canthomeatal (CM) line from +90 to +15 mm in 12–15 mm increments were done as quietly as possible with lights off in the scanner area. The slices were reconstructed (Buchs-

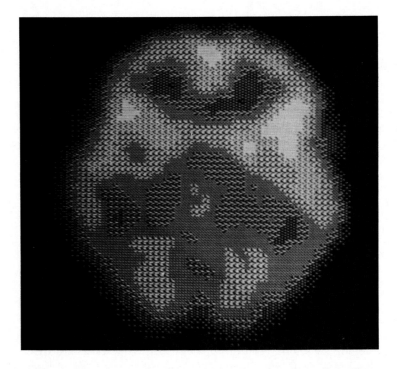

Fig. 1. Typical Positron Emission Tomography scan in normal volunteer resting with his eyes closed. A horizontal slice image is shown at about 45 mm above the canthomeatal line. The metabolic rate of glucose is represented by the gray scale with white being the highest and black the lowest. This subject shows the typical pattern of a high rate of glucose metabolism in the frontal areas (top) and low rate in the visual regions (bottom).

baum et al., 1982b) and raw counts of each PET image were transformed into glucose use in micromoles glucose per 100 g brain tissue per min (Buchsbaum et al., 1983). The mid-scan time for each slice was used as the decapitation time in the equation. Fig. 1 shows a typical PET scan.

EEG technique

EEG was recorded from 16 channels on the left hemisphere including all 10–20 system sites, midline F_z, P_z, C_z and O_z and four additional posterior locations (Buchsbaum et al., 1982c). Ten seconds epochs at 1-min intervals were digitized online at 102.4 Hz, low frequency subharmonics removed by autoregressive filter (Coppola, 1979), and epochs following [18]F-2DG injection were selected generally occurring (2–8 min post-injection) during the period of most rapid FDG uptake.

A standard Fast Fourier Transform was applied (Buchsbaum et al., 1982a) and power spectrum estimates computed at 0.1 Hz steps, 10 adjacent steps summed to yield 1 Hz resolution, and final estimates expressed as magnitude in microvolts (square root of power). Results from 1–20 Hz are shown in Fig. 2. Delta was 2–5 Hz, alpha was 8–12 Hz and beta 13–20 Hz for statistical summary; a mean amplitude alpha map is displayed in Fig. 3A.

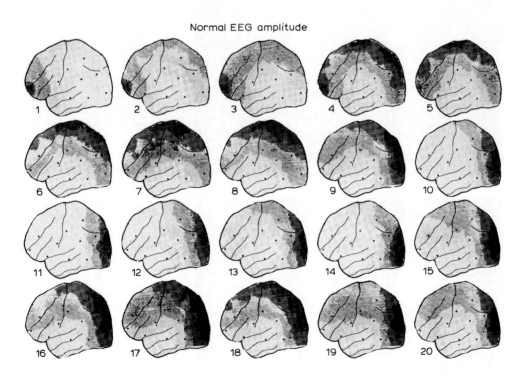

Fig. 2. Average topographic EEG amplitude maps in 16 normal volunteers. For each frequency (1–20 Hz) a map is presented and independently scaled into nine shades of gray so that the entire range is used. This series of maps demonstrates the shift of maximal brain electrical activity from the frontal regions (1–4 Hz) to the occipital regions (9–20 Hz).

A

B

C

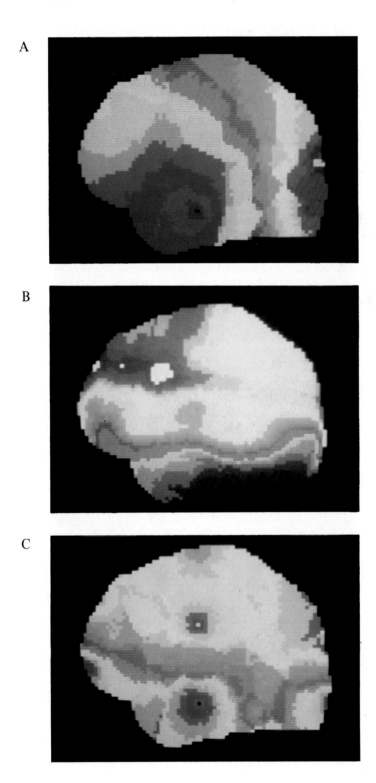

Fig. 3A. Mean EEG amplitude 8–12 Hz in 16 normal subjects. Scale in spectral sequence brown (highest), orange, yellow, green, blue, indigo and violet (lowest). B. Metabolic rate of glucose in a normal subject with brown highest and violet lowest. C. Correlation coefficients between alpha EEG amplitude and metabolic rate of glucose. Brown is positive and violet negative and significant. Note negative correlation at occiput. This indicates that individuals with low rates of occipital glucose metabolism had relatively high alpha and individuals with high occipital glucose metabolism had low amplitude alpha.

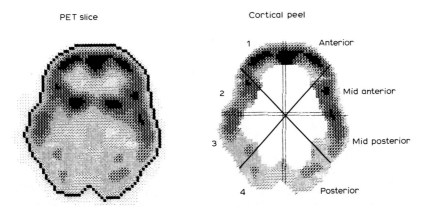

Fig. 4. Technique for measurement of regional glucose. PET image is outlined by boundary-finding algorithm (left) and vertical and horizontal meridians fitted by least squares. Next, a radial scan from their intersection defines a 2.3 cm thick peel which is divided into four sectors in each hemisphere, termed L1, L2, L3, and L4 for the left and R1, R2, R3 and R4 for the right. Typical localization of high glucose use cortical gray within this zone is seen (right). PET scan is presented as a 9-level dot-density gray scale.

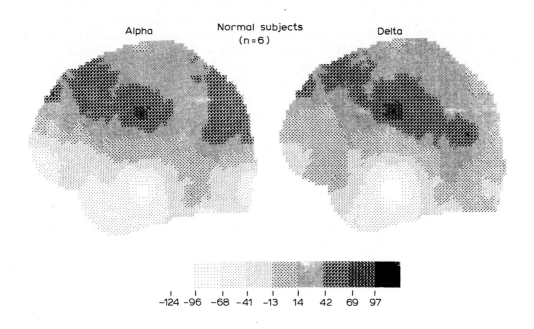

Fig. 5. Correlation coefficients between metabolic rate of glucose and alpha (see also Fig. 3C) and delta EEG amplitude respectively, calculated for each pixel on the lateral brain view. Scale shows product moment correlation coefficient z-transformed times 100. Note significant negative correlation at occiput for alpha rhythm. Both delta and alpha have negative correlation over temporal lobe.

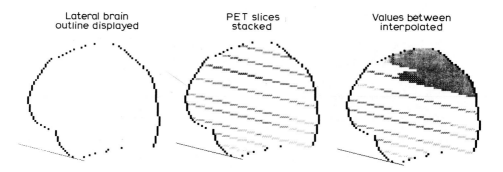

Fig. 6. Lateral cortex surface views are reconstructed on a brain lateral outline (left). Hemisphere cortical peels (see Fig. 3) are placed on the brain lateral outline (center) and values are interpolated between them.

Topographic mapping

The transverse PET glucose images were reconstructed into a lateral cortical equal area projection developed for EEG topographic mapping (Buchsbaum et al., 1984). First, each PET slice had a 2.5 cm (8 pixel) cortical strip peeled off the left hemisphere (Fig. 4) as described elsewhere (Buchsbaum et al., 1982a). Values were averaged across an 8-pixel depth. The proportional height of the slice from the CM line was calculated and the strip positioned and scaled anteroposteriorly on the lateral brain outline. Values between strips were interpolated forming a solid lateral view (Fig. 5). From the known EEG coordinate positions on this view, a glucose value was thus obtained for the cortex approximately underlying each of the 16 EEG leads; a glucose map was calculated from these values (Fig. 3B).

Statistical approach

As individual differences in mean slice glucose were greater than within slice differences, we also normalized each subject's glucose values. This was done by calculating the subjects mean and S.D. across the 16 positions and then expressing each value as the [absolute value/mean/S.D.]. Correlations were calculated between EEG power for the four frequency bands and the normalized glucose values, for $p < 0.05$, $r > 0.75$, 2-tailed. A negative association between beta amplitude and glucose use was observed, reaching statistical significance in the temporal lead ($r = 0.871$).

RESULTS AND CONCLUSIONS

A negative correlation between alpha and normalized glucose was observed at the occiput (O_z, $r = -0.76$) and temporal cortex ($r = -0.828$) positive correlations were seen in central cortex (C_3, $r = 0.805$) (Figs. 3C, 5). The relationship of the work of the brain to spontaneous EEG rhythms has previously been approached through examination of EEG change during behavioral tasks or through spatially limited blood flow studies. Here, the first direct and simultaneous measurement of glucose use and EEG revealed that individuals who clearly show the occipital alpha pattern at rest associated with no visual stimulation show regional lows in glucose use. The correlation was extremely similar to that reported by Jacquy ($r = -0.75$ in his report as in ours) despite his recording the REG from posterior but not occipital leads. An association between increased slow EEG (mainly delta) and low blood flow was noted by Ingvar et al. (1976) and Tolonen and Sulg (1981), although the latter findings were limited to patients' damaged hemispheres. Our finding that both positive and negative correlations appear in different cortical areas suggests that the physiological interpretation of these rhythms may differ from area to area. The harmlessness and repeatability and low cost of EEG topography give it some advantages over the high cost of PET or isotopic regional blood flow techniques. Extended studies will be necessary to further define regional relationships; simultaneous PET and EEG studies may be able to better characterize metabolic information available in scalp electrical activity.

SUMMARY

Simultaneous cerebral glucography with positron emission tomography and topographic quantitative electroencephalography was carried out in six normal volunteers. The presence of resting occipital alpha activity was associated with relatively low glucose use consistent with the phenomenon of alpha blocking with visual input. Higher EEG amplitude was associated with higher glucose use in some posterior and central regions.

REFERENCES

Buchsbaum, M.S., Cappelletti, J., Ball, R., Hazlett, E., King, A.C., Johnson, J., Wu, J., DeLisi, L.E., Holcomb, H.H., Zimmerman, S.D. and Kessler, R. (1984) PET image measurement in schizophrenia and affective disorders. *Ann. Neurol.*, 15 (Suppl.): S157–S165.
Buchsbaum, M.S., Cappelletti, J., Coppola, R., Regal, F., King, A.C. and van Kammen, D.P. (1982a) New methods to determine the CNS effects of antigeriatric compounds: EEG topography and glucose use. *Drug Devel. Res.*, 2: 489–496.
Buchsbaum, M.S., Holcomb, H.H., Johnson, J., King, A.C. and Kessler, R. (1983) Cerebral metabolic consequences of electrical cutaneous stimulation in normal individuals. *Hum. Neurobiol.*, 2: 35–38.
Buchsbaum, M.S., Ingvar, D.H., Kessler, R., Waters, R.N., Cappelletti, J., van Kammen, D.P., King, A.C., Johnson, J., Manning, R.G., Flynn, R.W., Mann, L.S., Bunney Jr., W.E. and Sokoloff, L. (1982b) Cerebral glucography with positron tomography. *Arc. gen. Psychiat.*, 39: 251–259.
Buchsbaum, M.S., Rigal, R., Coppola, R., Cappelletti, J., King, C. and Johnson, J. (1982c) A new system for gray-level surface distribution maps of electrical activity. *Electroenceph. clin. Neurophysiol.*, 53: 237–242.
Coppola, R. (1979) Isolating low frequency activity in EEG spectrum analysis. *Electroenceph. clin. Neurophysiol.*, 46: 224–226.
Ingvar, D.H., Sjolund, B. and Ardo, A. (1976) Correlation between dominant EEG frequency cerebral oxygen uptake and blood flow. *Electroenceph. clin. Neurophysiol.*, 41: 268–276.
Jacquy, J., Charles, P., Piraux, A. and Noel, G. (1980) Relationship between the electroencephalogram and the rheoencephalogram in the normal young adult. *Neuropsychobiology*, 6: 341–348.
Sokoloff, L. (1981) Relationships among local functional activity, energy metabolism, and blood flow in the central nervous system. *Fed. Proc.*, 40: 2311–2316.
Tolonen, U. and Sulg, I.A. (1981) Comparison of quantitative EEG parameters from four different analysis techniques in evaluation of relationships between EEG and CBF in brain infarction. *Electroenceph. clin. Neurophysiol.*, 51: 177–185.

Brain Ischemia: Quantitative EEG and Imaging Techniques, Progress in Brain Research, Vol. 62, edited by
G. Pfurtscheller, E.J. Jonkman and F.H. Lopes da Silva
©1984 Elsevier Science Publishers B.V.

Topographic Electroencephalographic Study of Ischemic Cerebrovascular Disease

KEN NAGATA[1], KAZUTA YUNOKI[2], GORO ARAKI[2], MASAHIRO MIZUKAMI[2] and
AKIO HYODO[2]

[1]*Department of Neurology, University of Colorado, Health Science Center, B-182, 4200 East Ninth Avenue,
Denver CO. 80220 (U.S.A.) and [2]Department of Neurology and Neurosurgery, Institute of Brain and Blood
Vessels, Mihara Memorial Hospital, 366 Oota-Machi, Isesaki, Gunma (Japan)*

INTRODUCTION

Quantitative and topographical representation of the electrical activities of the brain has been of great interest in clinical neurophysiology. The first topographical description of the human electroencephalogram was by Adrian and Yamagiwa (1935), who used a 4-channel polygraph to investigate the focus of the alpha rhythm. Walter and Shipton (1951) developed a 22-channel toposcope system that utilized brilliance-controlled tubes. Lehmann (1971) introduced a multichannel topography of the alpha field using a general-purpose computer with a 48-channel recording system. The results were shown in a semischematic map with equipotential contour lines sketched by hand. These earlier topographical display systems required many recording electrodes and considerable technical material.

Multichannel power spectral analysis was shown to be relevant for the localization of supratentorial lesions (Gotman et al., 1973), and polygons designating a ratio of slow to fast frequency wave components were topographically displayed in the canonogram (Gotman et al., 1975). Matsuoka et al. (1978) introduced a topographical display of the slow wave components with equipotential contour lines drawn by computer. They used the square root of the average power spectra as an equivalent potential over the given frequency band and displayed a map by interpolating the values between the scalp electrodes. Duffy et al. (1979) applied a color image of the EEG and evoked potential data to the study of dyslexic children.

The introduction of computer technology into clinical neurophysiology enabled scientists to make these topographical images of the EEG data which had been the method of display wished for by the first generation of EEG research workers. However, Petsche (1976) called a warning against drawing too many conclusions from the topographical representation of the EEG data, since there are considerable differences between the EEG derived from the scalp electrodes and the cortical electrical activities.

From the early days, electroencephalography had been employed in the studies of cerebrovascular disease as a parameter reflecting cerebral function, contrasting with the neuroradiological knowledge demonstrating anatomical lesions of the brain (Roseman et al., 1952; Birchfield et al., 1959). With the advancement of regional cerebral blood flow (rCBF) measurements, comparative studies were undertaken using EEG and rCBF measurements to clarify the pathophysiological relationship between cerebral function and circulation in brain ischemia (Obrist et al., 1963;

[271]

Ingvar, 1967; Mosmans et al., 1973). Computerized tomography (CT) soon made it possible to visualize ischemic lesions, and consequently less attention was paid to the clinical value of the EEG in cerebrovascular disease. In conventional reading of the EEG, one had to make a mental spatial image of the relationship between a large number of continuous wave forms. Thus the information derived from the conventional reading of the EEG was neither objective nor quantitative in comparison to CT and rCBF studies. Modern quantitative EEG analyses with computer, however, have been studied and compared with CT and rCBF measurements, and are now considered beneficial in correcting the previous problems in the conventional reading of the EEG (Ingvar et al., 1976; Tolonen and Sulg, 1981).

Our previous study (Nagata et al., 1982) presented a method of topographical representation of the EEG data: computed mapping of EEG (CME). We have shown that the CME provides additional useful information when correlated with CT and rCBF studies in ischemic cerebrovascular disease. The present study was designed to investigate the relationship between cerebral function, circulation, and anatomical lesions in ischemic cerebrovascular disease using CME, rCBF measurements, CT, cerebral angiography, and ultrasonic quantitative flow measurements (UQFM). Three different groups of patients were studied: (1) From the topographical point of view, we studied the localization of the lesions in patients with an aphasic syndrome due to an occlusive lesion in the left middle cerebral artery. (2) To investigate the pathophysiological mechanisms of a transient ischemic attack (TIA), we analyzed patients with TIAs in the territory of the internal carotid artery, with special reference to the reversibility of cerebral function. (3) To make an objective and non-invasive assessment of patients who underwent revascularization surgery, the clinical course was monitored by means of CME, rCBF measurements and UQFM.

SUBJECTS

The present study was based on 32 patients out of more than 2000 stroke patients who underwent an examination of topographic EEG using CME at the Institute of Brain and Blood Vessels, Mihara Memorial Hospital.

Twelve patients had an aphasic syndrome due to an occlusive lesion in the left middle cerebral artery. All of them were right-handed and their mean age was 60.6 years. They were admitted to the hospital within 2 weeks of onset and underwent cerebral angiography, CT, CME and rCBF measurements by the ^{133}Xe intra-arterial method. The evaluation of the aphasic syndrome was performed when the patients were thought to be alert.

Ten patients had transient ischemic attacks (TIAs) limited to the internal carotid system. Their mean age was 50.5 years. All of them underwent cerebral angiography, CT, CME and rCBF measurements by the ^{133}Xe intra-arterial method, from 6 h to 54 days after the last attack. They had been put on anti-platelet aggregation therapy and none of them developed further TIAs or completed strokes.

Ten patients underwent revascularization surgery (EC/IC bypass operation) for their occlusive cerebrovascular lesions. Their mean age was 53.8 years. The postoperative course was monitored using cerebral angiography, CT, CME and rCBF measurements by the ^{133}Xe inhalation method and UQFM. The bypassed arteries were all patent on the postoperative angiograms, and the postoperative clinical course was favorable in all patients.

METHODS

Computed mapping of EEG

The computed mapping of the EEG (CME) provided an equipotential topography of the EEG data by use of a computer. The system was designed according to the method of Ueno and Matsuoka (1976) and a detailed description was presented in our previous report (Nagata et al., 1982). The present system is based on three major functions: (1) the square root of the average power spectra was defined as an equivalent potential over the given frequency band; (2) interpolation was performed on the values between the scalp electrodes, and (3) the results were displayed in a schematic map in 11 different colors on color CRT as well as printed out in 11 characters.

The patients were examined lying on a bed in a relaxed state with eyes closed in a semi-darkened room. A referential derivation was used with the reference electrodes on both ear lobes or on the chin. EEGs were recorded from 16 scalp electrodes using the montage of the 10–20 method. A 17-channel EEG polygraph (1A56, San-ei Sokki) was used, which was connected to an online computer (CME-100 Japan System / Nissei Sangyo, modified 7T08 San-ei Sokki). The EEGs were checked to eliminate artifacts and eye movements on the polygraph during sampling epochs for the computation.

The EEG frequencies between 2.0 and 29.5 Hz were analyzed in this system and divided into six frequency bands: delta: 2.0–3.5 Hz, theta: 4.0–7.5 Hz, alpha-1: 8.0–9.5 Hz, alpha-2: 10.0–12.5 Hz, beta-1: 13.0–19.5 Hz, and beta-2: 20.0–29.5 Hz. Two-second EEG epochs were accumulated 60 times (120 sec) for the analyses. Fast Fourier transformation was used to calculate the power spectrum. The 10-20 system was rearranged onto a 25-point grid (5 points $\times$ 5 points). Using the EEGs recorded from the 16 scalp electrodes, the values of 16 points out of the 25-point grid were calculated; the values of the remaining 9 points were calculated from the average values of adjacent points. The values between the 25 points of the grid were interpolated with smooth contour lines, which were calculated from a combination of sinusoid curve and a convolution of a triangle. The calculated values were quantified into 11 different classes; the difference between two successive levels ranged from 0.5 to 2.0 μV. They were printed out in 11 characters by an online printer as well as displayed in 11 different colors on a color CRT. The calculated information was stored on small discs.

Neuroradiological examinations

The cerebral angiography was always performed on the internal carotid artery located on the side of the lesion and was occasionally performed on the opposite side as well. The collateral circulation was studied by four-vessel studies as indicated.

Regional cerebral blood flow was measured in patients with an aphasic syndrome and those with TIAs by the ^{133}Xe intra-arterial injection using a 16-channel multidetector system (Cerebrograph Meditronic) according to the initial slope index (ISI) method. The initial flow value was used: mCBF designating the mean value of all 16 channels, F designating the mean value of the left frontal 3 channels covering Broca's area, and T designating the mean value of the left temporal 3 channels covering Wernicke's area. The normal flow as measured with this system was (mean $\pm$

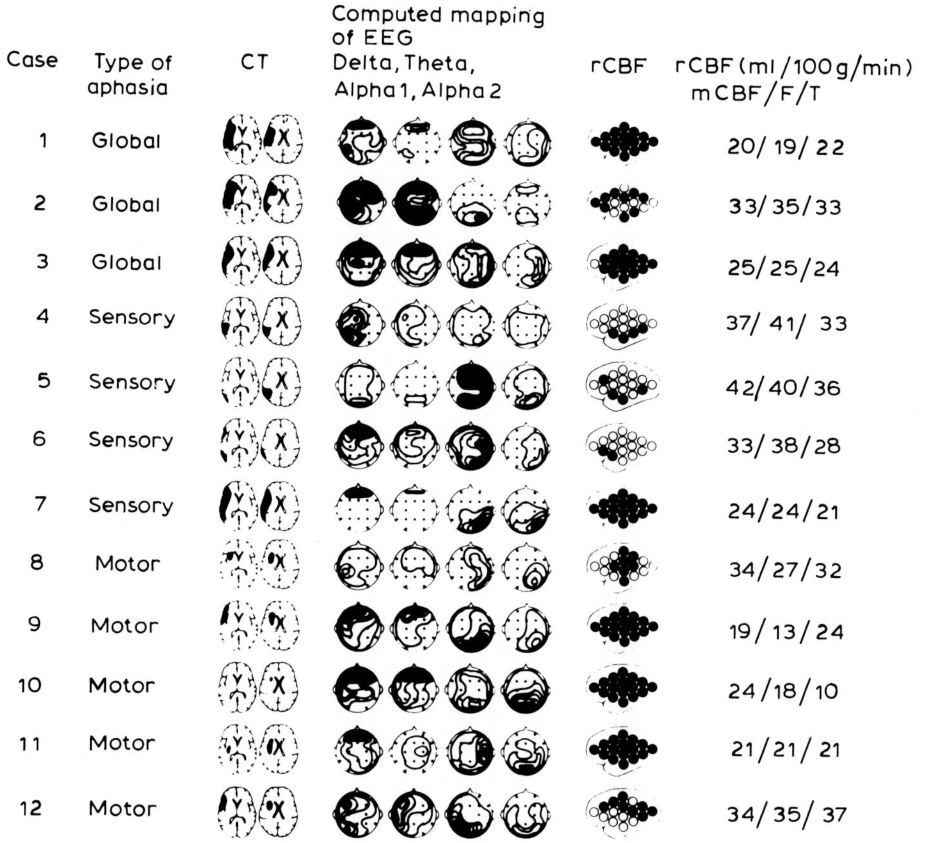

Case	Type of aphasia	CT	Computed mapping of EEG Delta, Theta, Alpha 1, Alpha 2	rCBF	rCBF (ml/100 g/min) mCBF/F/T
1	Global				20/19/22
2	Global				33/35/33
3	Global				25/25/24
4	Sensory				37/41/33
5	Sensory				42/40/36
6	Sensory				33/38/28
7	Sensory				24/24/21
8	Motor				34/27/32
9	Motor				19/13/24
10	Motor				24/18/10
11	Motor				21/21/21
12	Motor				34/35/37

Fig. 1. Twelve patients with different types of aphasic syndrome. Two CT cross-sections show the side and extent of the lesions represented in black. The next columns show computed maps of the equipotential lines of the EEG in 4 frequency bands; the dark areas represent those areas where the steepest gradients were found. The next column represents the results of CBF. A closed circle in the schemes of rCBF designates the blood flow below 60% of the normal flow value, which is considered to be a critical level for causing symptomatic cerebral infarction. The next column shows the values of the mean CBF (mCBF) of all 16 channels, of the mean value of the left frontal channels (F) and of the left temporal channels (T). (From Nagata et al., 1984, with permission.)

standard deviation): 62.3 ± 11.7 ml/100 g/min. In patients with revascularization surgery, a study was performed by the ^{133}Xe inhalation method with a 32-channel system (Cerebrograph Novo).

Ultrasonic quantitative flow measurements

Blood flow in the common carotid artery was measured following revascularization surgery using UQFMs which non-invasively provided an absolute value of the blood flow from the product of the vessel diameter measured by an ultrasonic Doppler method, and the blood velocity calculated by a pulse echo tracking method (Yamaguchi et al., 1981).

RESULTS

Patients with an aphasic syndrome

Figure 1 shows a summary of 12 patients with an aphasic syndrome. Three patients were diagnosed as having a global aphasia; 4 patients had sensory aphasia, and 5 patients had motor aphasia. In three patients with global aphasia, verbal communication was severely impaired in both comprehension and expression. The CT disclosed a large cortical infarct in the left frontal and temporal lobes. The CME revealed an extensive high voltage focus of slow wave components in the left hemisphere with an amplitude depression of alpha activities in the left hemisphere. Cerebral blood flow was markedly reduced and mCBF was less than 53% of the normal flow value in all patients. All these results indicated an extensive lesion in the left hemisphere in patients with global aphasia.

Four patients with sensory aphasia had fluent spontaneous speech with abundant paraphasia, but their verbal comprehension was severely impaired. A wedge-shaped localized low density area was found in the left temporoparietal region in the CT in three out of four patients, and an extensive low density area was found in one patient (case 7) who had a right hemiparesis in addition to the aphasic syndrome. A focus of delta activity was marked in the left temporoparietal region in the CME in one patient (case 4) who showed a focal ischemia in the corresponding region of the brain (Figs. 2 and 3). An asymmetrical distribution of alpha activities with a voltage depression in the

Case T.A. sensory aphasia

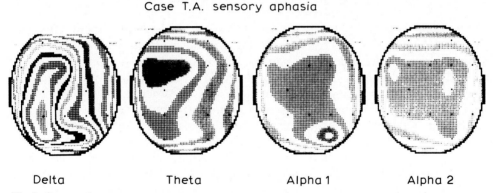

| Delta | Theta | Alpha 1 | Alpha 2 |

Fig. 2. Computed maps of EEG (CME) for 4 frequency bands in case 4 (T.A.). Eleven different classes of amplitudes are given in form of equipotential areas. (From Nagata et al., 1984, with permission.)

left hemisphere was seen in three patients who did not show a slow focus. The rCBF studies demonstrated a focal ischemia in the left temporal region in all four patients; the regional blood flow in the left temporal region (T) was lower than that in the left frontal region (F). The location of a focus of slow wave components showed a good correlation with the side of the lesions estimated using CT and rCBF studies in one patient with sensory aphasia.

Five patients were diagnosed as having a motor aphasia because their speech output was not fluent, in spite of a relatively preserved verbal comprehension. A cortical infarct was seen in the left frontal lobe in the CT in two patients, and a

276

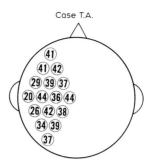

Case T.A.

Fig. 3. rCBF measurements in case 4 (T.A.); the left hemispheric mean flow value was 37 ml/100 g/min. (From Nagata et al., 1984, with permission.)

subcortical infarct was found in three patients. High amplitude foci of slow wave components were found in the left frontal region in three patients, including two patients with cortical involvement in the CT. Two patients without slow foci showed an asymmetrical distribution of alpha activities with voltage depression in the left hemisphere. Marked cerebral ischemia was demonstrated by rCBF studies and the left hemispheric mCBF was less than 60% of the normal flow value. Relative focal ischemia was observed in the left frontal region in four of five patients, F being lower than T. A focus of slow wave components correlated with the lesions in the CT and rCBF studies.

Patients with transient ischemic attacks (TIAs)

Table I shows a list of 10 patients with TIAs. Six patients had TIAs of left hemiparesis, and 4 patients had TIAs of right hemiparesis including 2 patients who had an aphasic syndrome in addition to hemiparesis. Cerebral angiography revealed no abnormality in 2 patients. A stenosis of the middle cerebral artery was found in 6 patients, an occlusion of the middle cerebral artery was found in 2 patients, and an occlusion of the internal carotid artery was seen in 2 patients. The CT scan disclosed no abnormality in all patients. Cerebral blood flow was normal in 7 patients, and it was moderately reduced in 3 patients who underwent rCBF measurements within 4 days of the last attack. Seven patients showed unilateral abnormalities in the CME that corresponded to the side of the lesions suspected through the clinical symptomatology of the TIAs. One patient with TIAs of left hemiparesis was shown to have a normal angiogram, CT, rCBF and CME.

A 44-year-old male (case K.I.) experienced a right hemiparesis when he was driving a car, which disappeared completely within one hour. Cerebral angiography revealed a mild stenotic lesion in the intracranial portion of the left internal carotid artery. The regional CBF study showed 62 ml/100 g/min for the left hemispheric mCBF (within normal limits), and the regional values were also normal. A CME taken 6 h after the TIA, however, showed an asymmetrical distribution of alpha activities (alpha-1 and alpha-2) with amplitude depression in the left hemisphere (Fig. 4A). After the attack the patient has been free of further TIAs or completed strokes. A series of CMEs revealed an asymmetrical distribution of amplitude depression in alpha activities at 10 days, 29 days, and 61 days after the attack. The CME was finally normalized with a symmetrical distribution of increased amplitude in both sides of the brain 149 days after the attack (Fig. 4E).

TABLE I

TEN PATIENTS WITH TIAs IN THE TERRITORY OF LEFT INTERNAL CAROTID ARTERY

*: Having TIAs of right hemiparesis in addition to the aphasic syndrome. ICA: internal carotid artery; MCA: middle cerebral artery; mean CBF: mean hemispheric cerebral blood flow values on the side of the lesion

Case	Age/sex (yrs)	Side of TIAs	Frequency of TIAs	Time to examination	Angiographic findings	CT findings	Mean rCBF	Lesion side on topographic EEG
1	44/m	right	1	6 h	left ICA stenosis	normal	62 ± 8.2	left (Alpha)
2	44/m	right*	4	6 h	left MCA stenosis	normal	43 ± 7.5	left (Alpha)
3	58/m	left	2	3 days	right MCA stenosis	normal	42 ± 5.0	right (Alpha)
4	78/f	right*	many	4 days	left MCA stenosis	normal	36 ± 5.2	left (Alpha)
5	50/f	left	1	4 days	normal	normal	64 ± 7.4	normal
6	52/m	left	3	9 days	right MCA stenosis	normal	63 ± 5.8	left (Alpha)
7	44/m	right	2	28 days	left MCA stenosis	normal	59 ± 2.8	left (Alpha)
8	42/m	left	2	37 days	normal	normal	61 ± 5.1	right (Theta)
9	47/m	left	2	50 days	right ICA stenosis	normal	57 ± 5.8	low voltage Beta
10	46/m	left	2	54 days	right MCA stenosis	normal	54 ± 9.0	diffuse slow Alpha
	51 ± 11 years			19 ± 21 days			54 ± 10.1 ml/100 g/min	

Patients with revascularization surgery

An extracranial-to-intracranial arterial anastomosis (EC/IC bypass) operation was performed on 10 patients who had occlusive cerebrovascular lesions. Table II shows a list of the 10 patients. Preoperative angiography showed a stenosis of the middle cerebral artery in 4 patients, an occlusion of the middle cerebral artery in 3 patients, and an occlusion of the internal carotid artery in 3 patients. All patients had a favorable recovery in clinical signs and symptoms after the operation. Seven patients showed an improvement in the CME findings: a disappearance or retraction of the focus of slow wave components and an increase of amplitude in alpha activities (alpha-1 and alpha-2) in both hemispheres. To estimate the efficiency of the revascularization surgery, the blood flow through the bypass was blocked during CME examination for approximately 2 min by compressing the superficial temporal artery (STA) which was the donor artery to the bypassed intracranial arteries. Five patients showed worsening of the CME findings during the compression of the STA, but later recovered to the same state as before compression. There was no particular change in the patients' clinical signs and symptoms during compression of the STA. The same

278

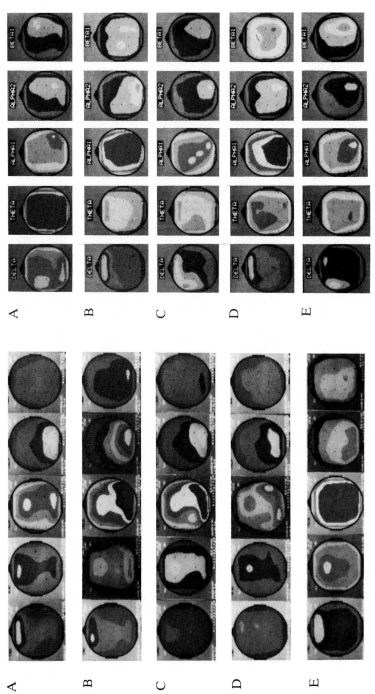

Fig. 4. Time course of CME findings in case K. I. who had TIA with right hemiparesis. From left to right: computed maps of equipotential lines in the frequency bands delta, theta, alpha-1, alpha-2 and beta-1; from top to bottom: 6 h (A), 10 days (B), 29 days (C), 61 days (D) and 149 days (E) after TIA. (From Nagata et al. 1984, with permission.)

Fig. 6. CME findings before and after EC/IC bypass operation in case T. S. From top to bottom: before operation (A), 135 days after operation with left STA free (B) and left STA compressed (C), 270 days after operation with left STA free (D) and left STA compressed (E). For further explanation see Figs. 2 and 4. (From Nagata et al. 1984, with permission.)

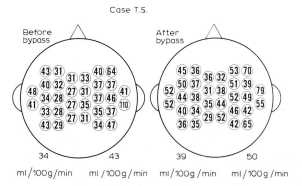

Fig. 5. rCBF measurements by the ^{133}Xe inhalation method before and following EC/IC bypass surgery in case T. S. (From Nagata et al., 1984, with permission.)

TABLE II

TEN PATIENTS WHO UNDERWENT REVASCULARIZATION SURGERY. POSTOPERATIVE ASSESSMENT WAS PERFORMED USING CME AND UQFM

				Topographic EEG		Common carotid flow in affected side		
Case	Age/sex	Angiographic findings	Outcome	improvement after bypass	during STA compression	STA free (ml/sec)	STA compression (ml/sec)	Reduced flow (%)
1	60/m	left ICA occlusion	good	improved	alpha(↓), delta(↑)	8.88	5.50	38.1
2	47/m	right MCA stenosis	good	improved	alpha(↓), delta(↑)	10.59	10.22	3.5
3	47/f	right MCA occlusion	good	improved	alpha(↓), delta(↑)	7.34	5.66	22.9
4	70/m	left MCA occlusion	good	improved	alpha(↓)	11.79	9.27	21.4
5	66/m	left MCA occlusion	good	improved	alpha(↓)	10.43	9.29	10.9
6	47/m	left MCA stenosis	good	unchanged	unchanged	6.92	6.12	11.6
7	48/m	right MCA stenosis	good	improved	unchanged	9.27	7.82	15.6
8	44/m	both ICAs occlusion	fair	improved	unchanged	6.32	3.57	43.5
9	49/f	left MCA stenosis	good	unchanged	unchanged	5.87	5.80	1.2
10	60/m	right ICA occlusion	good	unchanged	unchanged	8.02	3.95	50.7

procedure was performed to estimate the common carotid blood flow using UQFM. The common carotid blood flow was reduced during the compression of the STA in all patients, and the reduction of the blood flow ranged from 1.2 to 50.7% of that before the compression. No particular relationship was found between the degree of reduction of blood flow and clinical recovery after revascularization.

280

A 60-year-old male (case T.S.) had a right hemiparesis and a mild motor aphasia. Cerebral angiography revealed an occlusion of the left internal carotid artery in the extracranial portion. A localized low density area was found in the subcortex of the left frontal lobe in the CT. The patient underwent an EC/IC bypass operation on the left side of the brain and his postoperative course was very favorable. The cerebral blood flow was moderately reduced before operation; the left mCBF was 34 ml/100 g/min and the right mCBF was 43 ml/100 g/min. It increased in both hemispheres after the operation; the left mCBF was 39 ml/100 g/min and the right mCBF was 50 ml/100 g/min (Fig. 5). Before the operation a high amplitude focus of delta activity was seen in the left frontal region in the CME, and alpha activities were depressed in amplitude in the left hemisphere (Fig. 6A). There was an improvement in the CME findings 135 days after the operation; the delta focus disappeared and alpha activities were increased in amplitude on both sides. During compression of the left STA, the delta focus appeared again in the left frontal region and the alpha activities were depressed in amplitude in both hemispheres (Fig. 6C). At 270 days after the operation, there was also a good improvement in the CME findings; no slow foci but an asymmetrical distribution of alpha activities existed with a slight amplitude depression in the left hemisphere. During compression of the left STA, however, the high amplitude focus of delta activity appeared again on the left side (Fig. 6E).

The common carotid blood flow was 4.74 ml/sec in the left side, which was approximately one-half that in the right side (10.47 ml/sec) by UQFM. The left common carotid blood flow increased to be 9.82 ml/sec 135 days after the operation. It was reduced to 8.38 ml/sec during compression of the left STA. It was 8.88 ml/sec 270 days after the operation, and it decreased to 5.50 ml/sec on compression of the left STA (Table III).

TABLE III

COMPARISON OF BLOOD FLOW OF COMMON CAROTID ARTERY
PROVIDED BY UQFM BEFORE AND AFTER THE
REVASCULARIZATION SURGERY IN CASE T.S.

The common carotid blood flow was reduced during compression of the left
superficial temporal artery (STA), which was a feeding artery of the bypass

Case T.S.	Common carotid blood flow by UQFM		
	Right side	Left side	
	STA free	STA free	STA compressed (ml/min)
Before bypass	10.47	4.74	
135 days after bypass	9.65	9.82	8.38
270 days after bypass	10.78	8.88	5.50

DISCUSSION

A presence of slow wave components and slowing or amplitude depression of background activity on the ischemic side suggest a relationship between cerebral ischemia and the resulting electroencephalographic abnormalities. Polymorphic delta activity and an asymmetrical distribution of background activity were thought to be unilateral signs of the EEG abnormalities in ischemic cerebrovascular disease (Van der Drift, 1972). The incidences of the resulting EEG abnormalities have differed widely in various studies; these unilateral EEG abnormalities were found in 67.6% of the patients with unilateral cerebral infarction (Birchfield et al., 1959), in 85.7% of those with occlusive cerebrovascular disease (Carmon et al., 1966), and in 90.3% who had an infarct in the carotid or middle cerebral arterial territory (Paddison and Ferriss, 1961). These variations in the results are considered to depend on some basic factors. Jonkman (1981) indicated three important factors influencing the resulting EEG abnormalities in cerebral ischemia: (1) localization of the ischemia area, (2) the duration of the ischemia, and (3) the interval between the onset of ischemia and the recording of the EEG.

At first we analyzed the localization of the ischemic lesions in patients with an aphasic syndrome. The pathophysiology of the aphasic syndrome in cerebral ischemia has been studied using CT (Kertesz et al., 1979), and rCBF measurements (Soh et al., 1978; Tagawa et al., 1982). The results of these neuroradiological studies were consistent with the classical pathology of an aphasic syndrome.

The patients with global aphasia were suspected of having their causative ischemic lesions in the left frontal and temporal lobes. The extensive high amplitude focus of slow wave components in the left hemisphere corresponded well to the lesions in the CT and rCBF studies in patients with global aphasia. In one patient with sensory aphasia who had a slow focus in the left temporoparietal region in the CME, there was a good correlation of the localization of the lesions between CT, rCBF measurements and CME. Furthermore, in patients with motor aphasia the slow focus in the left frontal region corresponded to the CT and rCBF results. Consequently, the presence of a slow focus was considered to be a useful indicator of localization of functional impairment in cerebral ischemia. Loeb and Fieschi (1967) investigated 40 patients with ischemic cerebrovascular disorders. They found supporting evidence for our results in that, in the majority of cases, the location of the focal EEG abnormalities coincided with the area of rCBF reduction. Ingvar (1967) described that the degree of slowing of the EEG may represent the degree of metabolic depression as well as the reduction of mean cerebral blood flow except in the situation of a luxury perfusion syndrome.

In patients who did not display a slow focus there was an asymmetrical distribution of alpha activities with amplitude depression in the left hemisphere. In these cases the lesion side in the CME corresponded to their clinical symptoms, but the CME did not indicate the intrahemispheric localization of the lesions.

Roseman et al. (1952) reported that the appearance of delta activity may indicate a more superficial lesion, and that the depression of background activity in the absence of delta focus may indicate a deeper lesion in cerebrovascular disease. We likewise found that the presence of slow wave components in the CME correlated with the superficial brain lesion (cortical infarction) in the CT. Some patients who had cortical involvement in the CT did not, however, display slow wave components in the CME results throughout their course of cerebral ischemia. Contrary to the second conclusion made by Roseman et al. (1952), we found that the asymmetrical depression of background activity did not always represent a deep lesion of the brain.

The reversibility of cerebral function in cerebral ischemia has been studied using EEG and rCBF measurements. Enge et al. (1980) investigated 295 TIA patients and found EEG abnormalities in 56.3% of the patients during their symptom-free periods. In our results, 7 out of 10 patients with TIAs showed unilateral abnormalities in the CME even when they had completely recovered from neurological deficits; the CME abnormalities corresponded with their clinical signs and symptoms of TIAs. These results were considered to be a reflection of the residual impairment of cerebral function caused by a transient ischemic event.

From the results of 85 patients with TIAs, Kreindler et al. (1966) described that, when the EEG abnormalities were found following TIA, it was rather difficult to label them as occurring either before or after the attack. As atherosclerotic changes were commonly seen in the cerebral vessels of TIA patients, there is a possibility that the EEG abnormalities had already existed before the attack. However, the asymmetrical depression of alpha activities in the CME that had persisted since the first CME was normalized 149 days after the TIA in case I.K. Moreover, in our previous report (Nagata et al., 1981), fewer EEG abnormalities were found in the later examination period after the last attack. The above evidence may support the facts that one should take these EEG abnormalities as the results of a transient ischemic event.

In the earlier literature when EEGs were read conventionally, however, EEG changes were absent or slight in patients with transient or recurrent cerebral ischemia. The EEGs were considered to be normal in 57% of the patients with carotid insufficiency (Meyer et al., 1956), in 62% of those with recurrent focal cerebral ischemia (Paddison and Ferriss, 1961), and in 72% of those with recurrent cerebral ischemic attacks (Birchfield et al., 1959). Even though these early studies included some patients with persistent neurological deficits, these reports showed fewer EEG abnormalities. This discrepancy between the early literature and our results may be partly due to the accuracy of power spectral analysis over and beyond that of conventional reading of the EEG in detecting voltage asymmetries of background activity (Matousek and Petersen, 1973).

An asymmetrical amplitude depression of alpha activities was found in six patients who had intracranial atherosclerotic lesions in the angiogram but had normal CT findings. Three of them also had normal cerebral blood flow. They were suspected of having their ischemic process deep in the brain. Caplan and Young (1972) reported that the EEG abnormalities were minor or nonlocalizing in lacunar stroke syndrome. These results suggested some participation of small infarctions of the basal ganglia in the pathogenesis of TIA, which has been postulated from neuroradiological studies (Araki et al., 1983).

Postischemic blood flow appeared to be important in the recovery of neuronal function in experimental studies (Hossmann and Kleihues, 1970). However, a chronic disturbance of the cerebral circulation was found in TIA patients who had recovered completely from their neurological deficits (Rees et al., 1970; Wong et al., 1973; Yonekura et al., 1981). Skinhoj et al. (1970) substantiated that the cerebral circulation may recover after the clinical symptoms do in TIA. Three patients who underwent rCBF studies within 4 days of the last attack had reduced cerebral blood flows. Their mean hemispheric flow values (mCBF) ranged from 58% to 69% of the normal flow value. However, these values were higher than the critical flow level, which was assumed to cause symptomatic cerebral infarction (Kawase et al., 1980). A persistent disturbance of cerebral blood flow may be one of the important factors leading to further TIAs or completed strokes. From the view point of the hemodynamic theory of TIA, Bruens et al. (1960) described that the EEG abnormalities, caused by a relative ischemia of the Sylvian region, might be a useful indicator of an impending decompensation of cerebral circulation. Because of the persistent impairment of cerebral function and cerebral blood flow, TIA patients can easily have further TIAs or completed strokes when they are re-exposed to a global or focal ischemia.

Many diagnostic methods have been employed in the objective postoperative assessment of patients with revascularization surgery (Anderson et al., 1974; Austin et al., 1974). Most of them, however, have required traumatic procedures. A quantitative EEG analysis was thought to be an objective and non-invasive tool beneficial in repeated examinations. A mean hemispheric frequency of the EEG was used in the evaluation of the cerebral function following revascularization surgery (de Weerd et al., 1981; Pfurtscheller and Auer, 1983). In the present study, we monitored both localization of the lesions and their time course following revascularization.

In our results, seven patients showed an improvement in the CME findings accompanied by favorable recovery of their clinical symptoms and signs after revascularization. On the other hand, there was no particular change in CME findings in three patients in spite of their favorable recovery. This discrepancy between the CME findings and their clinical course might be partly due to the mild CME abnormalities found in the initial examination. Further functional recovery was nonetheless observed in these three patients, even though their CME findings had not improved.

In the previous studies, temporary deterioration of EEG findings occurred relatively shortly after the revascularization but an improvement became apparent on clinical recovery. It was considered to be a reflection of a temporary deterioration of cerebral function after the revascularization (Pfurtscheller and Auer, 1983). No deterioration was observed in the CME findings in our 10 patients who underwent CME examination from 6 to 65 months after the revascularization.

During compression of the STA, the CME findings worsened in 5 of the 10 patients but were not so extreme as to reveal neurological deterioration. The changes in CME findings included the appearance of delta activity in the appropriate hemisphere and amplitude depression of background activity in both hemispheres. In case T.S., the left frontal delta focus, which disappeared after revascularization, reappeared during compression of the left STA. This worsening of CME findings hypothetically reflects a temporary deterioration of cerebral function in the left frontal region by blocking the blood flow to the left frontal lobe through the bypass artery. Furthermore, the common carotid blood flow was reduced in all patients during compression of the STA. Although the degree of reduction in the blood flow ranged widely, this phenomenon may indicate the blood supply to the brain tissue through the bypass artery. Consequently, it would seem to be possible to estimate the functional reserve of revascularization, using CME and UQFM, by compressing the donor artery of the revascularization.

SUMMARY

Computed mapping of the EEG (CME) provided an equipotential topography of the square roots of the average power spectra over the given frequency band. To investigate the relationship between cerebral function, circulation and anatomical lesions in cerebral ischemia, 32 patients with ischemic cerebrovascular disease were studied using CME, rCBF measurements, ultrasonic quantitative flow measurements (UQFM), CT scan, and cerebral angiography.

In patients with an aphasic syndrome, a high amplitude focus of slow wave components correlated well with the localization of the lesions obtained with CT scan and rCBF measurements. In the patients without slow wave focus in the CME findings, the results did not indicate the intrahemispheric localization of the functional lesions.

Seven out of 10 patients with TIAs showed unilateral abnormalities with the CME when they had completely recovered from their neurological deficits, the CME abnormalities corresponding with the clinical symptomatology of TIAs. This result may indicate a reflection of the residual cerebral dysfunction caused by a transient ischemic event. It can be postulated that, because of the persistent impairment of cerebral function and blood flow, TIA patients can easily have further TIAs or completed stroke whenever they are re-exposed to a cerebral ischemia.

A series of CMEs demonstrated a recovery of cerebral function from cerebral infarction following the revascularization surgery. The worsening of the CME findings during compression of the superficial temporal artery may reflect a temporary deterioration of cerebral function by blocking of the blood flow to the brain tissue through the bypass feeding artery.

REFERENCES

Adrian, E.D. and Yamagiwa, K. (1935) The origin of the Berger rhythm. *Brain*, 58: 323–351.

Anderson, R.E., Riechman, H. and Davis, D.O. (1974) Radiological evaluation of temporal artery middle cerebral artery anastomosis. *Radiology*, 113: 73–79.

Araki, G., Mihara, H., Shizuka, M., Yunoki, K., Nagata, K., Yamaguchi, K., Mizukami, M., Kawase, T. and Tazawa, T. (1983) CT and angiographic comparison of transient ischemic attacks, correlation with small infarction of basal ganglia. *Stroke*, 14: 276–280.

Austin, G., Laffin, D. and Heyward, W. (1974) Physiological factors in the selection of patients for superficial temporal artery to middle cerebral artery anastomosis. *Surgery*, 15: 861–868.

Birchfield, R.I., Wilson, W.P. and Heyman, A. (1959) An evaluation of electroencephalography in cerebral infarction and ischemia due to arteriosclerosis. *Neurology (Minneap.)*, 9: 859–871.

Bruens, J.H., Gastaut, H. and Giove, G. (1960) Electroencephalographic study of the signs of chronic vascular insufficiency of the Sylvian region in aged people. *Electroenceph. clin. Neurophysiol.*, 12: 183–295.

Caplan, L.R. and Young, R.R. (1972) EEG findings in cerebral lacunar stroke syndrome. *Neurology*, 22: 204.

Carmon, A., Lavy, S. and Schwartz, A. (1966) Correlation between electroencephalography and angiography in cerebrovascular accidents. *Electroenceph. clin. Neurophysiol.*, 21: 71–76.

De Weerd, A.W., Van Huffelen, A.C. and Mosmans, P.C.M. (1981) Quantitative EEG and cerebral blood flow after surgery for cerebral ischemia. *Electroenceph. clin. Neurophysiol.*, 52: 78–79.

Duffy, F.H., Burchfield, J.L. and Lombroso, C.T. (1979) Brain electrical activity mapping (BEAM): a method for expanding the clinical utility of EEG and evoked potential data. *Ann. Neurol.*, 5: 309–321.

Enge, S., Lechner, H., Logar, C. and Ladurner, G. (1980) Clinical value of EEG in transient ischemic attacks. In H. Lechner and A. Aranibar (Eds.), *EEG and Clinical Neurophysiology*, Excerpta Medica, Amsterdam, pp.173–180.

Gotman, J., Skuce, D.R., Thompson, C.J., Gloor, P., Ives, J.R. and Ray, W.F. (1973) Clinical application of spectral analysis and extraction of features from electroencephalograms with slow wave in adult patients. *Electroenceph. clin. Neurophysiol.*, 35: 224–235.

Gotman, J., Gloor, P. and Ray, W.F. (1975) A quantitative comparison of traditional reading of the EEG and interpretation of computer-extracted features in patients with supratentorial brain lesions. *Electroenceph. clin. Neurophysiol.*, 38: 623–639.

Hossmann, K.A. and Kleihues, P. (1970) Reversibility of ischemic brain damage. *Arch. Neurol.*, 29: 375–384.

Ingvar, D.H. (1967) The pathophysiology of occlusive cerebrovascular disorders related to neuroradiological findings, EEG and measurements of regional cerebral blood flow. *Acta neurol. Scand.*, 43, Suppl. 31: 93–107.

Ingvar, D.H., Sjolund, B. and Arbo, A. (1976) Correlation between dominant EEG frequency, cerebral oxygen uptake and blood flow. *Electroenceph. clin. Neurophysiol.*, 41: 268–276.

Jonkman, E.J. (1981) Cerebral blood flow (CBF) and electrical activity (EEG). In J.H. Minderhoud (Ed.), *Cerebral Blood Flow, Basic Knowledge and Clinical Implications*, Excerpta Medica, Amsterdam–Oxford–Princeton, pp.202–222.

Kawase, T., Mizukami, M., Araki, G. and Nagata, K. (1980) Critical flow level in cerebral ischemia. I. Occlusive cerebrovascular disease. *Brain Nerve (Tokyo)*, 32: 1247–1255.

Kertesz, A., Harlock, W. and Coates, R. (1979) Computer tomographic localization, lesion size and prognosis in aphasia and non-verbal impairment. *Brain Language*, 8: 34–50.

Kreindler, A., Pollici, I. and Marinchesu, M. (1966) Electroencephalographic study of cerebral transient ischemic attacks. *Confin. Neurol.*, 28: 385–398.

Lehmann, D. (1971) Multichannel topography of human alpha fields. *Electroenceph. clin. Neurophysiol.*, 31: 439–449.

Loeb, C. and Fieschi, C. (1967) EEG and rCBF in cases of brain infarction. *Electroenceph. clin. Neurophysiol.*, 25, Suppl.: 111–118.

Matousek, M. and Petersen, I. (1973) Frequency analysis of the EEG in normal children and adolescents. In P. Kellaway and I. Petersen (Eds.), *Automation of Clinical Electroencephalography*, Raven Press, New York, pp.75–102.

Matsuoka, S., Aragaki, Y., Numaguchi, K. and Ueno, S. (1978) Effect of dexamethasone on electroencephalogram in patients with brain tumor. *J. Neurosurg.*, 48: 601–608.

Meyer, J.S., Leiderman, H. and Denny-Brown, D. (1956) Electroencephalographic study of insufficiency of the basilar and carotid arteries in man. *Neurology (Minneap.)*, 6: 455–477.

Mosmans, P.C.M., Jonkman, E.J., Magnus, O. and Van Huffelen, A.C. (1973) Regional cerebral blood flow and EEG. *Electroenceph. clin. Neurophysiol.*, 33: 122.

Nagata, K., Hirano, M., Araki, G. and Mizukami, M. (1981) Topographic electroencephalographic study of transient ischemic attacks in asymptomatic period. *Canad. J. neurol. Sci.*, 8: 187.

Nagata, K., Mizukami, M., Araki, G., Kawase, T. and Hirano, M. (1982) Topographic electroencephalographic study of cerebral infarction using computed mapping of the EEG (CME). *J. Cereb. Blood Flow Metab.*, 2: 79–88.

Nagata, K. Hyodo, A., Mizukami, M., Yunoki, K. and Araki, G. (1984) Topographic EEG and cerebral blood flow. In K. Matsumoto (Ed.), *Two Dimensional EEG Mapping in Clinical Testing: Proceedings of the Second Meeting of Japanese Society for Bidimensional Processing of Brain Electrical Activities*, Neuron, Tokyo, in press.

Obrist, W.D., Sokoloff, L., Lassen, N.A., Lane, M.H., Butler, R.N. and Feinberg, I. (1963) Relation of EEG to cerebral blood flow and metabolism in old age. *Electroenceph. clin. Neurophysiol.*, 15: 610–619.

Paddison, R.M. and Ferriss, G.S. (1961) The electroencephalogram in cerebrovascular disease. *Electroenceph. clin. Neurophysiol.*, 13: 99–110.

Petsche, H. (1976) Topography of the EEG, survey and prospect. *Clin. neurol. Neurosurg.*, 79: 15–28.

Pfurtscheller, G. and Auer, L.M. (1983) Frequency changes of sensorimotor EEG rhythm after revascularization surgery. *Electroenceph. clin. Neurophysiol.*, 55: 381–387.

Rees, J.H., du Boulay, G.H., Bull, J.W.B., Marshall, J., Russel, R.W.R. and Symon, L. (1970) Regional cerebral blood flow in transient ischemic attacks. *Lancet*, 2: 1210–1213.

Roseman, F., Schmidt, R.P. and Foltz, E.L. (1952) Serial electroencephalography in vascular lesions of the brain. *Neurology (Minneap.)*, 2: 311–331.

Skinhoj, E., Hoedt-Rasmussen, K., Paulson, O.B. and Lassen, N.A. (1970) Regional cerebral blood flow and its autoregulation in patients with transient focal cerebral ischemic attacks. *Neurology (Minneap.)*, 20: 485–493.

Soh, K., Larsen, K., Skinhoj, E. and Lassen, N.A. (1978) Regional cerebral blood flow in aphasia. *Arch. Neurol.*, 35: 625–632.

Tagawa, K., Sugimoto, K., Minematsu, K., Yamaguchi, T., Naritomi, H. and Sawada, T. (1982) Type of aphasia and regional cerebral blood flow, A study with 133-Xe inhalation method. *Neurol. Med. (Tokyo)*, 17: 454–459.

Tolonen, U. and Sulg, I.A. (1981) Comparison of quantitative EEG parameters from four different analysis techniques in evaluation of relationship between EEG and rCBF in brain infarction. *Electroenceph. clin. Neurophysiol.*, 51: 177–185.

Ueno, S. and Matsuoka, S. (1976) Topographic display of slow wave type of EEG abnormality in patients with brain lesion. *J. Med. Electr. Bio. Eng. (Tokyo)*, 14: 118–124.

Van der Drift, J.H.A. (1972) The EEG in cerebrovascular disease. In P.J. Vinken and G.W. Bruyn (Eds.), *Handbook of Clinical Neurology, Vol. 11*, Elsevier North-Holland, Amsterdam, pp.267–291.

Walter, W.G. and Shipton, H.W. (1951) A new toposcopic display system. *Electroenceph. clin. Neurophysiol.*, 3: 281–292.

Wong, E., Bull, J.W.B., du Boulay, G.H., Marshall, J., Russel, R.W.R. and Symon, L. (1973) Regional cerebral blood flow in completed stroke and transient ischemic attacks, a clinical correlation. *Neurology (Minneap.)*, 23: 949–952.

Yamaguchi, K., Yunoki, K., Nagata, K., Araki, G., Mizukami, M. and Katsunuma, H. (1981) Diagnosis of occlusive cerebrovascular disease using ultrasonic quantitative flow measurements (UQFM). *Brain Nerve (Tokyo)*, 33: 359–364.

Yonekura, M., Austin, G., Poll, N. and Hayward, W. (1981) Evaluation of regional cerebral blood flow in patients with transient ischemic attacks and minor strokes. *Surg. Neurol.*, 15: 58–65.

*Brain Ischemia: Quantitative EEG and Imaging Techniques, Progress in Brain Research, Vol. 62, edited by
G. Pfurtscheller, E.J. Jonkman and F.H. Lopes da Silva
©1984 Elsevier Science Publishers B.V.*

Brain Electrical Activity Mapping in Normal and Ischemic Brain

G. PFURTSCHELLER[1], G. LADURNER[2], H. MARESCH[1] and R. VOLLMER[3]

[1]*Department of Computing, Institute of Biomedical Engineering, Technical University of Graz, A-8010 Graz,* [2]*Department of Neurology and Psychiatry, University of Graz, A-8036 Graz and* [3]*Ludwig Boltzmann Institute of Clinical Neurobiology, A-1130 Vienna (Austria)*

INTRODUCTION

Metabolism and blood flow in the normal, nonischemic brain depend on the functional state of the brain tissue, and it has been shown that the bioelectrical activity under these circumstances correlates with the metabolic rate and cerebral blood flow (Sokoloff, 1981). The following measurements are used to study the functional brain activity pattern during conscious perception and behavioral reactions: regional cerebral blood flow (rCBF) with ^{133}Xe (Ingvar, 1979), CBF and cerebral blood volume (CBV) using CT scan (Ladurner et al., 1976; Meyer et al., 1981), and single photon emission tomography (Lassen, 1980); positron emission tomography (Frackowiak et al., 1980; Buchsbaum et al., 1982a; Phelps et al., 1982) gives CBF and CBV, as well as three-dimensional results for glucose and oxygen uptake. Most recently, nuclear magnetic resonance (NMR) appears to offer new insights into the relationship between cerebral metabolism and cerebral structures (Jolesz, 1983). The distribution of cortical steady state bioelectrical activity can be investigated by topographical display of EEG spectra in the form of EEG maps (Duffy et al., 1978; Duffy, 1981; Nagata et al., 1982; Buchsbaum et al., 1982b; Pfurtscheller, 1983).

The observation time used is an important factor in the two- and three-dimensional techniques of measuring and displaying brain activity patterns. So are the two-dimensional rCBF landscapes and the EEG maps obtained through averages over minutes, whereas emission tomography can measure oxygen uptake within just milliseconds. The time window in the range of minutes for EEG mapping is insufficient to study activation patterns during movement, speech or other types of conscious stimulus perception. We developed for that purpose a technique allowing us to study the topographical distribution of a special EEG parameter within a time window of milliseconds to seconds. Event-Related Desynchronization (ERD), a regional, brief blocking or attenuation of alpha- and beta-band activity, is a suitable parameter for this purpose.

This attenuation has a short duration and has been known since Berger (1929), who observed the typical blocking of the occipital rhythm after stimulation with light. Neither the rhythmical activity, however, nor the blocking reaction after peripheral stimulation is specific for the occipital cortex; moreover, attenuation of rhythmical background activity can also be observed during voluntary movements. In the early years of EEG recording, Jasper and Penfield (1949) observed some individuals with rhythmical activity over the central gyrus that was blocked by contralateral hand movements. Today it is well known that any voluntary movement is accompanied by slow changes of the DC potential (Bereitschaftspotential) and attenuation of the rhythmical activity, known as ERD. This has been shown by Kornhuber and Deecke (1964) for the "Bereitschaftspotential" and by Pfurtscheller and Aranibar (1977, 1980) for the ERD. Computer-assisted EEG analysis has revealed that more than 90% of the population have a central mu rhythm, which blocks with bilateral symmetry during hand movements (some years ago, such individuals were viewed as physiological variants).

There is evidence that the ERD is a very specific parameter for the local activation of different cortical areas, since visual stimulation selectively blocks the occipital alpha rhythm without having any affect whatsoever on the central mu rhythm, and vice versa. Thus, it is tempting to assume that each brain region has a rhythmic activity of its own that becomes desynchronized as soon as this special region is activated. The local distribution of ERD patterns after specific stimulation allows analysis of the ERD over the whole cortex and display of this measurement in the form of two-dimensional maps, representing cortical activation patterns within a time window of milliseconds to seconds.

The aim of this paper is first, to demonstrate the possibility of constructing computer topographical displays of short-lasting EEG changes in the form of ERD maps; secondly, to correlate these maps with the functional states during light perception, voluntary movement and spontaneous speech and, thirdly, to show ERD maps from patients with cerebral ischemia, and to compare these maps with clinical findings and computer tomography (CT).

METHODS

An event, either externally paced as light, somatosensory or auditory stimulus, or internally self-paced as voluntary movement or spontaneous speech, has to be repeated several times with intervals longer than 8 sec in order to obtain results of statistical validity. Data were recorded and processed shortly before, during and after each event.

Data acquisition

Two different electrode configurations were used to record from 16 EEG channels:
– Unipolar recordings with linked earlobes as reference (Fig. 1a);
– bipolar recordings in a transverse montage (Fig. 1b).
All experiments were done with collodion fixed surface electrodes according to the 10–20 system, or by using the Beckman electrode cap.

Within one task (external or self-paced events repeated 60 times), EEG epochs of 6 sec each were recorded and sampled (examples of raw data are displayed in Fig. 3). The first second was regarded as "reference period"; the externally paced events have a trigger after 3 sec and the self-paced events after 4 sec. The EEG from 0.5 to 1.5 sec after externally paced events and from −0.5 to 0.5 sec around the self-paced events was considered to be the "activity period" (Fig. 2).

All EEG signals were recorded with a time constant of $T = 0.1$ sec and a low-pass

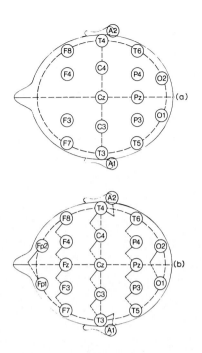

Fig. 1. a: Referential (monopolar) recording from 16 electrodes placed according to the 10–20 system used for EEG and ERD mapping; reference linked earlobes. b: Bipolar recording.

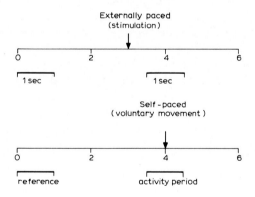

Fig. 2. Principle of data processing. Reference and activity period in externally paced and self-paced experiments.

filter cutoff frequency of 30 Hz. The sampling rate was 64/sec for each channel and the A/D converter accuracy 12 bits. The computer checked for artefacts, excluding all segments containing an A/D converter overflow.

The EEG recording, stimulation, trigger generation and data processing were done by an Eframed CCF 1601 system including a PDP 11/23 computer and a HMW color terminal (Pfurtscheller, 1983).

290

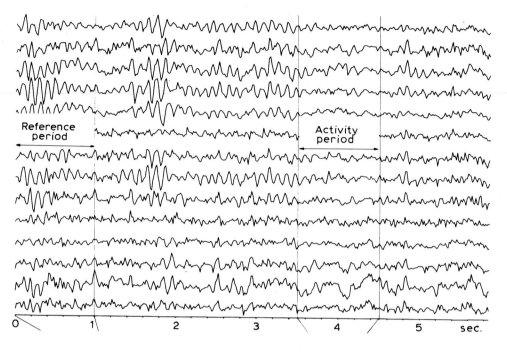

Fig. 3. Raw EEG data; the reference and activity periods are marked. Note the changed EEG pattern in the activity period.

Data processing

The Fast Fourier Transformation (FFT) was used to calculate the power spectra in the reference and activity periods, single spectra were averaged over all artefact-free segments. Figure 4a shows a typical example for both spectra superimposed. The power spectra can differ considerably in the alpha band, depending on the type of the event and the region recorded. These differences can also be checked by statistical methods, computing the confidence level for the ratio of the two spectra at a given level of significance (Jenkins and Watts, 1968). The power spectra were computed online for all 16 channels.

Two-dimensional presentation of data

Computation of the two-dimensional distribution. For computing the topographical presentation of the EEG parameters, a "potential-field"-like distribution of the variable U over the scalp is assumed. This permits the computation of the two-dimensional distribution over the head surface in the x and y directions as a solution of the potential equation (a partial differential equation of the second order)

$$\left(\frac{d^2}{dx^2} + \frac{d^2}{dy^2} \right) U = 0 ,$$

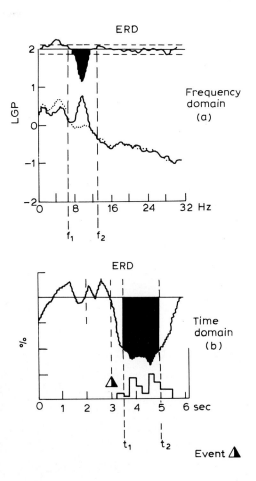

Fig. 4. Upper panel (a): power spectra calculated in the reference (full line) and the activity (stippled line) period. The black area indicates the integral over the difference of the two spectra in the frequency band limited by f_1 and f_2, used as ERD parameter for topographical presentation. Lower panel (b): power versus time curve calculated for the frequency band f_1–f_2. The black area within the time window t_1 and t_2 can be used as a measurement for the ERD. Statistical significance of the power decrease (black area) is indicated by the step function to be read on the right vertical scale ($p < 10^{-2}$, 10^{-6} and 10^{-10}).

with the 16 parameters as supporting values, located at the actual electrode positions for unipolar, or between the electrode positions for bipolar derivations. The potential equation is solved for a matrix (48*80 points) by an iterative algorithm (approximately 70 iterations), requiring approximately 5 sec computation time on a PDP 11/23 computer. The potential distribution is split up into 14 ranges, each represented by a separate color.

Photographs can be taken from the screen. A gray-scale presentation on a matrix printer and a plot output of the equipotential lines on an X–Y plotter are also available.

EEG mapping

The reference power spectrum is used for the parameter calculation. The integral over any chosen frequency band (e.g. 0–4 Hz, 4–8 Hz, 8–12 Hz, etc.) can be computed, giving a survey of the power (amplitude) distribution over the head surface. Figure 5 shows a typical example of an EEG map with dominant alpha activity over the occipital pole.

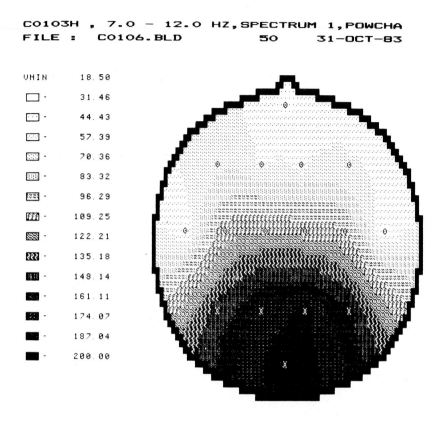

Fig. 5. EEG map representing alpha (7–12 Hz) power distribution during rest with eyes closed. The scale on the left side marks absolute power in μV^2. Bipolar EEG recording.

ERD mapping

As has been explained above, the difference in the power spectra between the reference and the activity period is the main interest and forms the parameter for the topographical display. These differences, especially a decrease in the EEG activity in the localized cortical areas due to an external or internal event, are known as event-related desynchronization and can be evaluated not only in the frequency domain (Fig. 4a), but also in the time domain (Pfurtscheller and Aranibar, 1977, 1980, Fig. 4b). For the former, the integral over the difference of the two spectra is computed in the alpha (beta) band and is displayed topographically. This results in an ERD map. A typical example is given in Fig. 6.

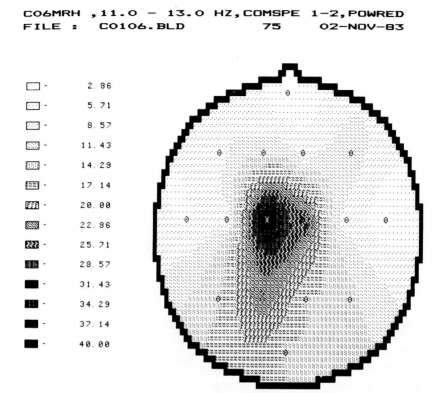

Fig. 6. ERD map calculated during voluntary self-paced movements of the right hand. The scale on the left marks power decrease (ERD) in percentage of the reference period. Bipolar recording.

Frequency mapping

The frequency of the highest spectral peak within the alpha band is an estimate of the alpha (mu) frequency and can also be displayed in the form of a map. In addition to those peak frequencies, the frequency changes between the reference and activity periods can also be calculated and displayed topographically.

EXAMPLES OF ELECTRICAL BRAIN ACTIVITY MAPPING

Normal brain function

Data from two normal subjects are displayed in Figs. 7 and 8. Theta and alpha distributions (EEG maps) demonstrate a high degree of hemispherical symmetry. In one subject (C. W., Fig. 7), the alpha band activity was maximal over the centroparieto-occipital region, in the other subject (J. K., Fig. 8) over both midcentral regions. In both subjects, unilateral voluntary hand movements resulted in a bilaterally symmetrical blocking response of the central mu rhythm, clearly localized over the sensorimotor cortex. Light stimulation resulted in the classical alpha blocking, maximal over

294

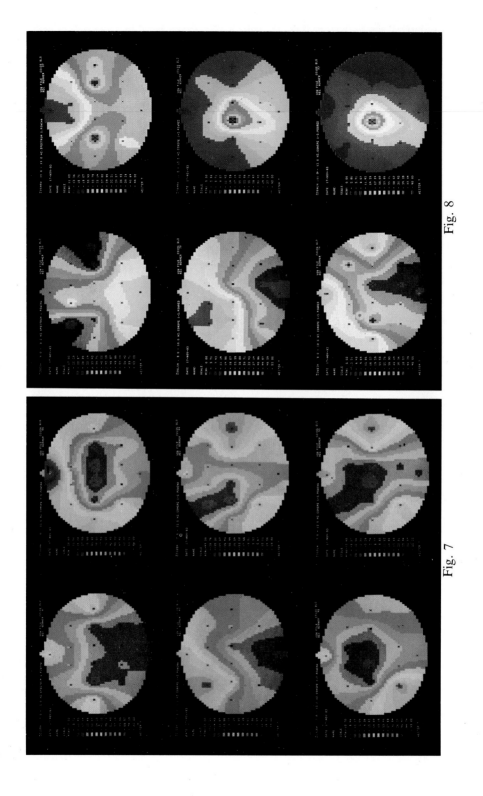

Fig. 8

Fig. 7

the occipital pole. The naming of simple figures presented by slide projection resulted in a more complex activation pattern involving occipital, sensorimotor and premotor areas as well. During voluntary speech or counting, however, the alpha band activity was blocked in the frontotemporal region.

These results demonstrate that the ERD, known as alpha blocking or mu blocking, is a strictly localized, short-lasting neuronal phenomenon, which probably indicates activated cortical fields. The ERD patterns during light perception, voluntary movement and speech are generally identical to the distributions of regional metabolic activity, as obtained by emission tomography (Lauritzen et al., 1981; Phelps et al., 1982).

Unilateral cerebral ischemia

Case 1: A 62-year old patient (F. G.) had a left arm paresis 4 weeks after suffering a stroke. The right internal carotid artery was occluded. The CT scan pictures demonstrated a recent right cortical infarction (Fig. 9), and the clinical EEG showed bilaterally symmetrical theta activity with small foci over both hemispheres. The EEG map in Fig. 10 demonstrates an alpha band activity only over the left parietal region, fully reactive to voluntary right-hand movements as seen in the ERD map. A clear blocking response of 46% in the left frontotemporal region was found during spontaneous speech. An atypical ERD pattern with increased alpha-band activity (negative ERD) was found during light perception. Summarizing this case, it can be said that there was a significantly reduced reactivity during movement and speech over the right parietotemporal region. The EEG and ERD map data correlated with the CT scan, but were in clear contradiction to the clinical EEG findings of bilateral slow-wave activity.

Case 2: A 59-year old patient (R. M.) had a left hemiparesis after a stroke. The angiogram revealed a subtotal stenosis of the right internal carotid artery and a recent right-sided cortical infarction was revealed in the CT scan (Fig. 11). The xenon inhalation method measurement showed reduced cerebral blood flow in both parietal regions. The clinical EEG findings showed minimal diffuse changes over the right

Fig. 7. Topographical display of alpha power (EEG map) during rest (reference period) in the left upper panel and phasic alpha power changes (ERD maps) in the other panels for different conditions. Voluntary left-hand movements (upper right), 1-sec light stimulation (middle left), spontaneous speech (middle right), spontaneous counting (lower left) and verbal image identification (lower right). The scale in the left side for the EEG map is absolute power in μV^2 and the scale for the other panels is the power decrease in percentage of the reference period. The same applies to all other ERD maps. "Violet" marks areas with highest alpha-band activity in the EEG map and maximal power decrease in the ERD maps; followed by red, brown, yellow, green, light blue; "dark blue" mark areas with smallest alpha-band activity and minimal power decrease, respectively; when a power increase (negative ERD) is measured, maximal increase is also indicated by "dark blue". Bipolar recordings; the black dots in each map mark the interelectrode positions. Data from a normal volunteer.

Fig. 8. EEG maps for theta (4–8 Hz) and alpha (11–13 Hz) power during rest (left and right upper panels, respectively) and alpha power decrease (ERD map) during light stimulation (middle left), voluntary right-hand movements (middle right), image identification (lower left) and left-hand movements (lower right). Data from another normal volunteer. Note the localized blocking response in central region during voluntary hand movements. For further explanation see Fig. 7.

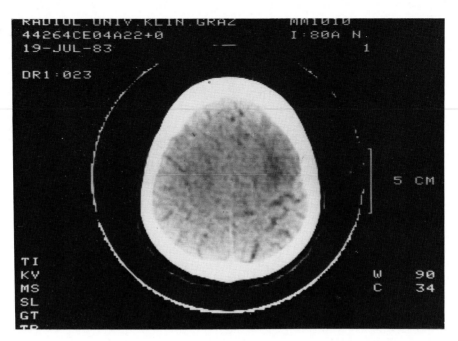

Fig. 9. CT image of a 62-year-old man (F. G.) with a hypodense area in the right hemisphere.

frontotemporal region.

Clear hemispheric asymmetries were found in the peak frequency map and in the ERD maps calculated during voluntary movement and speech. (Fig. 12). The frequency was up to 9.4 Hz over the left and down to 8.5 Hz over the right side; the blocking response due to movement reached 53% in the left parietal region. The blocking response to voluntary speech was very pronounced in the whole frontocentral and left parietal region, but not on the right side.

All these asymmetries in the reactivity pattern suggest severe regional dysfunction in the right hemisphere. In this example, CT scan, angiographic data, clinical EEG findings and the results of EEG and ERD mapping all had high correlations but were in contradiction to the rCBF findings, which showed symmetrically reduced flow.

Case 3: A 57-year-old patient (G. S.) had a transitory ischemic attack (TIA) with a left-sided sensory deficit. The angiogram showed a plaque in the right internal carotid artery and the clinical EEG revealed bilateral slow-wave activity. The CT scan was normal. A quantitative EEG was made 4 weeks after the TIA and it demonstrated a

---

Fig. 10. EEG map displaying square root of power in the 6–12 Hz band (left upper panel) and ERD maps demonstrating power decrease during voluntary right-hand movements and spontaneous speech, but a power increase during light stimulation in a 62-year-old man with left-side paresis. The black dots in each map mark the electrode position of the referential EEG recording. Further explanation see Fig. 7.

Fig. 12. EEG map displaying the square root of power within the 6–12 Hz band (left upper panel), ERD maps calculated during voluntary right-hand movements and spontaneous speech and topographical display of the peak frequency between 8.5 and 9.4 Hz (frequency map, "violet" marks areas with highest, "dark blue" areas with lowest peak frequency) in a 59-year-old patient with left-side paresis. Referential EEG recording.

297

Rest 6–12 Hz   Movement   Fig. 10

Light   Speech

Rest 6–12 Hz   Movement   Fig. 12

Frequency   Speech

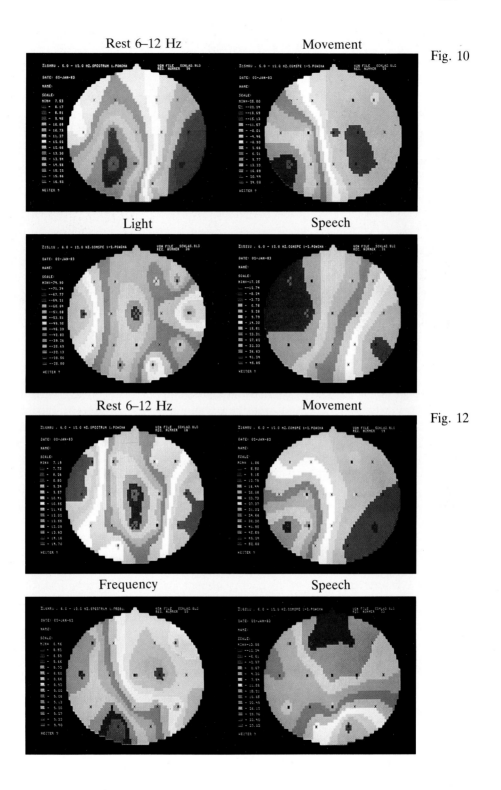

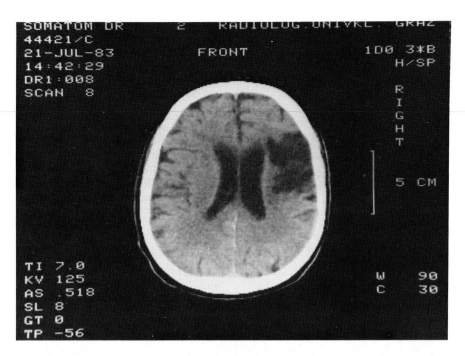

Fig. 11. CT image of a 59-year-old man (R. M.) with a hypodense area in the right centrotemporal region.

symmetrical alpha band activity distribution (left upper panel in Fig. 13) with an amplitude maximum in the centroparietal region, but an asymmetric blocking response to left-hand movement with a normal ERD of 50% over the left centroparietal region (right upper panel in Fig. 13). Hemispheric symmetry was found in the alpha peak frequency distribution with 10.4 Hz over the occipital pole; the frequency changes, however, during left-hand movements were clearly more pronounced over the left central region (0.45 Hz), indicating blocking of the low alpha-band activity in this region (right lower panel). It is interesting to note that the beta activity showed a bilaterally symmetric blocking response to movement and to spontaneous speech as well; although the movement pattern was more transverse (only centrally) and the speech pattern more anterior-posteriorly located (Fig. 14). This example suggests that minor brain dysfunction can be accompanied by a normal alpha band activity distribution but asymmetric ERD and frequency change pattern during hand movements. Furthermore, alpha- and beta-band activity can result in different reactivity patterns during hand movements: the beta ERD is more localized over the Rolandic region, whereas the ERD in the alpha band is more widespread.

Fig. 13. EEG map displaying the square root of power within the 6–12 Hz band (left upper panel), ERD maps during voluntary left-hand movements, frequency map between 8.7 and 10.4 Hz and topographical display of peak frequency increases Δf during voluntary movements (right lower panel), ("violet" marks areas with most pronounced peak frequency increase) in a 57-year-old woman (G. S.) with a TIA. Referential EEG recording.

Fig. 14. The same patient as in Fig. 13, but data from the 14–20 Hz (beta) band. EEG map with beta amplitude distribution (left upper panel) and ERD maps for beta blocking during spontaneous speech and voluntary movements of the right and the left hand.

Rest 6–12 Hz   Movement   Fig. 13

Frequency   Δf Movement

Rest 14–20 Hz   Speech   Fig. 14

left   (movement)   right

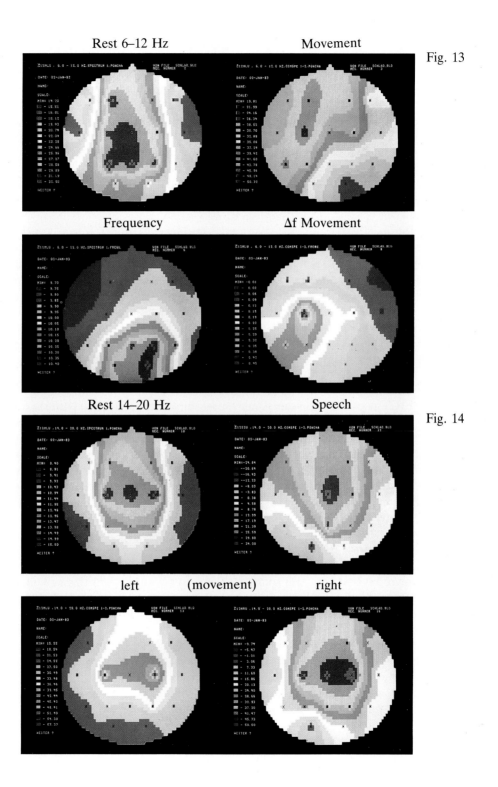

COMMENTS

Large parts of the brain are always active and the cortical activation pattern changes throughout life. This raises the question of the reliability and reproducibility of brain activity patterns calculated by computer methods. A prerequisite for all methods resulting in topographical display of brain activity pattern is, therefore, a controlled experimental condition resulting in a largely reproducible status of the brain. The "worst case" must then be the recording of brain electrical activity during "rest", with the patient thinking, fantasizing or becoming sleepy. This is a completely uncontrolled condition that can never be reproduced.

ERD mapping represents a first step toward obtaining reliable and reproducible maps of the brain activity pattern, whereby a given event is repeated several times so that a special brain status is established.

Repetition of externally paced stimulation, however, can result in a habituation effect of the neural response dependent on the stimulation condition. Internally paced movement or speech depends on emotional factors as well as the cooperation of the subject, on learning effects and the degree of automatization. Frequent hand squeezing, for example, can be done nearly automatically without extensive cortical involvement, while infrequent voluntary hand squeezing with long intervals in between is a much more complex task, where seconds can lie between the intention and the execution of each single movement (Kornhuber and Deecke, 1964). In this time period, the interfacing between the conscious mind, on the one hand, and the modules of the cerebral cortex concerned in planning and control of voluntary movements, on the other, takes place.

The ERD maps shown in this paper represent cortical activation patterns averaged over one second during sensory and motor behavioral processes. In principle, this time can be reduced to some milliseconds, when the ERD is not calculated in the frequency domain from spectra (compare Fig. 4a) but in the time domain from the band power versus time curve (compare Fig. 4b) and referring the band power decrease to the band power in the reference period only. The repetition of the event and the averaging process allow the use of statistical methods to verify significant changes in brain activity. ERD maps can therefore be computed only for statistically significant blocking responses in the EEG activity.

The figures presented have shown the development and some psychological and clinical applications of ERD mapping. Despite some spectacular pictures, it is worth mentioning that there are still some problems to be solved with this new technique. One major problem is the limited number of channels used for the calculation of ERD maps. In further studies, a greater number of channels will have to be used to obtain a higher resolution. The second problem concerns the question of referential versus bipolar recording. Referential recordings result in a distribution of EEG amplitudes (power) over the scalp more amenable to interpretation; transverse bipolar recordings result in a more pronounced ERD and are therefore better suited for ERD mapping. As early as 1938, Jasper and Andrews recommended bipolar derivations with closely spaced electrodes for studying localized blocking phenomena. Studies with calculated source derivations were also performed but did not succeed because of limited numbers of channels.

Another point of interest is the geometrical distortion of the cerebral anatomy. ERD maps show the head from above in a somewhat idealized manner. Sometimes it is difficult to coordinate regions with ERD with the correct anatomical structure. Here an approach as used by Buchsbaum et al. (1982b) should be helpful. And last but not least, it should be emphasized that the question of statistical validity is still an unsolved problem; that is, there must be further improvement in the control of the experimental situations. Nevertheless, ERD mapping seems to be a very promising new technique in applied brain research. The main advantages of this new technique are that it does not use radioactive isotopes, can be applied frequently without any danger to the patient, can be done in every modern EEG laboratory and finally, is very inexpensive. Considering all these facts, ERD mapping is a new tool for brain research offering interesting outlooks on the psychological and neurophysiological investigation of the human brain and can also be used to create a visual image of cortical regions with neuronal dysfunction after cerebrovascular insufficiency and a normal CT scan.

SUMMARY

This paper introduces a method that allows the topographical display of brief (seconds) EEG changes using multiple EEG recordings. These EEG changes occur in the form of an event-related desynchronization (ERD) or blocking of rhythmic activities within the alpha and beta bands. This ERD can be measured after externally paced events (e.g. light stimulation) or in parallel to internally self-paced events (e.g. voluntary hand movements, spontaneous speech). To obtain a reliable result, the event has to be repeated several times.

Using this technique for calculating an ERD map, local cortical activation can be visualized, e.g. over the occipital pole during light perception or over the sensorimotor region during voluntary hand movements. ERD maps therefore visualize event-related cortical activation patterns, similar to those obtained by regional blood flow measurements with isotopes (landscapes) or by positron emission tomography.

EEG maps (topographical display of alpha activity) and ERD maps from two normal volunteers and three patients with unilateral cerebral ischemia are presented and discussed. ERD maps are calculated during light perception, voluntary hand movements and spontaneous speech.

ACKNOWLEDGMENT

This investigation was supported by the "Fonds zur Förderung der wissenschaftlichen Forschung", project 4953, and the "Fonds zur Förderung der gewerblichen Wirtschaft". The authors gratefully acknowledge the assistance of Mrs. H. Blumenschein in preparing the speech experiments.

REFERENCES

Berger, H. (1929) Über das Elektroenkephalogramm des Menschen. *Arch. Psychiat. Nervenkr.*, 87: 527–570.

302

Buchsbaum, M. S., Ingvar, D. M., Kessler, R., Waters R. N., Cappelletti, J., van Kammen, D. P., King, A. C., Johnson, J. L., Manning, R. G., Flynn, R. W., Mann, L. S., Bunney, Jr., W. E. and Sokoloff, L. (1982a) Cerebral glucography with positron tomography. *Arch. Gen. Psychiatry*, 39: 251–259.

Buchsbaum, M. S., Rigal F., Coppola, R., Cappelletti, J., King, C. and Johnson, J. (1982b) A new system for grey-level surface distribution maps of electrical activity. *Electroenceph. clin. Neurophysiol.*, 53: 237–242.

Duffy, F. H. (1981) Brain electrical activity mapping (BEAM): Computerized access to complex brain function. *Int. J. Neurosci. eng.*, 13/1: 55–65.

Duffy, F. H., Burchfiel, J. L. and Lombroso, C. T. (1978) Brain Electrical Activity Mapping (BEAM): a method for extending the clinical utility of EEG and evoked potential data. *Ann. Neurol.*, 5: 309–321.

Frackowiak, R. S. J., Lenzi, G. L., Jones, T. and Heather, J. D. (1980) Quantitative measurement of regional blood flow and oxygen metabolism in man using ^{15}O and positron emission tomography: Theory, procedure, and normal values. *J. Comp. Ass. Tomogr.*, 4: 727–736.

Ingvar, D. H. (1979) "Hyperfrontal" distribution of cerebral grey matter flow in resting wakefulness; on the functional anatomy of the conscious state. *Acta. neurol. scand.*, 60: 12–25.

Jasper, H. and Andrews, H. L. (1938) Electro-encephalography. III. Normal differentiations of occipital and precentral regions in man. *Arch. Neurol. Psychiat. (Chic.)*, 39: 96–115.

Jasper, H. and Penfield, W. (1949) Electrocorticograms in man: Effect of voluntary movement upon the electrical activity of the precentral gyrus. *Arch. Psychiat. Z. Neurol.*, 183: 163–174.

Jenkins, G. M. and Watts, D. G. (1968) *Spectral Analysis and its Applications*, Holden-Day, San Francisco–Cambridge–London–Amsterdam.

Jolesz, F. A. (1983) Functional imaging of the brain. *Med. Instrum. (USA)*, 17: 59–62.

Kornhuber, H. H. and Deecke, L. (1964) Hirnpotential-änderungen beim Menschen vor und nach Willkürbewegungen, dargestellt mit Magnetbandspeicherung und Rückwärtsanalyse. *Pflügers Arch. ges. Physiol.*, 281: 52.

Ladurner, G., Zilkha, E., Iliff, L. D., Du Boulay, G., Marshal, J. (1976) Measurement of the regional cerebral blood volume by computerized axial tomography. *J. Neurol. Neurosurg. Psychiat.*, 39: 152–158.

Lassen, N. A. (1980) Regional cerebral blood flow measured with Xenon-133 inhalation using emission tomography. *Rev. E.E.G. Neuro-Physiol.Clin.*, 10/4: 407–411.

Lauritzen, M., Henriksen, L. and Lassen, N. A. (1981) Regional cerebral blood flow during rest and skilled hand movements by Xenon-133 inhalation and emission computerized tomography. *J. Cereb. Blood Flow Metab.*, 1: 385–389.

Meyer, J. S., Hayman, L. A., Amano, T., Nakajima, S., Shaw, T., Lauzon, P., Derman, S., Karacan, I. and Harati, Y. (1981) Mapping local blood flow of human brain by CT scanning during stable Xenon inhalation. *Stroke*, 12: 426–436.

Nagata, K., Mizukami, M., Araki, G., Kawase, T. and Hirano, M. (1982) Topographic electroencephalographic study of cerebral infarction using computed mapping of the EEG. *J. Cereb. Blood Flow Metab.*, 2: 79–88.

Phelps, E. M., Mazziotta, J. C. and Huang, S.-C. (1982) Review study of cerebral function with positron computed tomography. *J. Cereb. Blood Flow Metab.* 2: 113–162.

Pfurtscheller, G. (1983) *A new multifunctional system for investigation of brain dysfunction*. United Nations Seminar on Innovation in Biomedical Equipment, Budapest, Hungary, May 1983.

Pfurtscheller, G. and Aranibar, A. (1977) Event-related cortical desynchronization detected by power measurements of scalp EEG. *Electroenceph. clin. Neurophysiol.*, 42: 817–826.

Pfurtscheller, G. and Aranibar, A. (1980) Voluntary movement ERD: normative studies. In G. Pfurtscheller, P. Buser, F. H. Lopes da Silva and H. Petsche (Eds.), *Rhythmic EEG Activities and Cortical Functioning*, Elsevier, Amsterdam, pp.151–177.

Sokoloff, L. (1981) Relationships among local functional activity, energy metabolism, and blood flow in the cerebral nervous system, *Fed. Proc.*, 40/8: 2311–2316.

Brain Ischemia: Quantitative EEG and Imaging Techniques, Progress in Brain Research, Vol. 62, edited by
G. Pfurtscheller, E.J. Jonkman and F.H. Lopes da Silva

Comparison of Electrophysiologic and Metabolic Changes in the Human Epileptic Cortex

PETER K. H. WONG[1] and R. EUGENE RAMSAY[2]

[1]Department of Paediatrics, University of British Columbia, Vancouver, B.C. (Canada) and
[2]Department of Neurology, University of Miami, FL (USA)

INTRODUCTION

This study attempts to correlate several different diagnostic techniques in the investigation of patients with focal epilepsy. These include computed tomography (CT), electroencephalography (EEG), topographic evoked potential (TEP) recording, positron emission tomography (PET) and cortical surface redox state measurements using spectrophotometry (SP).

In general, patients with focal epileptic disorders first have a clinical examination and routine EEG. A CT scan may be carried out to demonstrate the presence of a focal anatomic lesion (Gastaut and Gastaut, 1976). The patient may ultimately proceed to surgery. The area for excision is usually defined by intra-operative electrocorticography (ECoG) (Falconer and Davidson, 1974; Engel et al., 1980).

Under certain situations, there may be significant error in the diagnosis of the lesion site. The CT scan may be non-contributory. Inter-ictal and ictal EEG recordings may show only bilaterally synchronous discharges, or present conflicting localization information. Depth recording may not always be possible or advantageous. Information about cerebral metabolism and blood flow can be obtained using PET techniques.

Inter-ictally, epileptic cortex is associated with regional hypometabolism (Kuhl et al., 1980; Engel et al., 1981). Despite its usefulness, PET remains a very expensive item and not commonly available in most centers. The use of TEP in a clinical group as described here has not been reported previously. Spectral measurements of EEG using topographic display techniques have been described in cerebral ischemia (Nagata et al., 1982), cerebral tumors (Duffy et al., 1979) and dyslexia (Duffy et al., 1980).

Direct intra-operative cortical metabolic measurements using spectrophotometry have been applied in both human and animal models. It is relatively non-invasive and allows estimation of oxidative metabolism and oxygen utilization. Preliminary results indicate that epileptic cortex can be distinguished from normal cortex by its response to electrical stimulation (Van Buren et al., 1978). Due to the fact that the measurement area is small, accurate intra-operative "mapping" of the exposed cortex may be carried out, complementing traditional ECoG.

[303]

MATERIAL AND METHODS

Patient population

The present series was made up of three patients. All had routine clinical examinations, several routine EEG investigations, video/EEG telemetry monitoring, routine X-rays, CT scan and TEP. Two had PET scans and two had intraoperative SP measurements. Intra-operative ECoGs were obtained in all. Table I provides a summary of the clinical information.

TABLE I

PATIENT SUMMARY

Patient	Age (yrs)	Clinical Seizure	EEG Focus	CT Scan	Topographic EP	Surgery	Follow-up
1	36 M	Partial complex-temporal ? (R)	(R) temporal	Normal	Hypoactive (R) frontal temporal area	(R) temporal lobe total resection	Seizure free – Working full-time
2	36 M	Psycho-motor-frontal or temporal (L)	(L) frontal	(L) frontal hypodensity and atrophy	Hypoactive (L) frontal (increased post-ictal)	(L) frontal – extensive	Seizure free
3	27 F	Partial complex-temporal ? (R)	(R) temporal	Bilateral frontal parasagittal atrophy	Extensive hypoactivity: (R) post. temp. > (R) parietal > (R) frontal	(R) temporal lobe, (R) orbital-frontal cortex	Seizure free

The major criteria in the selection of patients for surgical treatment were: (1) medical intractability despite adequate treatment with multiple anticonvulsant medication for over 2 years; (2) the seizures were judged to be devastating from a socioeconomic standpoint; (3) the seizures appeared focal in nature from clinical, X-ray and/or electrical evidence (scalp EEG and/or depth recording); (4) the focus was in a resectable region of the cerebral cortex.

EEG

Routine EEGs were obtained using at least 16 recording channels and sometimes 21 channels. Silver-silver chloride electrodes were applied with collodion using the international 10–20 electrode system. Both reference and bipolar montages were used. Electrode impedances were below 5 KOhms. A time constant of 0.3 sec and upper frequency cutoff of 70 Hz were generally used. Several inter-ictal recordings were obtained. Telemetry monitoring was carried out to obtain ictal EEG and simultaneous behavioral manifestations. A Grass model-8 electroencephalograph and a Telefactor split-screen video-EEG monitoring apparatus were used.

Topographic EP

TEP measurements were obtained using a microcomputer connected to the electroencephalograph using 21 EEG channels. The output from the EEG amplifiers was connected to an analog-to-digital converter. The conversion rate was 500 samples per second, at 8 bit precision. Artefacts were rejected by voltage overload sensing. Amplifier bandwidths were nominally set at 1–70 Hz. Stimulation (1 per second) was performed with diffuse light using a stroboscopic lamp (Grass Model PS1) placed approximately 12 inches in front of the patient in the midline. Two hundred samples were collected. Patients were instructed to keep their eyes closed and remain alert. At least two trials were obtained. Patient (2) had a seizure during the procedure; TEPs were thus obtained in the pre-ictal, ictal and post-ictal phases.

Online topographic maps of the EP were created using a digital-to-video graphics interface giving 16 gray tones. The topographic display consisted of the superimposition of the 21 electrode positions within a schematized head diagram (see Fig. 1). The maps are orientated as follows: each dot denotes an electrode position; the

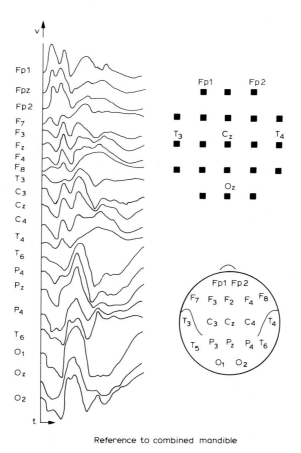

Reference to combined mandible

Fig. 1. Topographic map layout; reference to combined mandible. On the left a series of visual evoked potentials (0–512 ms).

anterior head is the top, the posterior head is the bottom, and right is the right side of the maps. The gray scale was set as follows: black represented maximal negative voltage, white represented maximal positive voltage, and medium gray represented zero voltage level. Nominally, each gray scale corresponded to approximately 10 μV. Thus, 16 gray levels could represent a voltage range of 160 μV. However, digital scaling of the averaged and digitized voltage values may be carried out, thus allowing a greater or lower digital sensitivity for the display. Conventional voltage versus time display of all channels was also possible online.

Each map consisted of 21 real values corresponding to each electrode position. All points between these electrode positions were computer calculated as the averaged value of the four nearest real electrode voltage values. These calculations were weighted by the distance from each of the four neighboring (nearest) electrodes. Thus a point near any one electrode would have a value close to it, while a point equidistant from its nearest four electrodes would have a mathematical average of these four real electrode values. There were 15 such interpolated points separating any two real electrodes. This interpolation "filled in" the unknown scalp voltage values between the real electrode grid and was necessary as the number of recording electrodes was limited. This linear interpolation guarded against possible statistical errors introduced by the use of non-linear techniques.

A TEP "scan" consisted of a "movie" of individual maps, each map (or frame) representing the scalp field at one instant in time. Maps were separated by two milliseconds of real time. The computer can play the movie rapidly at a rate of several frames per second, thus allowing a dynamic spatial-temporal display of cerebral electrical activity.

All sampled data were stored on floppy diskettes for later review. They also served as the basis for communicating data between the two principal investigators.

Another display format used for such TEP data was the "integrated map" (Fig. 2). This was obtained by integrating the "area under the curve" for each channel from 0–512 ms. Other time segments could be chosen instead to cover points of interest. After appropriate scaling, the integrated map was displayed. After integration, the + and − voltage values no longer had polarity significance, thus the black color then indicated low area value and white color high area value. This could be interpreted as "hypoactivity" or "hyperactivity", respectively.

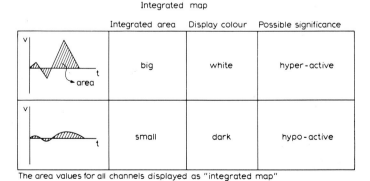

Fig. 2. Method used to obtain "integrated maps".

PET

A PET-V machine was used which had a seven slice capability; each slice was 15 mm thick. The isotopes used were: [^{11}C]deoxyglucose (DG) for absolute cerebral metabolic rate (MR), ^{15}O-labeled water for cerebral blood flow (CBF); ^{15}O-labeled CO_2 for cerebral blood volume, and ^{11}C-labeled valproic acid (VPA) for cerebral VPA uptake. Only the DG results will be discussed here. Sokoloff's rate constants were used for calculation of regional metabolic rate (Sokoloff, 1977). Approximately 12 points of each PET slice were quantified to yield average regional MR values. Overall hemispheric averages were obtained from these values. Comparison with normal values of regional and hemispheric MRs were then made. The range of normal values in our laboratory was 4.37–5.07 g/100 g/min, with a hemispheric asymmetry of < 10.2%.

Spectrophotometry (SP)

Dual wave length reflection SP of exposed cortex was carried out. Tissue was excited with light directed through a fiber-optic bundle, with the reflected light collected by a focused photo-multiplier tube. The light source was a 250-watt tungsten–halogen lamp with appropriate filtering to provide twin beams at 605 and 590 nm. The former wave length was chosen as it had the maximum absorption peak of cytochrome oxidase (cytochrome a, a_3). The latter wave length was chosen as it was off the absorption peak, and varied parallel to the 605 nm wave length when changes in tissue blood volume and oxygen saturation occurred. Details of the optical procedure are available elsewhere (Rosenthal et al., 1981).

Intra-operatively, electrical stimulation of the cortex under optical measurements was performed using an isolated constant voltage unit. Stimulation was applied through a pair of stainless-steel electrodes approximately 0.25 mm in diameter and 2 mm apart, placed on the cortical surface. Stimuli consisted of single pulses or pulse trains repeated at intervals. Generally, 1–2 sec pulse trains were used at a frequency of 10–20 Hz; each rectangular pulse had a duration of 0.5 msec. Photometric readings were then obtained to measure observable mitochondria redox shifts. ECoG, photometric response (oxidative or reductive), and stimulation pulses were recorded simultaneously. Measurements were taken over several areas, including both normal cortex and suspected epileptiform focus.

RESULTS

Table I summarizes both patient information and results of EEG, CT and TEP studies, together with the extent of surgery and brief follow-up notes. Patient (1) had the complete right temporal lobe removed. Patient (2) had an extensive removal of left frontal cortex. Both patients were seizure free on follow-up. The third patient underwent a removal of the right temporal lobe and also a partial removal of right orbital frontal cortex. There was complete cessation of seizures in the first postoperative month. The epileptic focus was localized in all patients on clinical grounds. Both routine EEG recordings and long term video/EEG telemetry provided information affirming the clinical localization. The CT scan was normal in the first patient and

308

showed focal abnormalities in the second and third patient. Focal atrophy was seen in patients (2) and (3), while extensive hypodensity was noted in patient (2) in addition.

TEP

TEP results (Fig. 3) were in agreement with the localization on clinical, EEG and CT grounds. (Due to the large number of individual maps comprising a TEP, only the integrated maps representing the entire epoch are shown). The integrated maps of patient (1) showed a large asymmetry in the temporal areas. There was extensive hypoactivity in the right temporal lobe, maximal in the anterior temporal-frontal areas. This was seen as an area of dark coloration in the map. In patient (2), the TEP was recorded prior to one of the patient's typical seizures, during the seizure, and 30 min thereafter. The pre-ictal integrated map showed an area of hypoactivity in the left frontal-anterior temporal areas. During the seizure, hypoactivity was seen in a more extensive region, maximal in the left central-midtemporal areas, but also present in the left frontal, anterior temporal, and posterior temporal areas. This hypoactivity was more significant than that on the pre-ictal map. The post-ictal map showed the same intense hypoactivity now maximal in the left mid-temporal area, although involving the left posterior temporal and left central areas as well. A comparison can be made between this patient's TEP maps and his CT scan shown in Fig. 4.

Patient (3) also had a markedly asymmetric TEP. He had an area of marked hypoactivity in the right posterior temporal-parietal areas, with extension to involve the entire right temporal lobe and right frontal-anterior temporal regions.

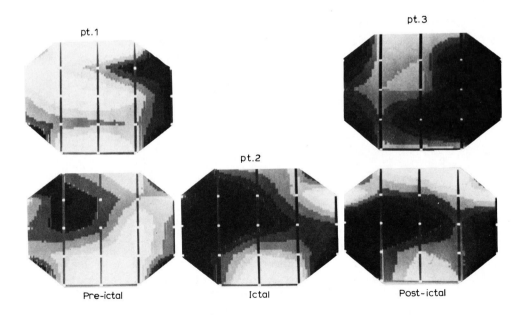

Fig. 3. Topographic evoked potentials (TEP) represented as integrated maps for three patients. For explanation see text, p. 306.

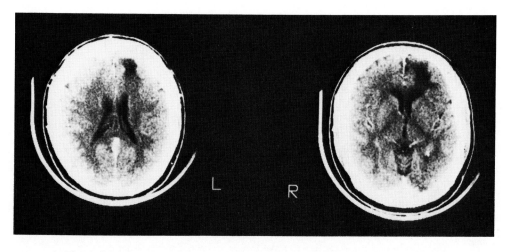

Fig. 4. CT scan of patient 2, showing hypodensity and atrophy of left frontal area.

PET

The regional CBF results using ^{11}O water were not encouraging. This may be due to the low resolution possible with this tracer. In contrast, the [^{11}C]DG studies were very encouraging. They are shown in Fig. 5. In patient (1), there was a hypometabolic "ring" in the anterior, medial and posterior regions of the right temporal lobe. Absolute metabolic rates of both patients (1) and (2) are presented in Table II.

Patient (2) had a markedly hypometabolic area in the left anterior frontal region, extending from the frontal pole posteriorly. There was also some extension to the left frontal-anterior temporal regions. Patient (3) did not have PET studies.

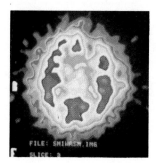
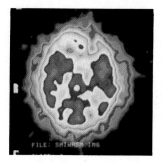
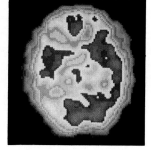

Fig. 5. PET [^{11}C]deoxyglucose (DG) images. As in Fig. 4 (CT scans) the left side of the patient is depicted on the right side of the slices. The two images on the left are from patient 1, and the right slice is from patient 2. Metabolic rate from brown (highest), yellow, green to blue (lowest): PET metabolic rates in g/glucose/100 g brain tissue/min. For explanation see above.

TABLE II

PET GLUCOSE METABOLIC RATES IN g/100 g BRAIN TISSUE/MIN.

Normal range 4.37–5.07; right–left asymmetry $< 10.2\%$

Area	Right	Left	Asymmetry (%)
Patient 1			
Normal temporal lobe	4.82	5.06	4.7
Anterior to normal temporal lobe	3.92	4.88	19.7
Posterior to normal temporal lobe	3.88	4.90	20.8
Patient 2			
Mean hemispheric	4.20	4.37	3.9
Frontal	3.49	2.62	24.8

Spectrophotometry

Figure 6 summarizes representative SP results from our patient material. The figure contains original traces recorded at two cortical sites. The upper trace at each site provides the difference between light reflected at 605 nm and at 590 nm, representing changes in the reduction/oxidation ratio of cytochrome a,a_3. Oxidative shifts were represented by a downward deflection in this signal, corresponding to decreased absorption at 605 nm. ECoG recordings were made in the approximate area of optical stimulation.

As shown in the figure in the traces labeled "Site 1", direct application of electrical stimulation pulses to the cortical surface (4 mA peak-to-peak) produced an oxidative shift. The stimulus train was indicated by the thickened ECoG artefact. This oxidative shift peaked within 5 sec following termination of the stimulus train and recovered to baseline within approximately 40 sec. Similar oxidative shifts were recorded with stimulus intensities from 1 to 5 mA. Such oxidative responses as obtained in this patient are consistent with the stimulus-evoked oxidative responses observed in animal experiments (Kreisman et al., 1981).

Results over the epileptic area are shown as "Site 2", which demonstrated a transient increase in reduction of cyctochrome a,a_3. This was the area of maximal afterdischarge upon electrical stimulation and was considered to be the center of the epileptic focus. Thus we have a reversal from the normal tissue recording: a reductive response to electrical stimulation rather than an oxidative response.

DISCUSSION

None of the investigative techniques produced disagreement on the localization of an epileptic focus. The CT scan was sometimes uninformative, as in patient (1), where three repeated CT studies were all normal. This may be due to the fact that an epileptic focus will not necessarily show up as an anatomic lesion.

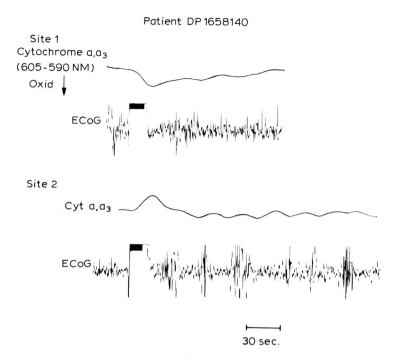

Patient DP 1658140

Site 1
Cytochrome a,a₃
(605-590 NM)
Oxid ↓

ECoG

Site 2

Cyt a,a₃

ECoG

30 sec.

Fig. 6. The electrocorticogram (ECoG) and the spectrophotometric measurements are shown for two cortical sides. The latter represents the changes in the reduction/oxidation ratio of cytochrome a,a_3. The ECoG artefact (black bar) is caused by the direct electrical stimulation of the cortical surface. For details see text, p. 310.

The TEP studies were very interesting. Analysis of the actual TEP "movie" of the entire epoch of 512 ms demonstrated the evolution of the evoked electrical activity in response to the visual stimuli. The integrated map was most convenient as a summary of the entire evoked potential. In one single frame, it allowed a graphic representation of areas of asymmetry. Our working hypothesis is that a low value of "area under the curve" of the voltage-time tracing correlates with a physiologically hypoactive cortical region. It is important to note that these areas of presumed TEP "hypoactivity" agreed well with the real hypometabolic regions as demonstrated by the PET scans.

One has to be careful in the comparison of these TEP maps and the PET scans. The former represent scalp voltage changes, while the PET scan images are actual horizontal slices through the cerebral hemisphere, demonstrating subcortical areas that are not generally accessible by scalp EEG recordings. We may view the TEP map as a "curved scalp slice" for purposes of comparison. It is thus subject to cartographic distortion when translation is done from a curved human scalp to a flat video display plane. In this case, the most lateral part of the convexity is under-represented.

The ictal TEP series in patient (2) is particularly impressive. It demonstrates an alternation of scalp responses during the progression from the pre-ictal to the post-ictal phase. By systematically studying more data, one may monitor the behavior of the cortical response in the resting and ictal phases, and at different times in the post-ictal phase. Knowledge of the ictal and recovery behavior may provide further insight on the epileptic focus.

312

For patients (1) and (2), the absolute MRs are shown in Table II. For patient (1), the MR of the relatively normal tissues in the right and the entire left temporal lobes were within normal limits. There was only a 4.7% asymmetry. However, the epileptic areas, anterior and posterior to the midtemporal region on the right, were hypometabolic. The relative asymmetry was approximately 20% (lower on the right side). There was no overall hemispheric abnormality. Patient (2) had a normal left hemispheric MR, but a minimally abnormal mean hemispheric MR on the right. The asymmetry was only 3.9%, and not significant. His frontal MR on the right and left were both diminished. The left frontal value was lower at 2.62 g glucose/100 g/min. Compared to the right frontal value of 3.49 (also low) the asymmetry was 24.8%. While the left frontal hypometabolism was expected, the slight low right frontal value was unexplainable.

The SP results were highly encouraging. All patients studied showed abnormal oxidative/reductive measurements over the epileptic areas. Furthermore, there was no disagreement between the SP determinations and the ECoG tracings. The method has shown itself to be relatively simple to use and complimentary in nature to other electrophysiologic measurements.

Close examination of the SP tracings from the abnormal area revealed that small increases in reduction appear to accompany spontaneous bursts of high-amplitude waves in the ECoG. It may be speculated that such epileptic areas may have an inappropriate response to increased energy demands. Thus, the results would suggest that there are basic metabolic differences between tissue of the normal cortex and of an epileptic focus.

CONCLUSION

Our small patient series has very much encouraged us to pursue our investigative protocol using these multiple techniques.

In particular, the TEP results appear exciting. TEP is very promising as a simple and non-invasive measure of physiologic function, potentially able to identify areas of cortical dysfunction.

SUMMARY

This study investigates the use of clinical electrophysiology (scalp- and cortical EEG, topographic evoked potential – TEP), computed tomography (CT) and positron emission tomography (PET) in patients undergoing epilepsy surgery. A PET-V machine was used with seven slice capability. The TEP mapping studies used a microcomputer utilizing 21 simultaneous EEG channels with online topographic display.

Patients were initially referred for intractable and socio-economically incapacitating seizures. All had a discrete focal epileptic area identified by routine scalp EEG and CT studies. The next step involved depth EEG recordings, PET studies of cerebral blood flow (CBF) and deoxyglucose (DG) uptake, and TEP using visual flash stimulus. Only those patients with a unilateral epileptic focus were then operated upon.

An attempt was also made to study the cortical metabolic state by intra-operative measurement of redox state changes, in both epileptic tissue and adjacent normal tissue, following brief electrical stimulation. Epileptic cortex correlated with decreased DG and/or CBF on PET, abnormal TEP maps and abnormal redox studies. Preliminary data are presented.

ACKNOWLEDGMENT

The authors wish to acknowledge the valuable assistance of C. Pennimpede, and the Biomedical Communications Department of UBC for preparation of the manuscript; Drs. M. Rosenthal, J. M. Van Buren and T. Sick for their part in the surgery and acquisition of data.

REFERENCES

Duffy, F. H., Burchfiel, J. L. and Lombroso, C. T. (1979) Brain electrical activity mapping (BEAM): a method for extending the clinical utility of EEG and evoked potential data. *Ann. Neurol.*, 5: 309–321.

Duffy, F. H., Denckla, M. B., Bartels, P. H. and Sardini, G. (1980) Dyslexia: regional differences in brain electrical activity by topographic mapping. *Ann. Neurol.*, 7: 412–420.

Engel, J., Rausch, R., Lieb, J. P., Kuhl, D. E. and Crandall, P. H. (1980) Re-evaluation of criteria for localizing epileptic foci in patients considered for surgical therapy of epilepsy. *Ann. Neurol.*, 9: 215–224.

Engel, J., Rausch, R., Lieb, J. P., Kuhl, D. E. and Crandall, P. H. (1981) Correlation of criteria used for localizing epileptic foci in patients considered for surgical therapy of epilepsy. *Ann. Neurol.*, 9: 215–224.

Falconer, M. A. and Davidson, S. (1974) The rationale of surgical treatment of temporal lobe epilepsy with particular reference to childhood and adolescence. In P. Harris and C. Mawdsley (Eds.); *Epilepsy, Proceedings of the Hans Berger Centenary Symposium*, Churchill/Livingstone, Edinburgh–London–New York, pp. 209–214.

Gastaut, H. and Gastaut, J. L. (1976) Computerized transverse axial tomography in epilepsy. *Epilepsia*, 17: 325–336.

Kreisman, N. R., Sick, T. J., LaManna, J. C. and Rosenthal, M. (1981) Local tissue oxygen tension-cytochrome a,a_3 redox relationships in rat cerebral cortex in vivo. *Brain Res.* 218: 161–174.

Kuhl, D. E., Engel, J., Phelps, M. E. and Selin, C. (1980) Epileptic patterns of local cerebral metabolism and perfusion in humans determined by emission computed tomography of ^{18}FDG and ^{13}NH$_3$. *Ann. Neurol.*, 8: 348–360.

Nagata, K., Mizukami, M., Araki, G., Kawase, T. and Hirano, M. (1982) Topographic EEG study of cerebral infarction using computed mapping of the EEG. *J. Cereb. Blood Flow Metab.*, 2: 79–88.

Rosenthal, M. and LaManna, J. C. (1981) Applications of optical techniques to brain physiology, In A. G. B. Kovach, E. Monosand and G. Rubanyi (Eds.), *Advances in Physiological Sciences, Vol 8, Cardiovascular Physiology: Heart, Peripheral Circulation and Methodology*, Pergamon Press, New York, pp. 343–352.

Sokoloff, L., Reivich, M. and Kennedy, C. et al. (1977) The [^{14}C]deoxyglucose method for the measurement of local cerebral glucose utilization: theory, procedure and normal values in the conscious and anesthetized albino rat. *J. Neurochem.*, 28: 897–916.

Van Buren, J. M., Lewis, D. V., Schuette, W. H., Whitehouse, W. C. and Marsan, C. A. (1978) Fluorometric monitoring of NADH levels in cerebral cortex: preliminary observations in human epilepsy. *Neurosurgery* 2: 114–121.

Subject Index

Activity time, 67
Acute ischemia, 8, 153
   stroke, 249
Adam–Stokes attacks, 75
Affected hemisphere, 46
Age, 5, 14, 34, 40, 70, 80, 124, 150
   dependency of frequency, 14
   factor, 71, 81
   normalized frequency, 34
   specific frequency, 34, 124
Alpha activity, 70, 76, 158, 165, 227, 275, 282, 292
   band, 11, 61, 67, 86, 154, 218, 273, 290
   blocking, 6, 150, 293
   mean frequency, 7, 54, 76
   peak frequency, 13, 17, 22, 123, 128, 155, 293,
      asymmetry, 13, 15, 17, 22, 126
      shift, 15
   power, 32, 108, 123, 218, 292
      asymmetry, 13, 17, 155
      reactivity, 24
   rhythm, 5, 55, 57, 99, 109, 124, 150, 288
Alzheimer's disease, 146
Anastomosis, 3, 30, 107, 121, 140, 146, 160, 203, 210, 235, 245, 272, 277
Anesthesia, 77, 86, 160, 176, 186, 202, 218, 225
Animal experiments, 86, 87, 148, 160, 175, 187, 201, 217, 239
Angiographic findings, 30, 89, 107, 123, 210, 236, 276
Anoxic damage, 149
Aphasia, 253, 272, 275, 281
Artifact rejection, 31, 123
Asymmetry measurements, 7, 11, 37, 58, 90, 113, 130, 139, 150, 156, 277, 280, 310
Atrioventricular block, 74
Autoradiography, 87, 160, 162, 203, 230
Autoregressive model, 32, 151
Averaged frequency, 52
   parameters, 34

Baboon, 153, 187
Band power, 13, 47, 108, 123, 150, 163, 292
   parameters, 16, 17
Barbiturate, 160, 217, 224
Basal ganglia, 115, 124, 153, 162, 211, 254, 256
Beta activity, 99, 227, 299
   power, 32, 86, 123, 154, 218, 273
Bipolar recording, 31, 88, 122, 187, 218, 288
Blood flow, 68, 74, 92, 109, 140, 153, 161, 191
Bootstrap, 44
Bradycardia, 75

Brain edema, 100, 140, 160, 202, 230
   electrolyte, 86
   infarction, 46, 76, 99, 126, 162, 201, 254, 281, 295
   metabolism, 29, 70, 79, 139, 162, 179, 254, 307
   stem, 195
   temperature, 229
   tumor, 71, 88, 96, 303
   water content, 86
Breach rhythm, 139
Broca's area, 248, 273, 296
Bypass operation, *see Anastomosis*

Canonogram, 7
Cardiac pacemaker, 73
Carotid endarterectomy, 3, 30, 91, 146, 235, 249
   artery occlusion, 91, 159, 198, 277
Cat, 87, 93, 148, 239
Central conduction time, 186, 198
   gyrus, 204, 212, 288, 298
Cerebral blood flow (CBF), 68, 86, 145, 152, 180, 185, 191, 230, 240, 275, 295
   asymmetry, 90, 113, 157, 248
   calculation, 87
   diaschisis, 147, 202
   measurement, 68, 87
   volume, 249, 307
Cerebral function monitor, 176
Cerebral infarction, 20, 61, 76, 98
Cerebral ischemia, 5, 20, 68, 225, 281
Cerebral metabolic rate for glucose, 256
Cerebral metabolism, 69, 175, 211, 307
Cerebral oxygen consumption, 78, 310
Cerebrovascular disease, 3, 9, 30, 52, 71, 88, 99, 107, 122, 153, 165, 245, 276, 296
Clinical outcome, 111, 124, 159, 282
   score, 154
Clusters, 34, 71
Coherence, 11, 23, 150
Completed stroke, 4, 30, 45, 110, 115, 246, 283
   ischemia, 175
Compression ischemia, 176
Computed mapping of EEG, 272, 292
Computerized tomography, 4, 6, 20, 30, 46, 124, 152, 245, 264, 272, 296, 304
   topography, 108, 268, 273, 292, 305
Conformation, 7, 14
Consciousness, 116, 138, 181, 253
Cortex, 124, 189, 202, 225, 311
Cortical electrodes, 153, 162, 187
   flow, 69

Cortical infarction, 46, 126, 212, 281, 295
  ischemia, 131
  necrosis, 181
  temperature, 227
Critical ischemia, 93, 99
Crossed cerebellar diaschisis, 249
Cross-validation, 44
Cytochrome oxidase, 307, 310

Deactivated tissue, 257
Delta activity, 6, 55, 75, 77, 80, 93, 99, 139, 146, 281
  band, 67, 70, 154, 273
  power, 32, 86, 108, 123, 206, 218, 227
Deoxyglucose, 160, 203, 240, 254, 307
Depth electrodes, 160, 190, 202, 240
Diaschisis, 116, 134, 147, 164, 166, 202, 249
Diffuse projection system, 80
Discriminant analysis, 33, 71
Dog, 217

Edema, *see Brain edema*
EEG asymmetries, 7, 13, 35, 40, 58, 60, 126, 139, 150, 156, 277, 280, 297, 310
  diaschisis, 134, 164, 166
  flattening, 227
  focus, 96, 280
  frequency, 73, 139, 148
    analysis, 86, 88
    index, 74, 94, 149
  intensity, 92
  map, 7, 108, 268, 273, 291
  mean power, 148
  reactivity, 7, 32, 293
  suppression, 94
  topography, 7, 108, 268, 275, 291
Electrocorticography, 185, 307, 311
Electrolyte, 86
  disturbances, 91
  homeostasis, 100
EMG, 77
Encephalitis, 79
Energy failure, 149, 175
  index, 67
  metabolism, 181
Equipotential map, 108, 275
Epileptic focus, 307
ERD asymmetry, 130
  map, 292, 300
Etomidate, 218
Event-related desynchronization (ERD), 32, 47, 116, 123, 150, 287
Evoked potential, 149, 175, 185, 201, 240, 305
  asymmetry 205
  topography 305
Experimental brain tumors, 95
  focal ischemia, 86, 100

  ischemia, 86, 99, 148, 152, 160, 175, 185
Extra-intracranial arterial bypass (EIAB) operation, *see Anastomosis*
Eyes opening, 11, 150

Fast Fourier Transform (FFT), 11, 32, 52, 76, 86, 108, 123, 150, 272, 290
Flow diaschisis, 166
Flunarizine, 225
Fluoro deoxyglucose, 254
Focal epilepsy, 303
  ischemia, 74, 79, 86, 88, 256, 276
Follow-up, 107, 121, 146, 159, 205
Frequency asymmetry index, 128
  index, 61, 67, 75, 86, 89, 97, 148
  map, 293, 297, 299
Frontal intermittent rhythmic delta activity, 5

Gamma camera, 76, 87, 246, 250
Gerbil, 86, 89
Glucose metabolism, 124, 257
  uptake, 162, 176, 210, 256, 264

Hand movement, 122, 138, 287
Head trauma, 96, 98
Hemiplegia, 160, 204, 210
Hemispheric flow, 280
  infarct, 160
  mean flow, 112
Hemodynamic, 249
Hemorrhage, 88, 98, 197, 217
High voltage slow focus, 110
Hill climbing, 11
Hjorth parameters, 52, 151
Hydrogen clearance, 153, 160, 186, 202
Hyperactivity, 306
Hyperglycemia, 180
Hypoactivity, 306
Hypometabolism, 312
Hypoperfusion, 248
Hypotension, 187, 193, 220
Hypovolemia, 176, 218
Hypoxia, 29, 60, 75, 79, 141, 225

Infarction acute, 97
  cerebral, 52, 98, 254
  cortical, 46, 126, 295
  hemispheric, 160
  model, 98
  non-cortical, 126, 276
Inhibitory phasing theory, 80
Initial slope index, 147, 153, 155
Integrated map, 306
Interhemispheric differences, 13, 35, 56, 125, 133, 157
Internal capsule, 12, 88, 124, 132, 197, 210, 248
  carotid artery, 107, 198, 238, 277

Intracerebral steal, 117
Intracranial pressure, 176, 225
Iodo-amphetamine, 245, 250
Ischemia acute, 97, 153
    cerebral, 5, 68, 249, 282, 204
    chronic, 165, 212, 235
    complete, 175
    compression, 176
    cortical, 131, 212, 275, 281
    critical, 93, 99
    experimental, 86, 148, 160, 175, 185, 201, 212
    focal, 74, 86, 88, 192, 235, 276, 282
    global incomplete, 225
    hypovolemic, 176
    incomplete, 175, 217
    mild, 116, 165
    minor, 4, 9
    non-critical, 93
    oligaemic, 217
    ·partial, 94
    recurrent, 282
    reversible, 4, 20
    selective, 190
    severe, 33, 115, 148, 178, 229, 253
    spontaneous, 146, 165
    subcortical, 131
    transient, 99
Ischemic penumbra, 149, 245
    stroke, 256
Isoelectric EEG, 223

Jackknife, 44

Kinetics, 257

Lactate, 176
Lacunar stroke, 282
Lacunes, 3, 4, 5
Local cerebral blood flow (lCBF), 87, 186, 202
Luxury perfusion syndrome, 69, 70, 78, 141, 281

Map, 108, 254, 268, 292, 305
    metabolic, 254, 264, 266, 309
Mean alpha frequency, 7
    amplitude, 77
    frequency, 52, 67, 73, 76, 88, 148, 151
    hemispheric CBF, 74
Medial lemniscus, 149, 188, 204
Metabolic rate, 257, 264, 307, 310
    recovery, 178
Metabolism, 29, 70, 79, 139, 152, 175, 257, 307
Microsphere technique, 87, 153
Middle cerebral artery, 87, 97, 107, 123, 148, 153, 160, 186, 202, 235, 248, 256, 272
Mild ischemia, 116, 165
Minor ischemia, 4, 9, 20
Misery perfusion, 249
Mode frequency, 80

Monitoring, 77, 146, 178, 198, 225
Monkey, 153, 160, 187, 201, 235
Movement, 7, 31, 42, 287
Multidimensional scoring, 151
Multi-infarct dementia, 146
Multiparametric asymmetry score, 40, 132, 135
Multivariable analysis, 20, 68
Multivariate linear discriminant analysis, 33
Mu peak frequency, 13, 16
    asymmetry, 13, 17
Mu rhythm, 6, 17, 23, 29, 33, 124, 116, 139, 150, 288, 293
    reactivity, 6, 29, 32, 123, 150

Neurological deficit, 30, 45, 115, 124, 153, 165, 210
    outcome, 76, 111, 124, 146
    symptoms, 94
Neuronal metabolism, 70
Neurotransmitter failure, 99
Noncompartment flow, 70, 79
Non-cortical infarction, 46, 126
Non-critical ischemia, 93
No-reflow phenomenon, 180
Normalized differences, 35
Normal perfusion-pressure breakthrough, 140
Nuclear magnetic resonance (NMR), 65, 287

Occlusion of cerebral artery, 18, 87, 91, 107, 123, 148, 159, 186, 192, 249
Open-heart surgery, 62, 75, 146, 151
Oxygen uptake, 78, 124, 224, 263, 287

Partial infarction, 249
    ischemia, 94
Partial nonprogressing stroke (PNS), 9
Peak frequency, 12, 34, 44, 53, 80, 125, 133, 150, 154
    parameters, 32
Pentobarbital, 219
Penumbra, 3, 121, 149, 235, 245
Perfusion pressure, 77, 140, 176, 185, 224, 249
Period and amplitude analysis, 52, 67
Phosphocreatinine, 176
Phosphorylation, 254
Photic stimulation, 6, 10, 18, 154, 295, 305
    driving, 6
Plasma, 257
Polygon-profile clustering analysis, 71
Positron emission tomography (PET), 116, 152, 253, 287, 307, 309
Potassium, 86, 91, 175, 230
Potential field, 290
Power spectrum, 11, 95, 148, 154, 203, 220, 271, 290
    parameters, 32, 34, 150
Prediction, 72

318

Primates, 149, 153, 185, 201, 235
Prolonged reversible ischemic neurological deficit (PRIND), 45, 51, 121

Radioisotopes, 245, 254, 301
Rat, 176
Ratio parameters, 58
Recirculation, 178
Recovery, 147, 181, 198, 235, 282
Recurrent ischemia, 282
Regional cerebral blood flow (rCBF), 68, 109, 139, 140, 147, 151, 248, 309
Relative alpha power asymmetry, 13
    asymmetry ratio, 7
    power asymmetry, 14
Revascularisation surgery, 110, 121, 140, 203, 235, 272, 283
Reversible ischemia, 4, 20
    ischemic neurological deficit (RIND), 9, 121
Risk factor, 139

Sensitivity, 19, 40, 44, 129,
Sensorimotor rhythm, 124, 139
Severe ischemia, 33, 115, 229
Single photon emission tomography, 65, 152, 245, 287
Slow-wave activity, 75, 88, 99, 166, 220, 281, 296
    focus, 109
Sodium, 91
Sokoloff model, 260
Somatosensory evoked potentials, 149, 177, 185, 201, 203, 240
Specificity, 19, 40, 44, 129, 151
Spectral band parameters, 59, 61, 150
    mean frequency, 57, 76
    peak parameters, 13, 17, 150
Spectrophotometry, 307
Speech, 248, 288
Stroke, 146, 155, 256
Subcortical ischemia, 131
Supratentorial cerebral infarction, 51, 76, 150

Survival time, 220
Symmetry index, 114
Systemic blood pressure, 186

Tactile stimulation, 8
Temperature, 86, 229
Thalamus, 149, 160, 186, 202, 210, 256
Theta activity, 55, 57, 70, 139
    band, 67, 154, 273
    power, 32, 86, 108, 123, 218
Theta/beta asymmetry, 39, 129
Thiopental, 219
Tomography, 152, 245, 253
Topographic evoked potential, 305
Topography, 108, 271, 268, 305
Total activity time, 67
    power, 11, 32, 86, 123
Transient cerebral ischemia, 99
    ischemic attack (TIA), 4, 9, 30, 45, 51, 110, 140, 154, 248, 272, 282, 296
Transorbital revascularisation, 238
Tumor, 48, 71, 88, 96, 303

Ultrasonic flow measurements, 274
Unilateral ischemia, 9, 29, 116, 281

Vasogenic brain edema, 100
Ventro postero-lateral nucleus (VPL), 160, 186, 189, 191, 202,
Visual evoked potential, 305
Voluntary movement, 31, 123

Wernicke's area, 248, 273
Wilk's Lambda, 42

Xenon-133, 68, 140, 246
    inhalation, 109, 147, 152, 246, 272
    intra-arterial injection, 147, 152, 272
    intravenous injection, 68, 76, 152

Zero-line crossing, 52, 146, 151